An Introduction to Human Language:
Fundamental Concepts in Linguistics

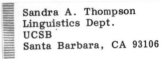

JAMES PAUL GEE
University of Southern California

PRENTICE HALL, Englewood Cliffs, New Jersey 07632

Library of Congress Cataloging-in-Publication Data

GEE, JAMES PAUL.
    An introduction to human language: fundamental concepts in
linguistics/James Paul Gee.
        p.   cm.
    Includes bibliographical references (p.   ) and index.
    ISBN 0-13-484528-5
    1. Linguistics. I. Title.
P121.G395 1993
410—dc20

92-7966
CIP

Acquisitions editor: Phil Miller

Editorial/production supervision
    and interior design: F. Hubert

Prepress buyer: Herb Klein

Manufacturing buyer: Patrice Fraccio

Cover design: Bruce Kenselaar

 © 1993 by Prentice-Hall, Inc.
A Division of Simon & Schuster
Englewood Cliffs, New Jersey 07632

Printed in the United States of America
10 9 8 7 6 5 4 3 2 1

ISBN   0-13-484528-5

PRENTICE-HALL INTERNATIONAL (UK) LIMITED, *London*
PRENTICE-HALL OF AUSTRALIA PTY. LIMITED, *Sydney*
PRENTICE-HALL CANADA INC., *Toronto*
PRENTICE-HALL HISPANOAMERICANA, S.A., *Mexico*
PRENTICE-HALL OF INDIA PRIVATE LIMITED, *New Delhi*
PRENTICE-HALL OF JAPAN, INC., *Tokyo*
SIMON & SCHUSTER ASIA PTE. LTD., *Singapore*
EDITORA PRENTICE-HALL DO BRASIL, LTDA., *Rio de Janeiro*

Contents

Preface   *vii*

    A NOTE ON USING THIS BOOK   *ix*

    ACKNOWLEDGMENTS   *x*

CHAPTER 1
Introduction: The Nature of Language   *1*

    1.1. HUMAN LANGUAGE   *1*

    1.2. ANIMAL COMMUNICATION   *2*

    1.3. LANGUAGE AND CULTURAL DISTINCTIONS   *7*

    1.4. DISCOURSE: LANGUAGE IN CONTEXT   *13*

    1.5. TYPES OF LANGUAGES   *15*

    1.6. LANGUAGE CHANGE   *18*

CHAPTER 2
Semantics: The Meaning of Language   *21*

    2.1. THE SIMPLIFIED PREDICATE LANGUAGE (SPL)   *21*

    2.2. PROBLEMS WITH SPL SEMANTICS   *31*

    2.3. POSSIBLE WORLDS   *38*

    2.4. PREDICATES AND ARGUMENTS   *40*

    2.5. FROM ENGLISH SENTENCES TO THEIR MEANINGS   *41*

    2.6. QUANTIFIERS   *48*

    2.7. LOGICAL PROPERTIES OF ENGLISH SENTENCES   *49*

    2.8. SEMANTIC ROLES   *51*

CHAPTER 3
Phonology: The Sound of Language *65*

    3.1. HUMAN-LIKE COMMUNICATION SYSTEMS *65*

    3.2. INDIVIDUAL SOUNDS AND THEIR RULES *73*

    3.3. THE RHYTHM OF SENTENCES *102*

CHAPTER 4
Phonetics: Description and Notation of Language Sounds *110*

    4.1. SYMBOLIZING SOUNDS *110*

    4.2. VOICED AND VOICELESS SOUNDS (IN FEATURE TERMS [+VOICE] AND [–VOICE]) *112*

    4.3. NASAL AND ORAL SOUNDS (IN FEATURE TERMS [+NASAL] AND [–NASAL]) *114*

    4.4. VOWELS AND CONSONANTS *115*

    4.5. STOPS (IN FEATURE TERMS [+CONTINUANT] AND [–CONTINUANT]) *118*

    4.6. SONORANTS AND OBSTRUENTS (IN FEATURE TERMS [+SONORANT] AND [–SONORANT]) *120*

    4.7. THE FEATURE [+STRIDENT] AND [–STRIDENT] *123*

    4.8. PLACES OF ARTICULATION (THE FEATURES [+ANTERIOR], [–ANTERIOR] AND [+CORONAL], [–CORONAL]) *123*

    4.9. FEATURES AND THE CLASSIFICATION OF SOUNDS *124*

    4.10. DISTINCTIVE AND NONDISTINCTIVE FEATURES *126*

    4.11. VOWELS *128*

    4.12. DESCRIBING VOWELS (THE FEATURES [+HIGH], [–HIGH], [+LOW], [–LOW], AND [+FRONT], [–FRONT] *129*

    4.13. THE SOUNDS OF ENGLISH *134*

CHAPTER 5
Morphology: The Shapes of Words *137*

    5.1. INVENTING GRAMMAR *137*

    5.2. WORDS *158*

    5.3. A FORM-BASED DEFINITION OF MORPHEMES *160*

    5.4. FROM MORPHEMES TO SENTENCES *162*

    5.5. WORD FORMATION RULES *164*

    5.6. WORD STRUCTURES *168*

    5.7. THE MENTAL LEXICON *172*

5.8. PRODUCTIVITY *173*

5.9. MORPHO-PHONOLOGICAL RULES *177*

CHAPTER 6
Syntax: The Structure of Language *185*

6.1. SENTENCES *185*

6.2. PHRASES *186*

6.3. CANONICAL PATTERNS AND RULES FOR CHANGING THEM *197*

6.4. GRAMMATICAL RELATIONS *218*

6.5. CASE AND GRAMMATICAL RELATIONS *224*

6.6. ARGUMENTS *228*

6.7. WORDS IN THE MIND *231*

6.8. BRINGING THE SYSTEM TOGETHER *237*

CHAPTER 7
Psycholinguistics: Processing Language in the Mind *245*

7.1. PSYCHOLINGUISTICS *245*

7.2. THE NATURE OF THE MIND *246*

7.3. RECOGNIZING WORDS IN THE STREAM OF SPEECH *250*

7.4. RECOGNIZING SENTENCES *254*

7.5. PARSING SENTENCES IN DISCOURSE CONTEXT *267*

7.6. THE MEANINGS OF WORDS *273*

7.7. LANGUAGE PRODUCTION *276*

7.8. BEYOND SENTENCES: STORIES *282*

CHAPTER 8
Language Acquisition: The Growth of Language in the Child *287*

8.1. INTRODUCTION *287*

8.2. GENERALIZATION: GOING BEYOND THE DATA *289*

8.3. LANGUAGE AS A FORMAL SYSTEM *302*

8.4. LANGUAGE AND COGNITION *305*

8.5. STAGES OF LANGUAGE ACQUISITION *312*

8.6. NOMINALS AND MEANING *320*

8.7. ACQUISITION OF MORE COMPLEX STRUCTURES: PASSIVES *324*

8.8. CHILD-DIRECTED SPEECH *326*

CHAPTER 9
Language, History, and Society   *333*

9.1. DIALECTS AND STANDARD LANGUAGE   *333*

9.2. VARIATION IN LANGUAGE AND THE SOCIAL HIERARCHY   *342*

9.3. COMMUNICATION AND SOCIETY   *349*

9.4. SOCIAL VARIATION AND HISTORICAL CHANGE   *355*

9.5. PIDGINS AND CREOLES   *359*

9.6. LANGUAGE CHANGE   *367*

9.7. LANGUAGE RECONSTRUCTION AND THE LANGUAGES OF THE WORLD   *370*

9.8. THE COMPLAINT TRADITION   *376*

CHAPTER 10
Discourse: Language in Context   *379*

10.1. THE NATURE OF DISCOURSE   *379*

10.2. PACKAGING INFORMATION WITHIN SENTENCES   *382*

10.3. WHAT SENTENCES ARE ABOUT   *393*

10.4. HOW GRAMMAR HELPS US TO FIT SENTENCES TO THEIR CONTEXTS   *399*

10.5. COHESION   *409*

10.6. PACKAGING BEYOND THE SENTENCE: THE ORGANIZATION OF CONNECTED DISCOURSES   *411*

10.7. SPEECH AND CONVERSATION AS SOCIAL ACTION   *420*

Index   *429*

Preface

Though this is not widely known, what scientists do is *play*. And like children, they have a lot of fun doing it. Experimental physicists play with giant pieces of equipment that cost millions of dollars. They race little particles round and round and smash them into other little particles. And this gives them the same glee children get out of smashing two trucks together. Archeologists play with picks and shovels, looking for little bits of old bone. When they find a particularly nice piece, they get as excited as a child unearthing a shell at the beach. Other scientists play with beakers of liquid and glass slides, having as much fun as children sloshing around in the kitchen. Astronomers look with awe through giant telescopes and, when they see something neat and fine, get as enthused as a child who sees her first giraffe.

And why do scientists and children play? Primarily because they enjoy it, because they discover new things, and because they find what they discover beautiful and wonderful. They think little creatures that float in jars, giant stars that whirl in space, and old bones that moulder in the dust are simply fascinating and mysterious.

Oddly, lots of adults, including lots of them going to college, unlike children and scientists, think that discovering things about the mind, the world, or other people is boring, hard, dry stuff. Someone or something has killed their desire to play with their minds and sold them a bill of goods that denies them some of the deepest pleasures life has to offer. Can you imagine a small child, faced with a world made up of "quarks" of different "colors" and "flavors," as is modern theoretical physics, who would not demand to know more? I cannot, though I can imagine many such adults.

Why should people think that science is boring and hard, when scientists have so much fun doing it? I don't know. I suppose we all have our theories about the matter. Some people have been sold this bill of goods because of poverty and horrible schools. Some people, neither poor nor in particularly bad schools, have willingly bought it. My favorite theory is that people who have power in a society where power is as poorly and unequally distributed as it is in ours are afraid of people discovering things and knowing things. They sense (what scientists and children know but some adults forget) that knowledge is power. They create a climate where knowing things is considered less valuable than owning them.

Language is as beautiful as any star or quark or hawk. Any human language is a wonderfully complicated, intricate thing, just the sort of thing that children and scientists love to rummage around in. There are always new things popping up. I once asked a seven-year-old who had acquired English as his first language and then, at six, spent a year in Italy and learned Italian, how he thought people learned languages. After all, at seven, he had done it twice. He thought for a while (he had not yet allowed anyone to take away his credentials as a seeker after knowledge, and so found my asking him perfectly reasonable). Then he said, "Well, I think it is like instinct in an animal. No one tells you, you just know. You hear the language and you just, after a while, know." I told him that Noam Chomsky, the founder of contemporary theoretical linguistics, had hit on much the same answer. He was not pleased, claiming that perhaps Chomsky had stolen it from him, and, in any case, it was unfair, because Chomsky, being older, had started first, and, after all, he, the seven-year-old, had only begun to think about the matter. He, like most scientists, made much too much about who had discovered things first.

As our seven-year-old saw, children are never overtly taught language. When adults try to instruct or correct them—and many children come from cultures where adults try no such thing—they pay little or no attention. They have mastered much of the language before they go to school. All of them master it, and like our seven-year-old, can do it again if they please. And if you have ever listened to a two-year-old babbling in her crib before bedtime, or little children bantering with their parents or each other, they obviously have immense fun doing it. It is an intellectual achievement that stuns and amazes linguists, or, for that matter, any adult who has sat through French class.

Like the knowledge that scientists gain, language is power and can be used for good or ill. We can use it to oppress others, to perpetuate lies, as an instrument of miscommunication giving rise to prejudice and hate. Or we can use it to bring people together, to break the hold of hate and oppression, and to discover new and wonderful things. We can use it to write poetry, to do science.

Linguists play with language, like children do, and like poets do. Their goal is to discover new things about it and about the creatures whose greatest possession it is, human beings. Linguists believe that language is the fountain-head of human creativity. They also believe that deep creativity exists in all human beings, and that it is a moral necessity that social environments be created where that creativity can be fulfilled and expressed by all people. Thus, they do not *just* study language as an intricate world of its own, like nature, or the cosmos, or the swarm of microscopic life in a jar of pond water, though this, indeed, they do. They also, like the small child who said the Emperor had no clothes on, unmask instances of linguistic social injustice and show the mastery, the creativity, and the sensefulness of victims of unjust social and linguistic prejudice. The black child who says, "My puppy, he always be following me," has not made a mistake but is speaking out of the linguistic creativity of her community, using a form familiar in many other languages, and the linguist will say so.

If you approach the material in this book with a sense of playfulness, you will have no trouble whatsoever mastering it, and, indeed, like our seven-year-old, you will go on to make up your own theories. If anyone or anything, including yourself, has taken away your credentials as a seeker after knowledge, take them back.

A NOTE ON USING THIS BOOK

This book is an introduction to fundamental concepts in the study of language. It seeks to develop ideas and arguments in enough detail and depth that the reader can gain a feeling for how they work and for their multiple interconnections. Serious and intelligent people have chosen to devote their lives to linguistics—they think it is beautiful, exciting, and important—and I hope this book will give some feeling for why that is so. I view linguistics, though it has many subareas, as an *integrated* discipline, and I seek to demonstrate this by bringing out connections across different areas. Thus, certain concerns (such as historical change, the social context of language, aspects of language acquisition and language development, the relationships between morphology, syntax, and discourse) are treated not only in separate sections and chapters, but throughout the book as a whole. This book treats theoretical linguistics, sociocultural concerns, and the study of discourse each as integral parts of a larger unified linguistics.

Each chapter is self-contained, and the chapters can be read in any order, though I have proposed a certain order in the way I have arranged them. People may also, to gain a feeling for the diversity and multisidedness of linguistics, want to read the chapters in pairs (say, Chapter 2 or 5 with Chapter 8; Chapter 3 with Chapter 9, and Chapter 6 with Chapter 10—this pairing allows one to read "theoretical linguistics" simultaneously with "sociocultural linguistics"). In fact, I have had good luck, when teaching long class sessions, dividing each session into halves, with a break, and teaching more theoretical work in the first half and more sociocultural work in the second. The chapter on Phonology (Chapter 3) has been written so that it can be read either before or after, or with or without reading Chapter 4 on Phonetics.

There is no need for a course to cover all the chapters in this book. Each chapter seeks, while covering the details of its area, to explicate major ideas about language in general, as well as to spell out connections to other areas of language study. Thus, any subset of the chapters will make for a substantive course of study. Furthermore, Chapter 2 (Semantics) and Chapter 5 (Morphology) can "trade off" for each other. Both are meant to get across some very fundamental ideas about language and start the thinking process going.

Each chapter is written in sections, each one of which is built around one basic idea. At the end of many sections are exercises designed to be done when one has read up to and through that section. (Chapter 1, the Introduction, has no exercises. It should be read without too much worry about details, to gain a feel for the issues involved.) Except where very specific answers are called for, ones that should always be clear if one has thought about the chapter thus far, exercises should be judged on the *thoughtfulness* with which they are done, since often there is no unique right answer, several good ones, and plenty of bad ones. "Recommended Further Readings" are listed at the end of each chapter. These are works the student can consult with profit after reading this book.

In each chapter, key terms are in boldface when they are first introduced. A good way to review the material in any chapter is to check whether you understand the meaning and the importance of the boldfaced terms in that chapter—not as a set of definitions, but in terms of the theories behind them. If you really understand the import of these boldfaced terms and their interconnections, you will be able to reconstruct most of the chapter for yourself.

I believe that one should call things by their real names and that it is pointless to hide every intricacy and technicality in the interest of "watering down" everything into soft, dull baby food. It is precisely the intricacies and technicalities that make language interesting and fun. I have tried to be as clear as I can be, and I intend that readers should be able to understand everything in this book (if they play with it). If you do not understand something, first assume it is your fault, and work and play at it. If you still do not understand it, it is my fault. No one is perfect.

ACKNOWLEDGMENTS

When John Isley asked me to do an introductory book for Prentice Hall, I said that if I was to write a linguistics text, I would want it to show linguistics as an integrated field built around interlocking fundamental ideas about language, thought, society, and human nature. He said he wanted such a book. I sincerely hope he has gotten it, though it was harder indeed in the making than in the desiring. At the least, I am grateful to him for his confidence and for the opportunity he gave me to try. I am grateful as well to Phil Miller of Prentice Hall, who took over the care and feeding of my ego after John moved on to other realms in the corporation. Without his support at a crucial point I would have given up. In addition, Patricia Daly did an excellent job copy editing the manuscript, and Frank Hubert adeptly guided the book and myself through the editing and production process.

Whatever may be good in this book, the vast majority of it is due to the fact that I was blessed with extraordinarily good teachers in my graduate work at Stanford: Joan Bresnan, Charles Ferguson, Jakko Hintikka, Dorothy Huntington, Joseph Greenberg, Richie Kayne, Will Leben, Julius Moravcsik, Elizabeth Closs Traugott, and Tom Wasow. I have been equally blessed throughout my career by deeply insightful colleagues: Mark Feinstein, Judy Kegl, Bill Marsh, Neil Stillings, and Chris Witherspoon in the School of Language and Communication at Hampshire College in Amherst, Massachusetts; Francois Grosjean, Harlan Lane, and Joanne Miller in the Department of Psychology at Northeastern University in Boston, Massachusetts; Maria Brisk, Katherine Demuth, Jean Berko Gleason, John Huchinson, Bob Hoffmeister, Lee Indrisano, Carol Neidle, Paula Menyuk, and Steve Molinsky in the School of Education and the Applied Linguistics Program at Boston University; and Elaine Andersen, Joseph Aoun, Bernard Comrie, Ed Finnegan, Jack Hawkins, and Steve Krashen in the Department of Linguistics at the University of Southern California. My students at all these places have been equally important in forming my views on and my love of language and linguistics.

Colleagues around the country have also played a major role in shaping my ideas and thus causing this book to have the shape it has: Courtney Cazden, Mary Catherine O'Connor, Henry Giroux, Jane Grimshaw, Donaldo Macedo, Sarah Michaels, Eliot Mischler, and Catherine Snow. As so many other linguists, I benefited immensely early in my career from the help of the late Adrian Akmaijian, one of the best linguists and most deeply decent human beings I have ever known. I hope this book has even a small bit of his spirit.

I gratefully acknowledge the input received from the following reviewers of the manuscript: Richard Veit, University of North Carolina, Wilmington; Janet Byron Anderson, Cleveland State University; David F. Marshall, University of North Dakota; Georgette Ioup, University of New Orleans; Eugene Smith, University of Washington; Roger C. Schlobin, Purdue University, North Central Campus; Alice S. Horning, Oakland University, Rochester, Minnesota.

I have been fortunate indeed that those I have turned to for support and encouragement as personal friends have sustained me with a good many ideas as well: Elaine Andersen, Tobey Berlin, François Grosjean, Darsie Minor Bowden, Emily Dexter, Randee Falk, Janie Simmons de Garcia, Laura Jappe, Donaldo Macedo, Bob Meagher, Sarah Michaels, Bea Mikulecky, Candy Mitchell, Steve Molinsky, Irma Rosenfield, Sylvia Sensiper, Kristine Strand, and Mary Ellen Vesprini.

Finally, I am indebted to both my twin brother, John, and my son, Justin Falk-Gee, for a great deal of illuminating discussion on issues germane to this book, and many others as well. Neither my father, Ernest Leffel Gee, nor my mother, Kathleen Bonner Gee, are here to see this book, though their firm belief in social justice informs many parts of this book and my interest in linguistics.

JAMES PAUL GEE

CHAPTER 1

Introduction

The Nature
of Language

1.1. HUMAN LANGUAGE

People have always been intrigued by questions about whether there are language universals, whether people who speak different languages think differently, whether some languages are better or worse than others, and what the first language might have looked like. Language has existed for tens of thousands, possibly hundreds of thousands of years, but it has been written down for at most only a few thousand years. Thus, we have no direct evidence of the origins of human language. There are thousands of languages that are acquired by children as first languages (what linguists call "native languages"). All of these languages are complex and fully developed. There are no "primitive" languages left in the world. Sanskrit, a language used in India for thousands of years and now only remaining in some sacred texts, is one of the oldest examples of a written language. The oldest Sanskrit writings are based on the language as it was spoken about 1200 B.C. Yet Sanskrit is one of the most elaborately structured languages we know.

All languages can communicate anything any human would want to communicate; any language can communicate what any other one can. However, this does not mean that it is as easy to articulate an idea in one language as it might be in another. Let me give one example out of many: Korean has a single word (*kkita*) for the following relationships (each of which is expressed by a different combination in English): *'put* a piece *in* a puzzle', *'put* a ring *on* a finger', and *'put* Lego ® pieces *together'*. English uses respectively 'put *in*', 'put *on*', and 'put *together';* the Korean word *kkita* means 'put into a relationship of tight fit or attachment'. So if you want to talk about what putting a piece in a puzzle, putting a ring on a finger, and putting Lego pieces together have in common, it is easier to do this in Korean than in English. Of course, this can be said perfectly well in English—it just takes more words and sounds somewhat odd. Furthermore, the English speaker can understand what the three relationships have in common and see that cutting up the world this way makes perfectly good sense.

Languages do just that: *cut up the world* in certain ways. But there are many different ways to cut up the world. Korean recognizes that 'putting a piece in a puzzle', 'putting a ring on a finger', and 'putting Lego pieces together' have something in common, and that makes perfect sense. On the other hand, English sees that 'putting a ring *on* a finger', 'putting a cup *on* a table', and 'putting a blanket *on* a bed' have something in common, and this also makes perfect sense. Each involves an object lying on a flat surface rather than being inside another object (for the latter, we use 'in'). English uses 'on' for each of these relationships (ring *on* finger, cup *on* table, blanket *on* bed) to capture this similarity; many other languages do not.

1.2. ANIMAL COMMUNICATION

Animals use various forms of communication, but only humans use language. A brief look at animal communication can throw light on the nature of human language. There are basically two types of animal communication systems: the first type is the remarkable system found in many species of bees; the second type is well represented by the calls of various monkeys and birds. Human language has something in common with each of these systems, but it differs in significant respects from both.

Point-by-Point (Unbounded Analog) System

The European honeybee is able to communicate the location of sources of food to its hive mates when it returns to the hive. The scout bee's message is communicated through a dance it does on the walls of the hive. There are two major types of dance, depending on the location of the food source with respect to the hive: the round dance, and the tail-wagging dance (different species of bees, or different groups within a species, have different dances or different versions of these two). If the source is within 10 meters of the hive, the bee performs the round dance. For distances greater than 100 meters, the bee performs the tail-wagging dance.

The tail-wagging dance is the more complicated and interesting. It consists of two roughly semicircular movements with a straight-line portion in between, during which the bee waggles. The bee first turns in a semicircle to the right, then waggles in a straight line, then turns in a semicircle to the left, and once again returns to the straight-line waggle, repeating this circuit over and over again. The dance communicates three sorts of information: (a) the direction in which the bees must fly; (b) the distance that must be flown; and (c) the richness of the source.

Since the surfaces inside the hive are vertical, but the bees have to fly horizontally to the food source, the dancing bee is not able to point directly toward the location of the food source. To indicate the direction of the food source, the bee uses its orientation in relation to the walls of the hive. There are three typical situations that the dancing bee faces. First, if the other bees are to fly along the ground in the direction of the sun, the straight-line portion of the tail-wagging dance points directly upward (head toward the top of the hive). Second, when the bees are to fly along the ground away from the sun, the dancing bee will orient the straight-line portion of the dance directly downward. Third, if, for example, the bees are to fly with the sun 80° to their right, the dance will be oriented 80° to the left of vertical. For other orientations, the bee adjusts its angle appropriately. In other words, the solar-oriented flight of the bees is systematically related to the orientation of the dancing bee on the wall of the hive.

The length of time the dancing bee spends in the straight-line portion of the tail-wagging dance (during which time it buzzes) represents the distance to the food source. The longer the bee spends in the tail-wagging portion of the dance, the farther the food source is from the hive. The length of time that the bee spends in the straight-line portion of the tail-wagging dance is also related to the number of complete circuits (circle-waggle-circle) the bee makes per unit of time. The fewer circuits per unit of time, the farther away the food source is. For example, if nine or ten circuits are made within a 15-second period, the distance to the food source is 100 meters; for six circuits per 15 seconds, the distance indicated is 500 meters; and if the number of circuits is four per 15 seconds, the distance is 1,500 meters (almost a mile). Bees can communicate distances up to 11 kilometers—almost 7 miles. The bee communicates the richness of the source of food (how much nectar is available) by its level of excitation as it dances. The greater its degree of excitement, the richer the source of food.

The bee type of communication (known as an unbounded analog system) is what I will call a **point-by-point** system. In such a system, each point along some real-world continuum (for example, distances or orientations in space) is associated with a point along a continuum of signals (for example, time spent in the straight-line portion of the dance, or orientation of the dancing bee in relation to the top of the hive). Such a system can be represented as in Figure 1-1.

In a point-by-point system, every little variation in the continuum of signals is potentially meaningful. Thus, in principle, the difference between being 80° and 79° to the left of vertical, or even between being 80° and 79.9° to the left of vertical, could be meaningful. Only the perceptual abilities of the bees (their ability to tell apart a difference between 80° and 60°, but not a difference between 79° and 80°, for instance) sets limits to the system. In principle, if not in actual practice, the system is unbounded in the number of distinctions it can make, and thus in the number of messages it can communicate.

Nonlinguistic dimension:
Distances from hive

Toward the sun	Sun 80° to right	Sun 60° to right	Sun 40° to right	etc.
↕	↕	↕	↕	↕
Bee points toward top of hive	Bee points 80° to left of vertical	Bee points 60° to left of vertical	Bee points 40° to left of vertical	etc. until bee is pointing downward to mean: away from the sun

Linguistic dimension:
Orientation of straight-line portion of dance to walls of hive

FIGURE 1-1. Unbounded Analog System

Bounded Discrete System

The second major type of animal communication system is well represented by the calls of various species of monkeys. For example, the vervet monkey (a semiterrestrial Old World monkey found in the grassy forests of southeast Africa) produces about thirty-six physically distinct sounds. Each of these sounds is evoked by different situations in the world around the monkey. Since some different situations evoke the same sound, and some situations evoke different sounds, the vervet's communicational system carries roughly twenty-two different messages. For example, a scream signals the approach of a strange male to an infant; a sound like "Eh, eh" signals a reunion of a mother and infant; a sound like "Uh!" signals the proximity of a minor mammalian predator; a sound like "Nyow!" signals a sudden movement of a minor mammalian or avian predator; and a sound like "Rraup" signals the initial perception of a major avian predator. Monkeys use several visual signals, both separate from and in combination with vocal signals, so they can communicate more than their vocal signals alone would indicate.

Many species of birds also use a repertoire of calls. Unlike the bee dance, the communicational system of monkeys and birds consists simply of a small vocabulary of distinct calls, which are not combined with each other in any systematic fashion. Such a system, called a **bounded discrete** system, can be represented as in Figure 1-2.

A bounded, discrete communication system has only a limited number of signals, each triggered by a certain condition in the world or by an internal state of the animal (like fear) and thus communicating that that condition or state holds. Such a system can, even in principle, communicate only a limited number of messages.

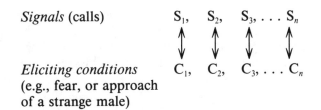

Signals (calls) $S_1, \quad S_2, \quad S_3, \ldots S_n$

Eliciting conditions $C_1, \quad C_2, \quad C_3, \ldots C_n$
(e.g., fear, or approach
of a strange male)

FIGURE 1-2.   Bounded Discrete System

Differences Between Human and Animal Languages

Human language is neither a point-by-point system like the bee's nor a bounded discrete system like the vervet's, but it shares something with each of these. Like a point-by-point system it can, in principle, communicate an unlimited number of messages. Unlike a point-by-point system, however, human language rarely varies its signs along a continuum to signal various points on a real-world continuum. For example, no human language would keep lengthening a word like 'far' to signal various distances between close to the speaker and far away from the speaker (as in 'far', 'faar', 'faaar', 'faaaar', 'faaaaar', etc.). Rather, a human language has to choose a certain number of discrete signs to signal a discrete number of distinctions (like the calls in vervet communication)—for example, 'near' versus 'far', or 'here' versus 'there' (some languages make a three-way distinction among being close to the speaker, being a middling distance away, and being far away). While we can say 'far', 'very far', 'very, very far', etc., which is something like bee communication, no language does this sort of thing regularly or systematically.

So how do human languages manage to have an unbounded number of messages, like bees, and unlike birds and monkeys? They do so by having **syntax.** English has a sign (word) 'red' for the color red, and a sign 'flower' for flowers. If we wanted to talk about red flowers, and had only a bounded, discrete system of communication (like monkeys and birds), we would have to add a new sign to refer to red flowers. But we don't do that; we *combine* the two signs 'red' and 'flower' into the phrase 'red flower', which serves as a complex sign for red flowers and saves us needing to invent and use a separate sign (for example, 'glub'). The meaning of the phrase 'red flower' is predictable to any speaker of English from knowing two things: first, the meanings of the words 'red' and 'flower', and, second, that 'red flower' counts as a unit or phrase in English that combines the meanings of these two separate words in a certain way (that is, we need to know that we are not referring to something red and some separate thing that is a flower). Saying a language has a syntax simply means that it has rules for combining discrete signs to produce more complex signs whose meanings are predictable from the meanings of the signs so combined.

A vervet monkey can utter one call after another, but the calls are always separate. The monkey cannot combine them to produce complex signs. Such combinatorial power gives rise to a potentially infinite set of messages. For example, we can now combine the complex sign 'red flower' with the sign 'dream' to get the more complex sign 'red flower dream', and we can combine this with the sign 'state' to get 'red flower dream state'. We could even combine this with 'dream' again to get 'red flower dream state dream'. There is obviously no end to this process. We are ensured of an infinite number of signs and, thus, an infinite number of things to talk about. But we get this infinity of things to talk about without having to deal with the continua the bees operate with. Such continua require acute powers of perception to discern small differences on the continuum, like 80° versus 79°, and thus ultimately limit the practical scope of what they can communicate. Furthermore, not everything we want to talk about comes in continua like distance, richness of food, and orientation to the sun.

Syntax is, however, only one key factor that differentiates human languages from animal communication systems. Another equally important factor is that human language is, unlike animal communication systems, stimulus free. What we talk about need not be triggered by any external stimulus in the world or any internal emotional state. A dog can understand that its master is at the door, and a dog can communicate that it is at the door and wants to be let into the house. But a dog cannot understand that its master will be home the day after tomorrow or communicate that it wants to come into the house only if it will be fed. Humans can communicate about things that don't or don't yet exist; thus, they can imagine new realities they have never experienced. Furthermore, human languages have signs not just for things in the world and for imaginary things (like unicorns), but they also have signs for signs themselves. I can use the word 'flower' to talk about flowers, but I can also use the phrase 'the word flower' (or *the word 'flower'*) to talk not about flowers but about the sign (word) 'flower' itself. This power makes language and thought infinitely self-reflexive: We humans can talk about talk and think about thinking, and thus only humans can ask what it means to communicate, to think, to be an animal, or to be human.

Obviously, the idiosyncratic course of human evolution gave rise to creatures (humans) capable of acquiring and using unbounded, discrete communication systems. It appears to have done so only once, since no other animal uses such a system in nature. There has been much interest over the last few years in attempts by scientists to teach chimpanzees, our closest and most intelligent relatives, American Sign Language (ASL), and other communicational systems (for example, placing differently shaped and colored chips on a magnetic board). While chimpanzees, given their vocal apparatus, cannot produce human-like sounds very well, they can produce the signs of sign language quite well. These scientists were interested ultimately in seeing whether chimps could acquire and use a discrete, unbounded communicational system. (Note: ASL, as used by deaf people, is just like any other human language—no worse, no better. Whether a language is spoken or signed is of little consequence.)

This research is now mired in great controversy (many scholars thought the research was not well carried out; many of the research people were not linguists and had quite different understandings of what language was). Nevertheless, it is clear from this research that chimps are capable of learning and using signs well beyond what they spontaneously do in the wild. They will make up novel combinations like 'sweet fruit' or 'water bird' from signs they already know (like 'sweet' and 'fruit', or 'water' and 'bird') and use them for things they do not have a sign for (such as a watermelon or a duck). They can learn to use fairly long combinations of signs like *you me go out hurry*. I see no reason to believe that this is not the rudimentary beginnings of syntax. However, even after many years of training, chimpanzees have relatively small vocabularies, and the combinatorial possibilities of their language do not remotely approach those of any human language even as used by a five-year-old child (for example, a five-year-old native signer of ASL).

   Human evolution has equipped human beings with a special capacity to acquire human-type languages, and this capacity makes the course of language acquisition in a child easier, with less variation in mastery among children, than comparably complex skills, like the acquisition of physics or chemistry, or learning to master a musical instrument. Chimpanzees, in all likelihood, acquire what language we humans can teach them by their general intelligence and problem-solving abilities. They do not have a special capacity for acquiring languages, because evolution never gave it to them. Lacking this capacity, they never reach anything comparable to even a five-year-old child. This is no indication that they are less intelligent than humans; their type of intelligence is just different. The quirks of evolution simply did not give them any characteristically *linguistic* intelligence, though it gave them a great deal of intelligence in other regards.

1.3. LANGUAGE AND CULTURAL DISTINCTIONS

Human languages are the products of a long course of human evolution. Each language cuts up the world in a characteristic way. However, while the ways in which different languages cut up the world are various, there are constraints on this process. Human languages differ because human cultures differ, but both languages and cultures have deep similarities because human beings are fundamentally similar: They all have the same sort of eye, the same sort of brain, the same basic biology. If there are Martians and they have language, even if there are many different Martian languages, none of them is likely to resemble human languages in any way. The course of Martian evolution (taking place in a very different world) has been quite different than the course of human evolution. Human evolution has shaped humans to acquire and use languages of certain types; Martian evolution has undoubtedly shaped Martians in different ways.

Color Terms Across Languages

To take a concrete example of how uniformity (language universals) and diversity (language difference) intermix in the study of language, let us consider for a moment color terms. In this area we see, in a particularly clear way, the interaction of diversity and universals across languages.[1]

Languages differ in how many basic (single-word) color terms they have. Some languages have only two basic color terms. For example, in Dugum Dani, which is spoken in the western half of New Guinea, the terms *modla* and *mili*, which roughly translate as 'light/bright' and 'dark/dull' respectively, are the only words that can be identified as basic color terms. On the other hand, like several other languages, English has eleven basic color terms: *black, white, red, yellow, blue, green, orange, brown, purple, pink,* and *gray*. Between these two extremes are languages with many different color term systems.

Despite this obvious diversity across languages, the human eye (a gift of human evolution) is everywhere the same. Humans beings (except those who are color blind) can see all the same colors. Color in the physical world is a spectrum of continuously graded shades running into each other with no discrete boundaries (we all have trouble telling where blue stops and purple begins, where red stops and orange begins, and so forth). In fact, some portions of the color spectrum that cannot be seen by human eyes are visible to the eyes of a bee.

Each language must choose where it will cut the color spectrum and how many times, with its discrete words. Dugum Dani divides it in half with two words and English makes eleven cuts, with eleven words; other languages make different numbers of cuts between these two extremes. Thus, there are differences across languages in regard to color terms. But the crucial question is this: Is this diversity constrained in any way? Can a language choose just any color terms it wants?

In every language there is a **prototype** (or typical instance) associated with every basic color term. For example, in English, the word 'blue' can be applied to all types and shades of blue, but most native speakers agree on what shade of blue constitutes the *most typical* or *best example* of blue. Such a prototypical shade is called the **focus** of the term. Interestingly, it turns out that there are only eleven possible color focuses, and all languages, regardless of how many basic color terms they have, choose terms that have as a focus one of these eleven colors. The focus of the Dugum Dani word that speakers of the language apply to all dark colors, for example, is the same as the focus of the English word 'black'; the focus of the Dugum Dani word that speakers of the language apply to bright colors is the same as the focus of the English word 'white'.

---

[1]For two recommended studies, see Brent Berlin and Paul Kay, *Basic Color Terms: Their Universality and Evolution* (Berkeley: University of California Press, 1969) and Paul Kay and Chad McDaniel, "The Linguistic Significance of the Meanings of Basic Color Terms," *Language,* 54 (1978) 610–46.

Actually, there is yet more order. If speakers of a language have fewer than eleven basic color terms, which colors they will have is determined by a set of universal principles. All languages that have only two basic color terms have one term whose focus (prototypical example) is black and one term whose focus is white (though, of course, the two terms will commonly be used to refer to all dark colors and all light colors, respectively). In languages that have three basic color terms, the focus of one term is black, the focus of the second term is white, and the focus of the third term is red. All languages with four basic color terms have a term whose focus is black, another whose focus is white, a third whose focus is red, and a fourth whose focus is yellow, green, or blue (typically, these languages have a single fourth term with two foci, one of which is green, the other of which is blue; that is, they have a single word meaning blue or green). A language with five color terms will typically have basic color words whose foci are black, white, red, blue/green, and yellow. A language with six basic color terms will distinguish blue and green with different terms, one having the focus green and the other having the focus blue. A language with seven basic color terms adds a term whose focus is brown to the terms in a language with six basic color terms. A language with more than seven terms adds terms with focuses for one or more of the following: purple, pink, orange, and gray.

These universal principles also constrain language change. That is, they limit how a language can change. Since any language with two basic color terms has terms whose focuses are black and white, and any language with three basic color terms has terms whose focuses are black, white, and red, no language can change from a two-term language to a three-term language except by adding a term for red. If it did otherwise (for example, by adding a term whose focus was brown), then it would be a three-term language that violated the universal principle that says three-term languages have terms whose focuses are black, white, and red.

We humans see eleven focal colors in the continuously graded color spectrum. That's just the way the eye is made. Other creatures—whether bees or Martians—whose eyes were differently made would see this spectrum differently. Languages pick some subset or all of these eleven focal colors, depending on the interests and needs of the culture. They then extend the color terms to apply to nonfocal shades (for example, a term whose focus is black is extended to talk about all dark and dull things; a term whose focus is blue is extended to talk about all shades of blue, many of them rather far from the prototype or focus). In this way, they can all talk about all the continuously graded shades of color in the spectrum.

Now we can ask: Do people from cultures with four basic color terms see the world differently, or think about it differently, than people from cultures with seven basic color terms? If you ask people from a culture with four color terms to sort colored chips into piles, they will initially sort them into four piles. Someone from a culture with seven terms will initially sort them into seven piles. This result once led psychologists to think that people with different languages saw and thought about colors differently. However, if you go on to tell each of these people to make more piles, that you want more distinctions, they will eventually come up with much the same piles. At some stage in the proceedings they quit using their language as a guide and just use the human eye—which is everywhere the same—as a guide.

These color chips are a good guide to how language, culture, and the human brain interact. Languages cut up the world in different ways. These ways are constrained, however, by the nature of the human body, the human eye, and the human brain. The way a language cuts up the world will influence how we *initially* think about something, but it does not determine how we *finish* thinking about it. Under pressure we can think about things outside the categories of our language, because we can find other people's ways of doing things senseful. We find them senseful because, at least where language is concerned, they are all chosen from the inventory of ways allowed by the human brain, which is, like the eye, everywhere the same across cultures.

Most linguists, confronted with diversity across languages, assume (as a working hypothesis until proven otherwise) that such diversity is in fact constrained and subject to universal principles that shape and limit the diversity. That is, they assume that the complex interplay between diversity and uniformity (or, put another way, the complex interplay between culture and common human nature), which we saw in the case of color is, in fact, typical. Admittedly, this is an article of faith in many cases. But it is a faith that gives a certain character to linguistics as a field.

Language Differences Not Explained by Culture

A language will have few or many color terms depending on the extent to which the culture in which the language is used needs more or less of these. The language used in a highly technological culture will add more and more color terms to cope with the demands of industry. But this is a superficial matter. After all, any language can borrow or make up new words if and when the need arises. What we need to know is whether there is any deeper sense in which culture shapes language.

It is often difficult to imagine that the distinctions a language makes are determined by, or even related to, the culture in which the language is spoken. For example, returning to the Korean example of *kkita,* it is hard to imagine what about Korean culture makes Koreans more interested in "putting things into a relationship of tight fit or attachment" (*kkita*) than members of another culture. What is it about the cultures where English is spoken that makes these speakers interested in flat surfaces versus three-dimensional spaces ('on' versus 'in')? These matters seem to have little or nothing to do with culture.

Of course, one can always invent some deep psychological reason or find something in the culture that appears to be figuratively connected somehow (for example, Koreans care a lot about family attachments). But there is no reason to believe such explanations. The Korean language's way of cutting up joining relationships is useful and senseful. Even if in the distant past there was some cultural reason why the linguistic ancestors of the Koreans cut up the world in this way, there is no reason why current Korean culture must have properties that motivate cutting up the world thus. Since it is a useful and senseful way to cut up the world, it could well have survived any cultural reason that originally motivated it. And, of course, English is a language used in hundreds of cultures across the world, but in each of them a distinction is made between 'in' versus 'on'.

For children learning a language in any culture, much of that language is a *form* or *structure* or *complex pattern* (however you want to phrase it) that is not related in any close way to the culture. In acquiring the language, the child is faced with a pure intellectual problem. Thus, language and the acquisition of language must be studied, to a certain extent, apart from studying culture (or, rather, nonlinguistic aspects of culture, since language is a part of culture).

The Influence of Culture on Syntax

To study the interaction of language and culture in any significant way, we must leave the level of what words a language has. Our question now is: Does culture influence language significantly in any other way than the interests of the culture determining (in part) how many and what words a language will have?

Consider an example from Navajo (an American Indian language). This example involves looking not at the words of Navajo, but at its syntax; that is, at the patterns or shapes of its phrases and sentences.[2] Consider the following sentences. These are all acceptable and normal sentences in English. However, the asterisk in front of sentence 4 indicates that this sentence is unacceptable in Navajo when it is directly translated into that language. I give a few examples of actual Navajo as well.

1. The horse kicked the mule.	*Líí'*	*dzannééz*	*yiztał*
	horse	mule	kicked
2. The mule kicked the horse.			
3. The man kicked the horse.			
4. *The horse kicked the man.	*Líí'*	*hastiin*	*yiztał*
	horse	man	kicked

The fact that it is unacceptable to say 'the horse kicked the man' in Navajo can be related to Navajo cultural practices and, in particular, to the Navajo world

---

[2]This discussion is based on Gary Witherspoon, *Language and Art in the Navajo Universe* (Ann Arbor: University of Michigan Press, 1977).

view, which distinguishes clearly who or what can control or dominate what or whom.

Navajos interpret sentence 1 to mean something like 'the horse controlled the action and kicked the mule without the mule's helping to bring this about; the horse dominated and controlled the mule'. Similar controlling actions are expressed in sentences 2 and 3. What is wrong with sentence 4 is not that it violates the normal pattern or structure of Navajo sentences, but rather that it is absurd to a Navajo. It claims that a horse can control and dominate a man without the man's consent, either openly given or inadvertently given through the man's carelessness. It means that the horse was intellectually dominating the man and had the man under its control, and the man was unable to resist. Such notions are absurd to the Navajo. Humans are more intelligent than horses in the Navajo view of the world, and thus, to them, horses cannot dominate and control humans without the human's consent (however tacit that may be). Horses cannot will and carry out actions against human beings without the action being stimulated or caused by the conscious will of the human being or by the human's careless and inadvertent behavior.

Many other aspects of sentences in Navajo are determined by who can control whom. Entities in the world are ranked in terms of degrees of intelligence, potency, animation, and activity. Entities that are higher in intelligence, potency, animation, or activity can control, but cannot be controlled by, entities that are less intelligent, less potent, inanimate, and stationary. For example, human babies who cannot speak, but who can call out and cry, are not classified as equal to human beings who have acquired the art of speaking. Thus, it is unacceptable to say the Navajo equivalent of the English 'the baby kicked the man' (you have to say something that roughly translates into English as 'the man let the baby kick him'). However, one can say both 'the baby kicked the horse' and 'the horse kicked the baby'. Human babies, who can only call out and cry, are thus considered to be approximately equal to animals, who can only call out and cry but do not speak.

To illustrate further the Navajo hierarchy of who can control whom or what can control what, consider how inanimate entities work in this scheme of things. A Navajo would not say 'thirst killed the tree'; he would say 'the tree let itself die by means of thirst'. This is so because in the Navajo world view inanimate entities with material, corporeal existence (such as rocks, trees, jewels, metals, and so on) are higher on the scale of what can control what than are inanimate abstractions without a material existence (such as hunger, thirst, ideas, emotions, and so on). Thus, an immaterial thing like thirst cannot control a material thing like a tree (so one cannot say 'thirst killed the tree').

A large part of Navajo ritual is based on the capacity of the people of the earth's surface (the Navajo) to control and compel the Holy People through ritual action, song, and prayer. The world in which Navajos live and act was brought into being by the *Diyin Dine'e*—gods, supernaturals, or Holy People, though the Navajo do not think of these beings as infinitely good and perfect. Who can act on whom or who can control whom is of basic interest and concern to Navajos and is one of the dominant perspectives in the Navajo world view.

However, once again, we must quickly counterpose to this example from Navajo the fact that much, probably most, of the structure or form of a language is in no obvious way related to the culture in which the language is spoken. Even in the case of Navajo, the considerations that we have looked at could stay in the language long past the time the cultural basis for them (in ritual, myth, and world view) had died out. They would then be just formal facts, facts that held of the form of the language, with no clear current reason why they held. Of course, the language could change when the culture did, but this is not necessary and does not always happen.

English orders words in its sentences in terms of the pattern SUBJECT/VERB/OBJECT ('The man kicked the mule'). Navajo has a different pattern: SUBJECT/OBJECT/VERB ('Man mule kicked'). There is no obvious cultural reason to explain this. Even if there were, there are thousands of languages in the world that use the Navajo pattern and thousands that use the English one, but the cultures in which these languages are spoken need have nothing much in common with Navajo culture or English culture (whatever that is). Rather, the word-order pattern (or lack of one in some languages) is just a pattern or form children are confronted with in learning the language.

1.4. DISCOURSE: LANGUAGE IN CONTEXT

The words and the syntax of particular languages and of language in general (language universals) are a large part of what linguists study. This study, referred to as **linguistic theory,** falls into several parts: **phonology** (the study of the sound structure in language); **morphology** (the study of words and their parts); **syntax** (the study of the structure of phrases and sentences, the combinatorial possibilities of language); and **semantics** (the study of how meaning is related to the words and syntax of a language). However, linguistics also involves moving beyond words and the syntax of phrases and sentences to study how language is *used* in real contexts.

For example, an upper-middle-class college woman (whom I will call Jane) was discussing a story with her parents at dinner. The story had been used in a college course about how people argue about values. In the story, a woman named Abigail wants to get across a river to see her lover, Gregory. A river boat captain (Sinbad) says he will take her only if she sleeps with him. In desperation she does so—only in order to see her true love. But when she arrives and tells Gregory what has happened, he rejects her and sends her away. There is more to the story (Abigail seeks revenge), but this is enough for our example.

In explaining to her parents why she thought Gregory was the worst character in the story, Jane said the following:

Well, when I thought about it,
I don't know,
it seemed to me that Gregory should be the most offensive.
He showed no understanding for Abigail
when she told him what she was forced to do.
He was callous.
He was hypocritical,
in the sense that he professed to love her,
then acted like that.

Earlier, Jane had told her boyfriend the same thing. This is what she said:

What an ass that guy was,
you know,
her boyfriend.
I should hope
if ever I did that to see you,
you would shoot the guy.
He uses her and he says he loves her.
Sinbad never lies,
you know what I mean?

It is apparent that Jane said much the same thing but in quite different ways to her parents and to her boyfriend. With her parents she uses a more tightly packaged, more formal, and more explicit language. With her boyfriend she uses a more loosely packaged, less formal, and less explicit language. In speaking to her boyfriend, she leaves several points to be drawn by inference whereas she spells them out more explicitly to her parents (for example, one must infer in the talk to the boyfriend that Gregory is being accused of being a hypocrite, since while Sinbad is bad, at least he does not lie, which Gregory did in claiming to love Abigail).

Language that is formal and more explicit is appropriate when one wants to show deference and respect for the hearer. Language that is informal and leaves much to inference is appropriate with those we regard as intimates and peers. In Jane's social group, a young woman addresses her parents at dinner with language that signals respect to them. This is not true in all social groups. Though all social groups may have deep respect for parents, in some groups parents are to be treated more as equals, at least in activities like dinner time.

This example demonstrates that each person, in fact, speaks more than one variety of a language (Jane has one variety for her parents at dinner and another for her boyfriend in private). Each person has different varieties for use in different contexts. Furthermore, different social groups, even in one society, use these different varieties in different ways (for example, they may not speak to their parents the way Jane does to hers).

1.5.   TYPES OF LANGUAGES

If two groups of people who speak the same language stop regularly communicating with one another, whether for social, political, or geographical reasons, the language they speak will change through time in different ways for each group. Two different dialects of the language will appear, and eventually the change may lead to what will be considered two different languages. This happened to Latin, for instance. As the Roman Empire fell apart, the diverse and far-flung groups of people who spoke Latin began to diverge more and more from a common model. This eventually gave rise to the so-called Romance languages (Catalan, French, Italian, Portuguese, Provençal, Romanian, Spanish, and others). In a similar way, both modern German and English grew out of fifth-century Germanic and are thus historically related to each other.

It is obvious that historically related languages—for example, English and German—will resemble each other to a certain degree. This is simply because they share the same parent language, a language from which they each diverged in the past. Linguists in the nineteenth century, however, became interested in how many different *types* of languages there were. They wondered if certain languages could resemble each other not because they were historically related, but just because they belonged to the same type of language. This interest instituted the study of *linguistic typology* (the study of types of languages).

One criteria that linguists have often used to place languages in types is the sort of words a language has. In many languages, including English, some or all words are complex; that is, they have meaningful parts. Take a word like 'unhelpful'. This word is made up of three meaningful parts: 'un' (meaning *not*), 'help', and 'ful' (meaning *full*). Such meaningful parts of a word are called **morphemes.** Thus, 'unhelpful' is said to be composed of three morphemes. The word 'boy' has only one morpheme, as do the words 'happy' and 'wonder'. That is, these words are not complex; they cannot be split further into meaningful parts. Some of them can be split into syllables, as 'wonder' can be split into 'won' and 'der', but syllables are not morphemes, because they are not in this word meaningful.

In some languages, most words contain many morphemes, while in some languages very few words contain more than one morpheme. Many other languages are somewhere in the middle. In English, most words do not contain many morphemes, though we can produce such things as 'institutionalization' (institute-tion-al-ize-ation). To speakers of some Eskimo languages, even this is "kid's stuff"; their words often contain many more morphemes than this (as we will see later).

To construct a typology (that is, a set of types) around morphology, we ask two questions about a language. First: How many morphemes per word (on the average, in the typical case) does the language have? Second: How clear and distinct within the word are these morphemes and the meanings they signal?

To clarify these questions, consider the word 'unhelpful'. As we saw, this word has three morphemes ('un', 'help', and 'ful'). Each of these morphemes has one clear meaning, and they are quite clearly separate from each other. On the other hand, the word 'likes' (as in the sentence 'John likes soup') has two morphemes ('like' and 's'). But the morpheme /s/ means two things: first, it means that the subject of the sentence is not the speaker or the hearer, but some third party; and second, it means that the subject of the sentence is singular and not plural. Furthermore, we cannot separate this /s/ into two parts, one of which signals the first meaning and the other of which signals the second. The two meanings are *fused* in the single morpheme /s/. Thus, we will want to know how many morphemes are typical in the words of a language, and how tightly fused together the meanings of these morphemes are.

In answer to our first question—what is the typical number of morphemes per word—we can set up a continuum ranging from languages (like Vietnamese) in which almost all words are only one morpheme long, to languages (like Greenlandic Eskimo) in which almost all words are many morphemes long. In languages like Vietnamese, a sentence is made up of many words; in some Eskimo languages a sentence is made up of one or two words, since each word contains so many morphemes, so much information.

As examples, consider the following sentences:[3]

5. *Vietnamese* (tone marks omitted)

com	nau	ngoai	troi	an	rat	nhat
rice	cook	out	sky	eat	very	tasteless

'Rice that is cooked in the open air is very tasteless'

6. *Greenlandic Eskimo*

silar	-luk	-ka	-u	-si	-qa	-lu	-ni	-lu
outside	bad	strongly	be	become	have	inf.	3rd	and
							sing.	

'and it becoming very apt to be bad weather'

In the Vietnamese example, every word is "simple"; that is, it has only one morpheme in it (the word itself). By contrast, the Greenlandic Eskimo sentence is only one word long, but that word contains many morphemes and is, in fact, the whole sentence. Notice that this is almost true of the English translation of the Vietnamese sentence ('Rice that is cooked in the open air is very tasteless'), where only 'cooked' (cook + ed) and 'tasteless' (taste + less) are complex words, and 'is' fuses together the meanings 'be' and *third-person subject* and *singular subject*).

Languages like Vietnamese, where almost every word is a single morpheme,

---

[3]This discussion is based on Bernard Comrie, *Language Universals and Linguistic Typology*, 2nd ed. (University of Chicago Press, 1989).

are known as **isolating** (or **analytic** languages). Languages like Greenlandic Eskimo, where most words have many morphemes (and thus where words often translate as sentences in English), are called **polysynthetic** languages. Most of the world's languages fall in between these two extremes, their words having more complexity than Vietnamese and less than Eskimo.

In answer to our second question—how clear and distinct within a word are its morphemes and the meanings they signal—we also get a continuum. At one end are languages (like Turkish) where each morpheme in a word has one clear meaning and is kept completely clear and separate in its "shape" (sound) from the other morphemes in the word. In such languages, each morpheme is like a differently colored block that is just glued to the others. For example, in the Turkish word *adamlarin,* the morphemes are *adam,* which means 'man', *lar,* which signals PLURAL (more than one), and *in,* meaning POSSESSOR ('of'); so the whole word translates 'of (belonging to) the men'. Each of these three morphemes has one clear meaning, and it always has this meaning regardless of what other morphemes it combines with. This sort of thing is typical and pervasive in Turkish.

At the other end of the continuum are languages (like Russian or Latin) in which the meanings of the morphemes in a word are often fused together and one morpheme can have several meanings, with no way to say that any particular part of the morpheme is associated with one of these meanings and another part with another one of them. For example, in the Russian word *stolov,* the morpheme *stol* means 'table', but the morpheme *ov* signifies two things: POSSESSOR ('of') and PLURAL (more than one); thus the whole word means 'of (belonging to) the tables'. We cannot say that separate parts of *ov* mean POSSESSOR and PLURAL, since *o* and *v* by themselves mean nothing in Russian (for example, in the word *stolom,* the morpheme *om* means INSTRUMENTAL ('with') and SINGULAR; thus the whole word means 'with the table'). The morpheme *ov* just fuses two meanings in one form (as *om* fuses two other meanings). This sort of thing is common in Russian.

Obviously, the Russian system is not as neat and clean as Turkish. Languages, like Russian, where a single morpheme can have several different meanings all at once, and where these meanings have blended into each other, are **fusional** (or **inflectional**) languages. Once again, many languages fall between the two extremes set by languages like Turkish and Russian, having some morphemes that are clear and separate (like English's 'unhelpful') and some that are not (like the *s* in 'likes', which means THIRD PERSON and SINGULAR). In fact, Russian is not as extremely fusional as some other languages, like classical Latin or ancient Sanskrit.

Ironically, when linguists in the nineteenth century became intensely interested in comparing languages, they held Latin and Greek, which are, like Russian, inflectional, to be "ideal languages." This was because these linguists confused their respect for the cultural achievements of the people who spoke these languages with the "goodness" of the languages themselves. It was also because the languages these scholars themselves spoke (e.g., German, French,

English) were historically related to Latin and Greek (all being Indo-European languages).

In any case, with regard to morphology, the Turkish language system is clearer than that used by Latin and Greek. In fact, children take quite some time to master the morphological system of fusional languages like Russian, Latin, or Greek, but master the morphological system of a language like Turkish quite quickly and effortlessly. We should, however, bear in mind that other parts of Turkish grammar are more complex and less neat than that of Latin or Greek, for instance. The grammars of all languages are so complex that we cannot say of any language *as a whole* that it is simpler or neater than another. We can only say this if we look at a particular part of the grammar of a given language.

1.6. LANGUAGE CHANGE

The foregoing typology can help illuminate the processes by which languages change over time from one type to another. It can also illuminate the processes by which children acquire languages, and in the act of acquiring them, change them. Humans make two demands on anything that they will accept as a native (first) language. (Actually, these demands stem from the biological inheritance with which every child is born thanks to the process of human evolution.) These two demands are that a native language (one acquired by children) be fast (quick and efficient) and clear (expressive and informative). It turns out that these two demands can, and often do, conflict with each other.

Humans are prone to speed up sentences like 'He is gone' and 'He has gone' to something like 'He's gone' (note the invention here of the complex word 'he's' with its two parts, *he* and *'s*). This latter version is faster, but less clear (because we cannot tell whether 's' means 'has' or 'is' here). If this second version became the only acceptable version (by being said so often that a new generation of children acquiring the language thought it the only version), the language would have changed, losing certain information but gaining speed.

The speeding-up process can continue, eventually producing perhaps 'He gone' instead of 'He's gone' (note that in this change we lose a morpheme, namely *'s,* and end up with the simple word 'he' again). Now a new generation of children may feel that the quickening-up process has gone far enough and begin to add back information for clarity, saying, perhaps, 'He done gone' for the meaning 'He has gone' and continuing to use 'He gone' for the meaning 'He is gone'. Now the language has regrown the original distinction (between the meanings 'He has gone' and 'He is gone') but has slowed down just a bit.

Such changes happen all the time in all languages. They can, over long periods of time, produce from an analytic language, with its simple words, a polysynthetic language, with its complex words (which might very well have been separate words in the past that have "collapsed" together into single complex words, like 'he + is' becoming 'he's'). Dropping sounds and morphemes from words, can also produce analytic languages from polysynthetic ones. Languages move in an ever-changing circle through these various types, driven by the demands that humans make for clear, but quick, native languages. If a language gets too slow, children in acquiring the language speed it up; if it gets too unclear, they slow it down. In the process, they continually change it over thousands of years. A language is never "perfect," but always a compromise between these two forces, as well as various forces stemming from history and culture. But this compromise is always played out within the limits set by the human biological specification for language.

RECOMMENDED FURTHER READING

CHOMSKY, NOAM (1972). *Language and Mind,* enlarged edition. New York: Harcourt Brace Jovanovich. (An early classic by the founder of contemporary theoretical linguistics explicating the philosophical underpinnings of his view of language.)

CHOMSKY, NOAM (1986). *Knowledge of Language: Its Nature, Origin, and Use.* New York: Praeger. (Chapters 1 and 2 are a relatively accessible statement of Chomsky's current views on the nature of language and the enterprise of linguistics.)

GOODALL, JANE (1986). *The Chimpanzees of Gombe: Patterns of Behavior.* Cambridge, Mass.: Harvard University Press. (A masterpiece of descriptive science studying the behavior of chimpanzees in the wild).

MELLOR, D. H., ED. (1990). *Ways of Communicating.* Cambridge: Cambridge University Press. (An excellent set of essays covering diverse aspects of communication, each written by a leading scholar in the area. See in particular, Horace Barlow on "Communication and Representation within the Brain," pp. 14–34; Patrick Bateson on "Animal Communication," pp. 35–55; and Noam Chomsky on "Language and Mind," pp. 56–80.)

OSHERSON, DANIEL N. & LASNIK, HOWARD, EDS. (1990). *Language: An Invitation to Cognitive Science: Vol. 1.* Cambridge, Mass.: MIT Press. (Contains excellent introductory articles on many aspects of linguistics, each chapter written by a well-known expert in the field).

PREMACK, DAVID (1985). *Gavagai! On the Future History of the Animal Language Controversy.* Cambridge, Mass.: MIT Press. (A fascinating book by a psychologist who has worked extensively trying to teach chimpanzees human-like language systems.)

SAPIR, EDWARD (1921). *Language: An Introduction to the Study of Speech.* New York: Harcourt, Brace & World. (A classic work by one of the greatest linguists of the twentieth century.)

TANNEN, DEBORAH (1990). *You Just Don't Understand.* New York: Marrow. (A readable and fascinating discussion of problems in communication, especially between men and women.)

VON FRISCH, KARL (1967). *The Dance Language and Orientation of Bees,* trans. L. E. Chadwick. Cambridge, Mass.: Harvard University Press. (A classic work by one of the greatest students of animal behavior of the twentieth century.)

NOTE: There are a number of new encyclopedias devoted to language and linguistics which have entries relevant to almost all the issues discussed in this book. See especially, *International Encyclopedia of Linguistics,* Oxford: Oxford University Press, 1992, and *The Encyclopedia of Language and Linguistics,* New York: Pergamon Press and Aberdeen University Press, 1992.

CHAPTER 2

Semantics

The Meaning
of Language

Every human language is so intricate and complex that we will never "see the forest for the trees" if we begin our exploration with a real human language. Instead, we will use a very simple "made-up" language that will help us describe and explain actual human languages like English. What is important in our discussion of making up a simplified language is to see how one can "play" with language and to see the interesting philosophical issues that arise when we try to do this.

2.1. THE SIMPLIFIED PREDICATE LANGUAGE (SPL)

We call our made-up language the **Simplified Predicate Language,** SPL for short, because it views sentences as made up of two parts, **names** and **predicates.** In SPL, names name *things* in the world, like people or objects (whereas in English nouns also name ideas like honor, democracy, and freedom). Predicates label **properties** of these things, like their being *red* or *tall,* or **relations** between the things (like their being *in love with* or *taller than* another thing).

Names and Predicates

The English sentence 'John is happy' says of the person named 'John' that he has the property of being happy. The sentence 'John fell' attributes to John the property of having fallen. Notice that, in English, both adjectives and verbs can attribute or ascribe a property to an individual; thus they both count as predicates. Some verbs attribute not a property to a single person or thing, but rather name a relation between two or more things. For example, in 'John loves Mary', the verb 'loves' names a relation between two persons, John and Mary. We say that 'love' is a predicate that attributes the relation(ship) of love to John and Mary. The sentence 'Mary hit John' attributes the relation of hitting to John and Mary; that is, it says that John and Mary are related to each other through an act of hitting.

———————————————— **E X E R C I S E** ————————————————

Exercise A. For each sentence below, state whether each italicized word is a name or a predicate. If it is a predicate, state whether it designates a property (attribute, quality) of an individual or a relation between two or more individuals. (The sample answer is provided as a guide.)

Example Answer. Consider sentence 7. 'John' is a name, 'put' is a predicate, 'the book' is a name, and 'the table' is a name. The predicate 'put' is a relation between three things; in this sentence the three things are a *person,* a *book,* and a *place* (on the table).

1. *Mary* was *crying.*
2. *John loves wine.*
3. *The girl* is *happy.*
4. *John admires honesty.*
5. *Wind* is *powerful.*
6. John *gave a book* to *Mary.*
7. *John put the book* on *the table.*

———

The Lexicon (Dictionary) of SPL

SPL is simple enough that its vocabulary and structure can be described completely, something that cannot yet be done for any human language. We will carry out our description in a step-by-step fashion.

First, I give the **lexicon** of SPL; that is, its set of words. Initially, this will just be a list of symbols, which you are informed are words in the language. At first you will know nothing more about the matter than that. It's as if I told you that *ngalek* is a word in the Palauan (a language spoken in Micronesia). You have no idea what it means; all you now know is that it is a word. However, to help you, I will cheat a bit: Though SPL has nothing particularly to do with English, I will "translate" it into English, just to make my description easier to follow. But until we get to the semantics of SPL (that is, the rules for determining the meanings of the words and sentences of the language), you have to pretend you don't see these translations.

The lexicon of SPL is listed below. The predicate words look odd, perhaps, but not much odder than *ngalek* to English eyes (by the way, *ngalek* means 'child'). The term **functors** stands for the little grammatical words in English such as 'and', 'or', 'the', or 'if':

LEXICON FOR SPL

NAMES:	*a*	like the name 'Aaron' in English
	b	like the name 'Bill' in English
	c	like the name 'Cathy' in English
PREDICATES:	*S__*	like the word 'smile' in English
	T__	like the word 'tall' in English
	H__	like the word 'happy' in English
	L___	like the word 'love' in English
	K___	like the word 'kick' in English
FUNCTORS:	and	like the word 'and' in English
	or	like the word 'or' in English
	not	like the word 'not' in English

The symbols for names and functors in SPL have no parts; that is, the name *'b'* and the functor 'and' are like the word 'help' in English, not like the word 'unhelpful', which has three parts ('un', 'help', 'ful'). The predicate symbols *do* have parts; for instance, the capital letter *L* in '*L___*' is one part and the little fill-in blanks are each another part. These little fill-in blanks are called **places.**

The Syntax of SPL (Rules 1 and 2)

We are ready now to say what counts as a sentence in SPL; that is, to give its **syntax.** This is done by stating the rules that show how the words in the lexicon of SPL can be combined to make up sentences.

Consider first the symbols called "predicates" in the lexicon above. The "places" after the capital letters can be "filled" by the symbols called "names" in the lexicon. Thus, a predicate like '*S__*' has one place and a name like '*a*' can "fill" it to yield: '*Sa*' (which will eventually mean something like 'Aaron smiles'). And a predicate like '*L___*' has two places that can be filled by two names to yield '*Lac*' (which will eventually be seen to mean something like 'Aaron loves Cathy'). Below is the first rule for what counts as a sentence in SPL, and a sample sentence to illustrate each formulation shown.

RULE 1. Any predicate symbol with all its places filled by names counts as a sentence.

Ta	*T__* plus *a*	Aaron is tall
Hc	*H__* plus *c*	Cathy is happy
Lcb	*L___* plus *c* & *b*	Cathy loves Bill
Kba	*K___* plus *b* & *a*	Bill kicked Aaron

According to Rule 1, the combination *'Lc___'* is ungrammatical (not a sentence) because predicate *L* has two places and one of them is left unfilled.

Next, we add new rules stating how anything that counts as a sentence in virtue of Rule 1 can be combined with the symbols labeled as *functors* in the lexicon ('not', 'and', 'or') to produce more complicated sentences. Rule 2 has three parts, one for each functor:

RULE 2a (The *not* rule). Any sentence in SPL can have 'not' placed in front of it, and the result also counts as a sentence of SPL. We will put parentheses around the result to make it clear that the whole thing (that is, 'not' plus the sentence it is in front of) is itself a bigger sentence.

EXAMPLE: 'Lcb' ('Cathy loves Bill') is a sentence of SPL according to Rule 1, so then '(not *Lcb*)' is also a sentence of SPL, according to Rule 2a: ('It's not the case that Cathy loves Bill').

RULE 2b (The *and* rule). Any two sentences of SPL can have 'and' put between them, and the result will also count as a sentence of SPL. Again, we will put parentheses around the result to make it clear that the whole thing (that is, a sentence plus 'and' plus another sentence) is itself a bigger sentence.

EXAMPLE: 'Lcb' ('Cathy loves Bill') is a sentence of SPL and so is *'Kbc'* ('Bill kicks Cathy') according to Rule 1. Thus, combining these two sentences together with 'and' in between is also a sentence, according to Rule 2b: '(*Lcb* and *Kbc*)' ('Cathy loves Bill and Bill kicks Cathy').

RULE 2c (The *or* rule). Any two sentences of SPL can have 'or' put between them, and the result will also count as a sentence of SPL. Again, we will put parentheses around the result to make it clear that the whole thing (that is, a sentence plus 'or' plus another sentence) is itself a bigger sentence.

EXAMPLE: 'Lcb' is a sentence of SPL and so is *'Kbc'* according to Rule 1. Thus, combining these two sentences with 'or' in between is also a sentence, according to Rule 2c: *'(Lcb* or *Kbc)'* ('Cathy loves Bill or Bill kicks Cathy').

Summary of SPL Syntax Rules

To summarize the rules for the syntax of SPL, we let SENT stand for 'sentence'. Then, Rules 1 and 2a–c can be represented as follows:

Rule 1.	SENT	→	PREDICATE LETTER plus NAME FILLING EACH PLACE
Rule 2a.	SENT	→	(*not* SENT)
Rule 2b.	SENT	→	(SENT *and* SENT)
Rule 2c.	SENT	→	(SENT *or* SENT)

Rule 1 means "A sentence in SPL can be made up of a predicate letter (the capital letters in the predicate symbols) plus names filling each place in the predicate symbol (each little blank)." Rule 2a means "A sentence in SPL can be made up of the word 'not' followed by any sentence of SPL" (with the whole thing enclosed in parentheses). Rule 2b means "A sentence of SPL can be made up of any sentence of SPL followed by 'and' followed by any sentence of SPL" (with the whole thing enclosed in parentheses). Rule 2c means "A sentence of SPL can be made up of any sentence of SPL followed by 'or' followed by any sentence of SPL" (with the whole thing enclosed in parentheses). Alternatively, we can explain Rule 2c by saying that a sentence like '(*Lcb* or *Kbc*)' ('Cathy loves Bill or Bill kicks Cathy') is composed of the parts '*Lcb*', 'or', and '*Kbc*' (and the parentheses we use to enclose the bigger sentence). When rules are written in this form, they are called **phrase structure rules,** because they tell us the parts, that is, the "phrases," out of which the sentence is made.

SPL Has an Infinite Number of Sentences. The syntactic rules of SPL have an interesting property. They can create an infinite number of sentences. To see this, consider the following. Both '*Lcb*' and '*Kbc*' count as sentences by Rule 1. They can be combined into a bigger sentence by putting 'and' between them according to Rule 2b. This gives us '(Lcb and Kbc)'. This counts as a sentence by Rule 2b just as much as simpler sentences like '*Lcb*' count as sentences by virtue of Rule 1. Now this bigger sentence itself can be combined with another sentence, such as '*Ha*' ('Aaron is happy'), by placing 'and' between them (by Rule 2b again; see Example 1a, below) or by placing 'or' between them (by Rule 2c, see Example 1b). Or we could simply place 'not' in front of 'Lcb and Kbc' (by Rule 2a; see Example 1c). This will get us yet bigger sentences, as is seen in these examples:

1a. ((*Lcb* and *Kbc*) and *Ha*)
    (Cathy loves Bill and Bill kicks Cathy) and Aaron is happy
1b. ((*Lcb* and *Kbc*) or *Ha*)
    (Cathy loves Bill and Bill kicks Cathy) or Aaron is happy
1c. (not (*Lcb* and *Kbc*))
    It is not the case that (Cathy loves Bill and Bill kicks Cathy)

Notice how the various sets of parentheses in 1a–c make clear how the smaller sentences are combined into the bigger ones; for example, the two sets of parentheses in 1b make clear that the smaller sentence '*Lcb* and *Kbc*' (already itself made up of two even smaller sentences) is combined by means of 'or' with the sentence '*Ha*' to make a yet bigger sentence.

There is obviously no end to the process we have started here. For instance, we can take the whole sentence in 1b and combine it by Rule 2b, with another sentence, say '*Sc*' ('Cathy smiles'), by placing 'and' between them. This would generate sentence 1d, which contains all of 1b, shown enclosed in brackets.

1d. (((*Lcb* and *Kbc*) or *Ha*) and *Sc*)
  [(Cathy loves Bill and Bill kicks Cathy) or Aaron is happy] and Cathy smiles

We could now take all of 1d (it's a sentence) and combine it with another sentence by Rule 2b or 2c, or we could place 'not' in front of it by Rule 2a, in either case getting a yet longer sentence.

The process is open ended, and the sentences keep getting longer and more complicated. But whether you can figure them out or not, the rules of SPL tell you they are sentences. As for the meaning of these sentences, you will learn that when we get to semantics.

SPL's Rules Are Recursive. Having seen that there is no longest sentence in SPL, we can conclude that SPL has an *infinite number* of sentences. When a set of rules (like those in Rule 1 and Rules 2a–c) can produce an infinite number of sentences, they are said to be **recursive**. This means that such rules can produce sentences that are too long and complicated for any human to utter, write down, or comprehend, yet according to the rules they are sentences. All human languages are governed by recursive rules.

Competence Versus Performance. When someone or something (like a computer) knows rules like 1 and 2 in SPL, linguists say that this knowledge represents his, her, or its **competence**. Knowledge of such rules need not be conscious; it could be tacit or unconscious knowledge (such as the data stored in a computer program). Since one could know these rules yet still be unable to utter or write a sentence that the rules say is grammatical (because it is too long or complicated), there is a real sense in which such knowledge "outruns" ability. Linguists call abilities to perform (utter, write down, or figure out a sentence) **performance.** So we see that competence can very well exceed performance. When linguists study the phonological, syntactic, or semantic rules of a language (that is, its grammar), they are studying human linguistic competence, not performance.

───────────── **E X E R C I S E S** ─────────────

Exercise B. State which of the strings of symbols below are sentences in SPL. For any that is not a sentence, state why it is not. For any that is a sentence, show how the rules apply to make the sentence.

Example Answer. Consider #11: '(not (*Ta* or *Tb*))'. This is a sentence because it obeys the rules for constructing sentences in SPL. We can show this as follows: '*Ta*' is a sentence by Rule 1, which says any predicate symbol with all its places filled by names is a sentence. The predicate symbol '*T*__' has one place and here it is filled by the name *'a'*. The same is true of *'Tb'*, except that here it is the name *'b'* that fills the place of the predicate symbol. The larger string '(*Ta* or *Tb*)' is a sentence by Rule 2c, which says that the result of placing 'or' between any two sentences (with parentheses around the whole thing) is itself a sentence. The whole string '(not (*Ta* or *Tb*))' is also a sentence, this time by Rule 2a, which says that the result of placing 'not' in front of any sentence (with the whole thing placed in parentheses) is also a sentence itself.

NOTE: To prove something is a sentence, first show that the smallest parts are sentences, here *'Ta'* and *'Tb'*; then show that the material in the smallest parentheses is a sentence, here '(*Ta* and *Tb*); and then that the material in the next larger parentheses is a sentence, until you have worked your way up to the whole thing enclosed in the widest set of parentheses.

1. *T__*	**5.** *Tab*	**9.** (*Ta* or *Tb*)
2. *Ta*	**6.** (not *Ta*)	**10.** ((*Ta* or (not *Tb*))
3. *Lc__*	**7.** (*Kbc* and *Lcb*)	**11.** (not (*Ta* or *Tb*))
4. *Lcb*	**8.** (*K* not *bc*)	**12.** ((*Ta* or *Lcb*) and *Tc*)

Exercise C.   What is the difference in SPL between these two sentences:

1. (not (*Ta* and *Lcb*))
2. ((not *Ta*) and *Lcb*)

Exercise D.   Demonstrate that English has an infinite number of sentences.

The Semantics of SPL (Rules 3, 4, and 5)

The semantics of SPL are the rules for determining what its words and sentences mean. A language means nothing unless it is somehow hooked up with a world of things (persons or objects) to "talk about." This world we call the **universe of discourse.** For human languages the universe of discourse starts with the real world in which we all live and breathe, but it does not end there, as we can also talk about what does not exist in the real world, but is, for instance, imaginary, existing in the world of our human imaginations.

So, to give the semantics for SPL, we must first identify its universe of discourse. We will assume for now that, unlike human languages, SPL will talk only about its "real world." The nature of that world is indicated below (it is, indeed, a very small world). For simplicity's sake, we ignore time in that world, whether something happened in the past or is happening in the present, treating events as if they existed timelessly, once and for all.

UNIVERSE OF DISCOURSE FOR SPL

People in the World

A man named *a* (known as 'Aaron' in English)

A man named *b* (known as 'Bill' in English)

A woman named *c* (known as 'Cathy' in English)

Properties of the People

Aaron smiles (is smiling)
Aaron is tall
Aaron is not happy

Bill smiles (is smiling)
Bill is not tall
Bill is happy

Cathy is not smiling
Cathy is tall
Cathy is happy

Relationships Between the People

Aaron loves Aaron (himself)
Aaron loves Bill
Aaron does not love Cathy
Aaron does not kick Aaron (himself)
Aaron does not kick Cathy
Aaron does not kick Bill

Bill loves Bill (himself)
Bill loves Aaron
Bill does not love Cathy
Bill does not kick Bill (himself)
Bill does not kick Aaron
Bill does not kick Cathy

Cathy loves Cathy (herself)
Cathy does not love Aaron
Cathy does not love Bill
Cathy does not kick herself
Cathy kicks Aaron
Cathy kicks Bill

This universe of discourse is all there is in the entire world of SPL (even such a small world takes a lot of space to describe). But now giving the semantics of SPL is quite straightforward. In stating the semantic rules, I will use the word 'denotes' for the way in which a name or predicate hooks up to the world. Thus, I will say that a name like 'Bill' in English or *'b'* in SPL *denotes* (names) the person Bill. And I will say that a predicate like 'happy' in English or *'H'* in SPL *denotes* (names) the group of people who are happy. I will also use the phrase *'is true of an individual'* in regard to predicates. Thus, I will say that the predicate 'is happy' in English or *'H'* in SPL is true of the individual Bill just so long as Bill is in the set (group) of people who are happy. And the predicate 'loves' is true of the individuals Aaron and Bill just so long as Aaron and Bill are in a relationship such that the first (Aaron) loves the second (Bill). Sentences hook up to the world by being *true* or *not true (false)*—terms that will be defined in the rules below.

SEMANTICS OF SPL:

RULE 3 (Semantics of Names).   A name denotes the person it is assigned to on the following list:

a denotes Aaron
b denotes Bill
c denotes Cathy

RULE 4 (Semantics of Predicates).   Each predicate symbol denotes the set (group) of individuals (persons named by the names above) that the predicate is true of according to the following cases:

The predicate *'S__'* denotes the set (group) of people who smile (consulting the world given above, we see this is Aaron and Bill).

The predicate *'T__'* denotes the set (group) of people who are tall (consulting the world given above, we see this is Aaron and Cathy).

The predicate *'H__'* denotes the set (group) of people who are happy (consulting the world given above, we see this is Bill and Cathy).

The predicate *'L___'* denotes all the *pairs* of people such that the first loves the second (consulting our world, we find that these pairs are Aaron and Aaron; Aaron and Bill; Bill and Bill; Bill and Aaron; Cathy and Cathy).

The predicate *'K___'* denotes the *pairs* of people such that the first kicked the second (consulting our world, we find that these pairs are Cathy and Aaron; Cathy and Bill).

RULE 5 (Semantics of Sentences)

Rule 5a. Any sentence made up of only a one-place predicate with its one place filled by a name is true just so long as the person denoted by the name is in the set (group) denoted by the predicate. Thus, for example, *'Sa'* ('Aaron smiles') is true just so long as Aaron is in the set of people who are smiling. Since we find that he is when we consult our world above, the sentence is true.

Rule 5b. Any sentence made up of only a two-place predicate with both its places filled by names is true just so long as the two people denoted by the names are one of the pairs denoted by the predicate. Thus, for example, *'Lab'* is true just so long as Aaron and Bill are among the pairs of people such that the first loves the second. Consulting our world, we see that they are, so the sentence is true.

Rule 5c. Any sentence of the form '(not SENTENCE)' is true just so long as the SENTENCE following 'not' is not true. Thus, for example, '(not *Tc*)' ('It is not the case that Cathy is tall') is true just so long as *'Tc'* ('Cathy is tall') is not true (because saying that something that is not true is not true is true!). Since *'Tc'* is not true, '(not *Tc*)' is true.

Rule 5d. Any sentence of the form '(SENTENCE and SENTENCE)' is true just so long as the first sentence is true and the second sentence is true (so long as both of the sentences connected by 'and' are true). Thus, for example, '(*Ta* and *Tb*)' ('Aaron is tall and Bill is tall') is true just so long as both *'Ta'* ('Aaron is tall') and *'Tb'* ('Bill is tall') are true. Since we find that both of them are indeed true in our world, the sentence combining them with 'and' ('(*Ta* and *Tb*)') is true.

Rule 5e. Any sentence of the form '(SENT or SENT)' is true just so long as at least one of the sentences combined by 'or' is true. Thus, for example, '(*Ta* or *Tc*)' ('Aaron is tall or Cathy is tall') is true just so long as at least one of *'Ta'* ('Aaron is tall') or *'Tc'* ('Cathy is tall') is true. Since one is true (*'Ta'*), even though the other is not true (*'Tc'*), the whole sentence '(*Ta* or *Tc*)' counts as true.

Computing Whether a Sentence in SPL Is True or Not. Using the foregoing semantic rules, we are able to compute whether any sentence in SPL is true or not. Let's examine a sentence like the following:

2. ((*Lcb* or *Lab*) and *Hb*)
     ((Cathy loves Bill or Aaron loves Bill) and Bill is happy)

We will take the sentence apart piece by piece. Consider first '(*Lcb* or *Lab*)'. According to Rule 4 (the rule for predicates), *'Lcb'* (the first part of this sentence) is false because in our SPL world Cathy does not love Bill. But, also according to Rule 4, *'Lab'* (the second part) is true because Aaron does love Bill. Thus, according to Rule 5e (the rule for 'or') the bigger sentence '(*Lcb* or *Lab*)', made up of these two sentences, is true because at least one of the littler sentences it is made up of is true (*'Lab'* is true), and that is what Rule 5e requires.

Now, having seen that the big sentence '(*Lcb* or *Lab*)' is true, we check *'Hb'*. According to our universe of discourse, *'Hb'* ('Bill is happy') is true. Thus, both of the sentences combined by 'and' in sentence 1 are true, and this means that the whole big sentence is itself true (since Rule 5d, which gives the semantics of 'and', says that any sentence with 'and' is true just so long as both the sentences that 'and' combines are true).

Thus, no matter how complicated or long a sentence in SPL might be, with enough time, paper, and pencils (or computers) we could compute whether it was true or false. Of course, if the sentence was long enough, there wouldn't be enough time, because humans do not live forever. That is, as we pointed out above, our performance does not always match our competence, and the semantic rules are competence rules.

─────────────── **E X E R C I S E S** ───────────────

Exercise E. Following the procedure just explained, demonstrate that the sentence in 1 below is true in SPL and the sentence in 2 is false (not true):

1. (*Lcb* or (*Lab* and *Hb*))
2. (*Lcb* and (*Lab* and *Hb*))

Exercise F. According to Rule 5e, any sentence in SPL containing 'or' is true so long as at least one of the sentences connected by 'or' is true. Thus, in SPL a sentence like '(*Hb* or *Ta*)' ('Bill is happy or Aaron is tall') is true if *'Hb'* or *'Ta'* or both of them are true. Is this how English 'or' works? In answering this question, consider the following English sentences:

1. Johnny is going to mow the lawn *or* he's not getting his allowance.
2. John is there by now *or* he's late.
3. Either the President signed the bill last night *or* he vetoed it.

───

2.2. PROBLEMS WITH SPL SEMANTICS

There are several complaints one could make against the semantic rules for SPL presented in the previous section. Dealing with these complaints will give us a deeper insight into the nature of meaning. One such complaint may be stated as follows:

COMPLAINT 1: All along you indicated in the English translations of SPL that a predicate like 'S—' can be translated by the English word 'smile'. Now, Rule 4 says that a predicate symbol denotes the group of individuals that the predicate is true of. So, for example, the predicate 'S—' denotes the set of people who smile. But this is surely not what the word 'smile' means in English. The word 'smile' doesn't mean the *people* who just happen to be smiling; surely it has something to do with having a certain look on one's face. Just because Aaron and Bill happen to be smiling doesn't mean that 'smile' *means* Aaron and Bill. If they stopped smiling and other people started to smile, the word would not change its meaning. So either 'S___' doesn't translate as 'smile', or you haven't really said anything about its meaning, or for that matter, about meaning at all.

This complaint is completely well taken. I have really been talking about what words *denote* (stand for, name); that is, which individuals in the world they apply to, not what they *mean*. And while we will see that denotation is part of what is involved in meaning, it is not itself the meaning of a word.

Validity (Valid Argument)

SPL is a simplified version of a language used by logicians and mathematicians. The language in its fuller (but still fairly simple) form is called "The Predicate Calculus," which I will call PC for short. Logicians and mathematicians are less interested in what words actually mean than they are in knowing what **deductions** they can make from a particular statement or set of statements taken as **premises** in an **argument.** For example, consider the following argument:

ARGUMENT 1

PREMISE 1:   All humans are mortal
PREMISE 2:   Aaron is a human
CONCLUSION: Aaron is mortal

Arguments like Argument 1 are called **deductive arguments.** The best way to see what 'valid' means is to see why this argument is valid. To say that an argument is valid is to say that its premises could never be true while its conclusion was false. That is, you are guaranteed that *if* the premises are true, then you may logically *deduce* that the conclusion is true.

Argument 1 is valid, and we can see this as follows: The first premise says that every human (no matter how many of them there are in the world we choose to be talking about) is mortal. So imagine mortality as a big circle that encloses all beings who are mortal. The first premise then says you should place all humans inside this big circle (since all of them are mortal). The second premise says that Aaron is a human. Therefore, you must have placed him inside the big mortality circle when you put all the humans in there. So Aaron must be mortal, otherwise he would be outside the mortality circle. Since all humans are inside it, he couldn't be a human. But Premise 2 says he is a human. So he must be in the circle. No matter how you think about it, you cannot imagine the premises being true and the conclusion—that Aaron is mortal—false. That is exactly what it means to say that the argument is valid.

Logicians seek to formulate the rules by which we can determine of any argument whether or not it is valid, and they use PC to help them in this task. There is a very interesting thing about Argument 1. It does not rely at all on what words like 'human' and 'mortal' *mean,* but rather it relies on the *form* of the argument. Thus, we can switch these words to others and the argument remains valid:

A VALID ARGUMENT

PREMISE 1:	All swans are white
PREMISE 2:	Sandy is a swan
CONCLUSION:	Therefore Sandy is white

It does not matter whether the premises are *actually* true or not (in fact, Premise 1 is false; there are black swans). All that matters is that you cannot imagine the premises being true and the conclusion being false. *If* all swans *were* white and Sandy *was* a swan, then the world could not be otherwise than that Sandy is white.

What all this amounts to is that you could substitute *any* words into the argument above and get a valid argument. It turns out that it is the *form* of the argument (that is, the arrangement of the words in the argument together with the meanings of its little words like 'all' and 'is') that make it valid, *not* the meanings of the big words like 'human' and 'mortal'. The big words can be replaced by any other big words and the argument remains valid.

So we can in fact state the argument as a schema or pattern or form, as below:

PREMISE 1:	all X are Y
PREMISE 2:	Z is X
CONCLUSION:	Z is Y

This type of argument form is called a **syllogism.** Several types of syllogisms were formulated by the ancient Greek philosopher Aristotle. There is no need to worry about what X, Y, Z actually *mean;* whatever words we substitute for X, Y, and Z, the argument will remain valid. The argument form we have looked at here is a deductive argument because you can validly deduce its conclusion from its premises. Not all arguments are deductive. Consider the following argument:

ARGUMENT 2

PREMISE 1:	Most swans are white
PREMISE 2:	Sally is a swan
CONCLUSION:	Sally is white

This is not a valid argument. The premises of this argument could be true (Most swans *are* in fact white, and Sally could indeed be a swan), but its conclusion could still be false (Sally may happen to be one of those rare black swans). Of course, if most swans are white, it is probable that Sally is white, but you can't be sure of it the way you could with a valid argument. Arguments like Argument 2, where the premises lead you to conclude that the conclusion is *likely* or *probable,* but where you cannot deduce with logical certainty that the conclusion is true, are called **inductive arguments.**

————————————————— E X E R C I S E —————————————————

Exercise G. One of the arguments below is valid and one is not. Which one is not valid? Why? Which one is valid? Why? Give another version (with different words) of the valid argument. Give an abstract schema that can characterize this valid argument form.

Example Answer. The following argument is valid:

> Premise 1: All humans are animals
> Premise 2: All animals are mortal
> Conclusion: All humans are mortal

This argument is valid because if we draw a circle that contains all the animals in the world, the first premise says that all humans are inside that circle. The second premise says that all animals are inside an even bigger circle containing all mortal things (so the animal circle is inside the mortal things circle). Since all humans were inside the animal circle and the animal circle is inside the mortal circle, then all humans must also be inside the mortal circle. Another example of an argument using the same logical form, but with different words is

> Premise 1: All elephants are big (things)
> Premise 2: All big things are happy
> Conclusion: All elephants are happy

The abstract schema that characterizes this sort of argument is

> Premise 1: All X are Y
> Premise 2: All Y are Z
> Conclusion: All X are Z

No matter what one substitutes for X, Y, and Z in this argument, the argument will remain valid. Now, you do the ones below:

1. Premise 1: All humans are mortal
   Premise 2: Rover is mortal
   Conclusion: Rover is human
2. Premise 1: All ducks are animals
   Premise 2: All ducks are birds
   Conclusion: Some animals are birds

Sense and Denotation

The complaint that 'smile' doesn't mean the people who just happen to be smiling, but rather has something to do with a certain look on the face, is still not answered. The word 'meaning' itself has many meanings. This is how we will define it:

> The **meaning** of a word in a language (for example, English) is *the information in the head of the speaker* of that language that allows him or her to identify the set of individuals which the word denotes.

Thus, the meaning of 'smile' in English is the information in your head (which you obtained in learning the language) that allows you to identify the set of people who are, at any given time, smiling; that is, to know when it is correct to say that someone or something is smiling. The meaning of the word 'love' in English is the information in your head that allows you to identify people who are in love; that is, to know when it is correct to say of one person that that person loves another person.

Obviously, the key question is, "Exactly what *is* this information?" Unfortunately, that turns out to be a very hard question, one to which we do not yet know the answer, though there has been much fruitful speculation about the matter in psychology, linguistics, and philosophy. For some words, however, the answer is easy. Take a word like 'bachelor'. It is clear that the information that allows you to identify the people that the word 'bachelor' denotes is something like UNMARRIED MALE. And there are various social tests (criteria) for whether someone is married (for example, the existence of a marriage license) and various social and biological tests (criteria) for whether someone is a male. These tests stand behind your knowledge of what it means to be unmarried and what it means to be male, and they could be used to test whether someone belongs in the set of bachelors or not. By writing these words in capital letters, we signify that they are to stand for *concepts, ideas,* or pieces of mental information in your head, not English words. The concepts UNMARRIED and MALE combined together are the meaning of the word 'bachelor'. (Chapter 7 on psycholinguistics will modify this a bit.)

Because the word 'meaning' has so many meanings, philosophers often substitute the term 'sense'; I will hereafter use these words interchangeably. A word is said to have both a sense and a denotation. The sense of 'bachelor' is UNMARRIED MALE, and its denotation is the set of people who are picked out by the word 'bachelor'. The sense is the information we use to identify the denotation of the word.

Philosophers sometimes use the word 'reference' instead of 'denotation', but I will *not* do this; rather I will use 'reference' for what people actually do when they use language. For example, the word 'boy' denotes the set of boys, but when Mr. Smith says of Johnny Jones "That boy is going to get in trouble," he is using 'that boy' to refer to Johnny Jones. For me, words *denote* things, but people *refer* to things.

Complaint 2. The Language–Metalanguage Distinction

Another complaint that one could justly lodge against the semantic rules for SPL is the following:

> **COMPLAINT 2.** The semantic rules for SPL are given in English, and to understand them one has to know what English means. We were dealing with SPL because it was supposed to be easier than English, but now it turns out that one has to understand English to understand SPL. Does this get us anywhere?

This complaint brings up a profound problem in dealing with language. To give the meaning of a word or sentence in any language, you have to use a language. Now obviously, I can give the meanings of some English words by defining them in terms of other English words. For example, I can define 'bachelor' as meaning *unmarried male* or 'nepotism' as *undue favoritism to relatives.* But then you must know the meanings of 'unmarried' and 'male' and of 'favoritism' and 'relatives'. Sooner or later I must give the meanings of some words without using English words or the whole process is circular (you have to know English already to say what English means). Of course, I could give the meanings of these English words in Russian, but then I would be assuming that you know Russian. And we would still face the paradox that to give the meanings of words in a language like English, one already has to know some other language (like Russian).

Some people are tempted to say, "To give the meaning of a word, you can just point to something that is part of the denotation of the word." But that won't work. Most things can't be pointed to: Imagine trying to point to honesty or democracy. And even when one can point, the learner would have to know already what to look for. If I point to a horse and say 'horse', how do you know I am denoting the horse and not its color, shape, size, gender, or type?

When one gives the meaning of a word or sentence in a language L1 (say, English) in terms of another language, L2 (say, Russian), the first language (L1) is called the **object language** and the second one (L2) is called the **metalanguage.** If you define 'bachelor' as 'unmarried male' you are using English as its own metalanguage. Earlier, when I treated UNMARRIED and MALE (in capitals) as mental concepts, not as English words, I was assuming that concepts make up a *mental language* (what we might call the **language of thought**), and so I was treating this mental language (L2) as a metalanguage for the object language, English (L1). Before that we were using English as a metalanguage to describe SPL as an object language, which is what gave rise to Complaint 2 in the first place.

There is no way out of this paradox. Linguists simply have to hope that once they have used English or some other human language (as a metalanguage) to construct and understand a clear and precise technical language like SPL (as an object language), they can turn around and explicate the nature of English (as an object language) by using SPL (as a metalanguage). But other scientists face a similar problem. Physicists use technical languages (several branches of mathematics) to understand the world because they believe that human languages are not clear and precise enough for this task. But they had to use English originally or some other human language to construct and come to understand these technical languages.

The metalanguage paradox arises not just for scientists but for children as well. If one cannot understand one language without using another one as a metalanguage, how do children learn the meanings of words when they start the language acquisition process? How can they represent to themselves the meanings of English words when they have no other language into which they can translate them? We are forced, I believe, to conclude that children *do* know a language already, when they start learning their first human language, and that they use this language to represent the meanings of the human language they are learning. This language children already know is the *language of thought,* some of which they build up through their sensory-motor awareness of the world before language acquisition starts and some of which they are born knowing as part of the biological birthright of human intelligence.

I will assume that some of the most basic words in any human language (for example, words like 'alive', 'dead', 'kill') can have their meanings (senses) specified in terms of concepts drawn from this language of thought. For example, the meaning of a word like 'kill' would be something like CAUSE SOMETHING TO GO FROM BEING ALIVE TO BEING NOT ALIVE, where these capitalized words stand for 'words' (concepts) in a language of thought which is part of a common human inheritance stemming from our biology or our early prelinguistic experiences of the physical and social worlds. Many less basic words can then be given meanings in terms of definitions constructed out of these basic words, which are explicated through concepts in the language of thought.

We have no complete idea what the language of thought looks like, though there is some research that bears on the matter. We will progressively build on this idea of a language of thought, gradually, we hope, making the idea more plausible.

--------------------------------- **E X E R C I S E S** ---------------------------------

Exercise H. People whom we call 'bachelors' are unmarried and male and are sometimes thought of as DESIRABLE. People we call 'spinsters' are unmarried and female and are sometimes thought of as UNDESIRABLE. Using the word 'meaning' ('sense') as we are in this chapter, is BEING DESIRABLE part of the meaning of the word 'bachelor'; is BEING UNDESIRABLE part of the meaning of the word 'spinster'? Why do these words have these values or attitudes associated with them?

Exercise I. Values or attitudes like those associated with 'bachelor' and 'spinster', or with the things the words denote, which we considered in Exercise H, are often called the **connotations** of a word. For the words listed below, give their meaning (sense), their denotation, and some of their connotations (you may consult a dictionary to help you with the sense of the word, but be careful: Dictionaries sometimes mix up sense and connotation).

Example Answer. Take the word 'skunk'. The sense of this word is something like "a small black and white furry animal in the weasel family which is capable of ejecting a smelly fluid" (I found the weasel family description in a dictionary). The denotation of the word 'skunk' is the set of skunks. Some connotations include 'smelly thing', 'dangerous', 'to be avoided', 'suspicious'. Because of these connotations, the word can be used figuratively to mean a contemptible person (as in "He's a real skunk").

    rat
    tiger
    poem
    blond
    smog

2.3. POSSIBLE WORLDS

Language is used to talk about not just the "real world," but also about worlds that do not exist, worlds built up in our imaginations or through our theories about reality (which are not, of course, always true). Consider a sentence like the following:

3. Mary believes that *the king of France takes bribes.*

Since there is no king of France in the real world, the italicized portion ('the king of France takes bribes') is not true. (Some philosophers would say it is false;

others consider it neither true nor false. What do you think?) However, the whole sentence can be true just so long as Mary does believe that the king of France takes bribes (every human can believe false things).

One way we can understand sentence 3 is to say that, while it happens that there is no king of France in the real world, in Mary's **belief worlds** there is a king of France and he takes bribes. Mary's belief worlds are all the possible worlds compatible with everything that Mary believes to be true in the real world.

There are, in fact, many such belief worlds for Mary (and, indeed, for each of us). This is so because Mary does not have beliefs about everything. For example, Mary has no belief about the truth or falsity of the sentence 'There are mountain lions in California'. It is true in the real world that there are mountain lions in California. But since Mary has no belief about the matter, then a world in which there are mountain lions in California and one in which there are no mountain lions in California are both compatible with Mary's beliefs in the real world, and thus possible worlds as far as Mary's beliefs are concerned. Indeed, there are a huge number of worlds compatible with everything that Mary believes in the real world.

Note that since Mary believes the king of France takes bribes, but in fact, in the real world there is no king of France, the real world is not compatible with Mary's beliefs. Thus, the real world is, in this sense, not a possible world as far as Mary's beliefs are concerned. In fact, since all of us have beliefs that are not true, this is the case for all of us fallible mortals (though we all think the real world is the way we believe it to be). Let us call any description of a world that fits with Mary's beliefs one of her "belief worlds." We have seen there are many of these, since the description of a world in which there are no mountain lions in California and the description of a world in which there are mountain lions in California are both worlds compatible with what Mary believes, both "Mary belief worlds."

To give the meaning of sentence 3, we must, then, talk about Mary's belief worlds, not just the real world. To explicate the meaning of sentence 3, we must say something like the following:

4. 'Mary believes the king of France takes bribes' means that in all of 'Mary's belief worlds,' that is, in all the worlds that are compatible with what Mary believes in the real world, there is a king of France and he takes bribes.

In sentence 3, it is the word 'believe' that cues us into considering possible worlds (here, Mary's belief worlds), and not just real ones; it is, so to speak, a **worlds creating** word. Many words can do this. Consider, for instance, the following sentences, all of which encompass more than the real world:

5a. It's *possible* the mayor of Boston will be President in 1996.
5b. It's *likely* that Ray Flynn will be President in 1996.

5c. I can't *imagine* Mary ever marrying Sam.

5d. John *saw* a pink elephant.

5e. Mary is *looking for* (*seeking*) a unicorn.

5f. John *hopes* that he will win the race on Friday.

─────────────────── **E X E R C I S E S** ───────────────────

Exercise J.   For three of the sentences in 5a–f above, suggest why they involve us in thinking about possible worlds and not just the real world.

Exercise K.   The following sentence is ambiguous (has two different meanings):

Mary is looking for a friend.

This sentence can mean that Mary is looking for any friend, it doesn't matter who it is (she wants a friend), or it can mean that she is looking for a specific person who, in fact, is a friend of hers (say, Sam Smith). How would you account for this ambiguity in terms of talking about possible worlds? (NOTE: One can also look for things that don't exist, like unicorns.)

2.4.   PREDICATES AND ARGUMENTS

We have seen how in SPL each predicate has one or more places that can be filled by names. Names filling the places of predicates are often called the *arguments* of the predicate (the word 'argument' here has nothing to do with the key term **argument** as used in Section 2.2 to talk about deductive and inductive arguments). When the right number of arguments are put in the predicate's places (the number required by the predicate), we get the sentences of SPL shown in 6:

6a. $K\_\_ + b$ and $a = Kba$ Bill kicks Aaron

6b. $S\_ + c = Sc$ Cathy smiles

6c. $H\_ + a = Ha$ Aaron is happy

English verbs and adjectives behave just like SPL predicates. They require one or more arguments to make up a sentence. These arguments can be proper names, as in 7:

7a. *Bill* kicked *Aaron*   =   'kicked' + 'Bill' and 'Aaron'

7b. *Cathy* smiled   =   'smiled' + 'Cathy'

7c. *Aaron* is happy   =   'is happy' + 'Aaron'

The arguments can also be NOUN PHRASES, that is, a set of words meaningful-ly organized around a NOUN (Chapter 6 explains further the concept of the noun phrase). In fact, if a string of words can replace the proper names in sentences like 7a–c, it indicates that this string of words is a noun phrase. Thus, the sentences in 8 contain full noun phrases where the sentences in 7 have proper names:

8a. *The old man* kicked *the little puppy* =
'kicked' + 'the old man' and 'the little puppy'

8b. *The young girl from Brooklyn* smiled =
'smiled' + 'the young girl from Brooklyn'

8c. *That tall young man with a smile on his face* is happy =
'is happy' + 'that tall young man with a smile on his face'

To have a term covering both proper names (like 'Bill') and full noun phrases (like 'the young girl'), both of which can serve as arguments to predicates, I will call them both NOMINALS. For the time being, I make no distinction between verbs like 'kick' and 'smile' and adjectives like 'happy'. They are all predicates which take nominals to make sentences.

All of the examples above are either ONE-PLACE PREDICATES (like 'smile'), which have only one place and thus take only one nominal to make up a whole sentence, or TWO-PLACE PREDICATES (like 'kick'), which have two places and thus take two nominals to make up a sentence. English also has some THREE-PLACE PREDICATES, that is, verbs that have three places and thus take three nominals (arguments) to make up a sentence. For example, 'give' has three places, one for a giver, one for a gift, and one for the recipient. It is a property of English that if a predicate takes more than two nominals to fill its places, then the third nominal is usually preceded by a preposition. With the verb 'give' this preposition is 'to'. A verb like 'put' is also a three-place predicate, and its third argument must be preceded by some preposition that names a location or a direction:

9. *Mary* gave *the book* to *John*

10a. *Mary* put *the flowers* in *the vase*
10b. *John* put *the money* on *the table*
10c. *The child* put *her toys* under *the table*

2.5.   FROM ENGLISH SENTENCES TO THEIR MEANINGS

It is time now for us to see how English sentences can be related to their meanings. We assume that English sentences are ultimately given meaning by being translated into the language of thought. But this translation will not be direct. We will do it in two stages. First, we will translate the English sentence into an expanded version of SPL (expanded by adding more names and predicates). Second, we will translate the SPL translation into the language of thought.

Translating into SPL

In many cases, we do not yet know enough about the language of thought to go beyond the SPL translation to the language of thought. However, the SPL translation itself gives us good information about the meaning of the sentence, both because we understand SPL better than we understand English, and because SPL's structure is simpler and more transparent than any human language. Further, it may be that SPL resembles the language of thought in its structure more than any human language does. We will see, however, that there are many types of English sentences that have no translation in SPL, because SPL is too simple. These types of English sentences require us to enrich SPL if it is to serve as a language for **semantic representation** (translation of human languages).

The attempt to translate English into SPL immediately gives rise to an interesting discovery. Almost all English sentences, no matter how simple they are, translate into *several* SPL sentences. To see this, consider the one sort of case where this doesn't happen. To translate an English sentence into SPL, we treat each verb or adjective in the sentence as a predicate of SPL, and each proper name as a name in SPL. Thus, the English sentences in 11 translate as shown:

11a. Mary kicked John = *Kmj* (Mary = *m*, John = *j*, kicked = *K___*)
11b. Mary is tall = *Tm* (Mary = *m*, tall = *T__*)

But when the argument positions of a verb or adjective are filled not by proper names, but full noun phrases, something quite different happens. Consider sentence 12:

12. The tall man lit his awful cigar

Each word in this sentence actually contributes a predicate to its SPL translation. The adjective 'tall' still translates as the predicate TALL even though it is now in front of a noun and not after a copula (verb 'to be'). 'Tall' here contributes the information that something IS TALL. The noun 'man' contributes the information that something IS A MAN. The adjective 'awful' contributes the information that something IS AWFUL, and the noun 'cigar' that something IS A CIGAR. Even the little words 'the' and 'his' contribute predicates to the meaning of this sentence. 'The' contributes the information that something IS KNOWN (already identifiable from previous knowledge or the prior discourse). 'His' contributes the information that something BELONGS TO someone. And, of course, the main verb 'lit' is the main predicate in the sentence, taking two arguments ('the tall man' and 'the awful cigar').

To translate sentence 12 into SPL we need to introduce one more element of the fuller language PC, namely *indefinite names* or *variables*. Let x and y be VARIABLES for individuals (persons or things) in the universe of discourse. They mean what the English words 'someone' or 'something' mean. Or better, treat x as if it means *some person or thing, call it x, since we don't know or care what its name is,* and treat y as if it means *some person or thing, call it y (a different person or thing from x), since we don't know or care what its* NAME *is.*

Listed in 13a are the translations of each word in the English sentence in 12 in terms of variables and predicates in SPL, where the SPL predicates will be represented as English words in small capital letters; 13b puts all these elements together to give a full translation of 12:

13a. the = KNOWNx = x is KNOWN
tall = TALLx = x is TALL
man = MANx = x is a MAN
lit = LITxy = x LIT y
the = KNOWNy = y is KNOWN
awful = AWFULy = y is AWFUL
his = BELONGyx = y BELONGS TO x
cigar = CIGARy = y is a CIGAR

13b. KNOWNx and TALLx and MANx and LITxy and KNOWNy and AWFULy and BELONGyx and CIGARy

We read 13b as follows: 'x is KNOWN and x is TALL and x is a MAN and xLITy and y is KNOWN and y is AWFUL and y is a CIGAR and y BELONGS to x'. Sometimes I will write 'KNOWNx' (the "correct" word order in SPL as I have defined it) and sometimes 'x is KNOWN' (just because the latter is easier for English speakers to read). Each piece of information contributed by each word in sentence 12 is connected to the other pieces by 'and', and the order of the pieces in 13b does not really matter since in SPL the word 'and' does not care in what order the two things it connects are put (in SPL 'Sa and Tb' and 'Tb and Sa' amount to the same thing). We will just agree to keep the pieces of our translations in much the same order as they appeared in the English sentence. This will make them easier to read.

This translation process shows that English sentences usually package in one sentence what is actually a large number of discrete pieces of information (in terms of claims about what predicates are said to be true of what arguments). Of course, one could say something like sentence 14 in English, where the information that is tightly packaged in sentence 12 is unraveled into several separate sentences (note that the pronouns 'he' and 'it' function much like x and y, except that they contain information about the GENDER—male, female, or neither—of the thing which they name):

14. There's this man. He is tall. He lit something. It was a cigar. It was his. It was awful.

Obviously, communication would be slow indeed if we had to communicate as in 14, though we will see in Chapter 10, on discourse, that there are circumstances when people do begin to communicate in a fashion not far removed from this.

In summary, then, simple English sentences usually translate into a series of simple SPL sentences (connected together by 'and'). Each simple SPL sentence (like 'Kx' or 'Lxy') is called a PREDICATE-ARGUMENT STRUCTURE and is said to communicate a PROPOSITION. 'Proposition' is a term from philosophy that (very roughly) is used for the smallest sentence-like unitary ideas expressed by SPL, PC or, by extension, any language. The English sentence 12 is seen to express and combine eight separate propositions.

It is important to see also that the translation in 13b makes clear also how the various propositions in the meaning of sentence 12 are fit together or combined together. The main predicate 'lit' has two places. One is filled by x and the other by y. Every other predicate in 13b which has x in one of its places is tied to the x position of 'lit' (gives more information about this thing x), and every one that has y in one of its places is tied to the y position of 'lit' (gives more information about this thing y).

_____ **E X E R C I S E** _____

Exercise L.   Translate the following sentences into their SPL representations (as we did for example sentence 12) and say how many propositions there are in each translation. Treat English "gives" in sentence 3 as a three-place predicate 'GIVExyz' in SPL meaning 'x GIVES y TO z'; thus 'John gave Rover to Sue' would translate as 'GIVEjrs', where j is an SPL name for John, r is an SPL name for Rover, and s is an SPL name for Sue.

Example Answer.   Consider sentence 4 below. This would translate as 'UNKNOWNx and HAPPYx and GIRLx and HITxj' (where j is an SPL name for John and UNKNOWNx translates the English word 'a'). The sentence translates into four propositions (the translation means the same as 'x is UNKNOWN and x is HAPPY and x is a GIRL and x HIT j').

1. The happy boy loves the girl with blue eyes.
2. John is not happy.
3. John gives a big cookie to a small boy.
4. A happy girl hit John.

Problems in Translation

If we are concerned with a phrase like 'the tall man', it works perfectly to say that the meaning of this phrase is made up of the combination of the meanings 'x is KNOWN', 'x IS TALL', and 'x is a MAN', combined together by 'and' as in sentence 15a below. However, the phrase 'the alleged burglar' surely cannot be a simple combination of 'x is KNOWN' (the contribution of 'the'), 'x is ALLEGED' (the contribution of 'alleged'), and 'x is a BURGLAR' (the contribution of 'burglar'), since alleged burglars may very well turn out to be innocent and thus not burglars at all. Thus, a translation for 'the alleged burglar' along the same lines as the translation of 'the tall man' in 15a is out of the question:

15a. the tall man = KNOWNx and TALLx and MANx

15b. the alleged burglar = KNOWNx and ALLEGEDx and BURGLARx
(*wrong* because an alleged burglar need not be a burglar)

A phrase like 'fake gun' gives rise to the same problem. This surely cannot be translated as 'x is FAKE and x is a GUN' because fake guns precisely are *not* guns, just things that look like guns.

The trouble here is once again the difference between SENSE and DENOTATION. In a phrase like 'the alleged burglar', we are concerned not with the things 'burglar' denotes (the group of burglars), but just with its sense (the sorts of tests that go into determining what constitutes a burglar). Likewise for a 'fake gun'. Here we are concerned not with the denotation of 'gun' (the set of guns), but just with its sense (the tests which something must pass to be a gun). 'Alleged burglar' says that some x is *claimed* to fit the sense of burglar, but we cannot be sure x really does. 'Fake gun' says something only *looks* to fit the sense of 'gun', but in fact it does not (and therefore is not, in fact, in the denotation of 'gun').

What is involved here are, once again, *possible worlds*. 'Alleged burglar' says that someone is in the denotation of 'burglar' in a possible world but not necessarily in the actual world, and 'fake gun' says something is in the denotation of 'gun' only in some perceptual world, a world compatible with how guns look, not with what they really are (it could *possibly* be taken *as* a gun from the *look* of it). Whenever possible worlds are involved in meaning, SPL cannot handle the translation. In fact, we need a more powerful language. I will not detail that language here, but just to give the flavor of it, I offer translations of sentences with words like 'fake' and 'alleged':

15c. The alleged burglar smiled = x is KNOWN in the real world and x is ACCUSED OF A CRIME in the real world and x is a BURGLAR in a possible world compatible with all the evidence against x in the real world and x SMILED

15d. The fake gun is big = x is KNOWN in the real world and x is a FAKE OBJECT in the real world and x is a GUN in some possible world compatible with the way guns look in the real world (perceptual worlds = worlds just like the real world, save in these worlds things really are what they look like) and x is BIG

These translations bring out the fact that someone could not be an alleged burglar if there were no imaginable circumstances under which it is reasonable to conclude he or she is a burglar. And something could not be a fake gun if there were no imaginable circumstances under which people would conclude by looking at it that it was a gun. The problem with 'alleged' and 'fake' is the same one we saw with words like 'believe', which of necessity involve going beyond the way things *are* to considering the way things *could be,* or *look to be.* Just for completeness I will offer one possible translation of a sentence with 'believe':

15e. Mary believes that the tall man died = (KNOWNx and TALLx and MANx and DIEDx) is true in the possible worlds compatible with what Mary believes to be true, though not necessarily in the real world

Another Problem in Translation. Words that involve us in consideration of possibilities are not the only ones that give rise to problems in translation from English to SPL. Consider a sentence like 'A big mouse is a small animal'. It may appear that this sentence should be translated as follows:

16a. x is BIG and x is a MOUSE and x is SMALL and x is AN ANIMAL

This is obviously a contradiction. How can x be BIG and x be SMALL at the same time?

Phrases like 'the big elephant' and 'the big mouse' cannot really be translated as 'x is KNOWN and x is BIG and x is AN ELEPHANT' and 'y is KNOWN and y is BIG and y is A MOUSE' respectively. The trouble is that even a big mouse is a small thing compared to even a small elephant. Thus, BIG in 16a cannot mean (its sense cannot be) something like 'OF LARGE SIZE', since no mice are of large size compared to elephants, yet there are big mice. Obviously, 'the big mouse' means that this particular mouse is big by the standards of normal size for mice. And 'the big elephant' means that this particular elephant is big by the standards for normal size for elephants. Thus, 'big' must translate as something like 'x is LARGE IN COMPARISON TO THE NORMAL SIZE FOR THINGS OF TYPE___', where the blank must be filled in with information given by the word that 'big' modifies (either elephant or mouse in the examples above). 'Big' (and 'small') is, then, an inherently *comparative* word. Thus, the real translation of our sentence is

16b. x is BIG IN COMPARISON TO THE NORMAL SIZE FOR MICE and x is a MOUSE and x is SMALL IN COMPARISON TO THE NORMAL SIZE FOR ANIMALS and x is an ANIMAL

There are many words that are inherently comparative. The word 'good' is a particularly interesting case. A good knife is one that cuts well, a good book is one that reads well, a good car is one that drives well. 'Good' must translate as a predicate like 'PERFORMS WELL THE FUNCTION THAT A __ TYPICALLY PERFORMS', where once again the blank is filled in by information from the word that 'good' modifies ('knife', 'book', and 'car' in our examples). It is particularly interesting to think about what a phrase like 'a good person' means. Thinking about such meanings goes well beyond semantics into the realm of values, ethics, and philosophy.

From SPL Translations to the Language of Thought

Consider the English sentence in 17a and its translation into SPL in 17b:

17a. A woman killed a bachelor

17b. x is A WOMAN and x KILLED y and y is a BACHELOR

The translation in 17b contains the predicates WOMAN, KILLED, and BACHELOR. But these are just English words being treated as SPL predicates. To finish the job of giving the meaning of the English sentence, we have to translate these SPL predicates into the language of thought, the language in terms of which we assume meanings are represented for human beings.

In our earlier discussion of the language of thought, we represented its words in small capital letters (as we have also been doing in the case of SPL words), and we took its words to name concepts or ideas in our minds. These are the basic concepts in terms of which human beings represent their experience of the world and the meanings of their languages. While it is the job of psychology to discover what the language of thought looks like, and while we do not know much about the matter yet, let's assume that the SPL translation in 17b could be translated into the language of thought as in 17c:

17c. x is FEMALE and x is ADULT (this is the contribution or translation of 'woman') and x DID SOMETHING and THAT SOMETHING CAUSED y to GO FROM BEING ALIVE TO BEING NOT ALIVE (this is the contribution or translation of 'kill') and y is MALE and y is ADULT and y is NOT MARRIED (this is the contribution of 'bachelor')

It is quite possible that some of these concepts (for example, MARRIED) are not yet basic enough and should really be reduced to (translated into) yet more basic concepts. But this will at least give the flavor of the idea. Since we know so little about the language of thought, in many cases when we explicate the meanings of English sentences we just stop with the SPL translation.

A word like 'bachelor' can be defined fairly straightforwardly in terms of more basic concepts (like MALE and ADULT and NOT MARRIED, which may not be the most basic ones we could discover), but not all words reduce so easily. Take a word like 'bird'. Some psychologists have suggested that the way in which humans think about the meaning of the word 'bird' is in terms of a prototype bird or a typical bird (for many people something like a robin is very close to a typical bird). The more something shares with the typical bird, the more bird-like it is judged to be; the less it shares with the typical bird, the less bird-like it is judged to be. Thus, canaries and sparrows are judged to be very bird-like; chickens, turkeys, and penguins progressively less so (though close enough to count as birds); and flying squirrels and flying fish are so far from the typical bird that they don't count as birds at all. The concept BIRD may be represented in someone's head as a list of features or properties of a PROTOTYPICAL bird (for example, SMALL, FEATHERED, FLIES, SINGS, LOOKS LIKE) against which other things are compared when judging their "birdhood". There is also a sense in which we defer to scientists: If we are unsure whether or not something counts as a bird, we know (or think) that scientists have tests (perhaps based on genetic structure) that will determine whether or not something is a bird.

Other sorts of concepts may be thought of in different ways (consider 'CHAIR', 'GAME', 'BACHELOR', and 'GOLD' as examples of concepts that may be thought of in different ways from each other and from 'BIRD'). Ultimately, there must be some concepts that we know just because we were born with them or because all humans become familiar with them through their early sensory exploration of the world through vision and their other senses (for example, MALE, ALIVE, RED, GREEN, ACTION). We will take up this question further in Chapter 7, on the psychology of language.

2.6. QUANTIFIERS

We mentioned earlier that SPL is a simplified version of a language used by logicians. This language, which I have called PC, goes by various names, including "first-order logic" and "the predicate calculus." As we have developed SPL, it cannot translate sentences with words like 'all' or 'some' (called quantifiers) in them (for example, *'All* humans are mortal', *'Some* humans are male'). The language PC has the words ALL and SOME to handle cases like these.

To understand how ALL and SOME function in PC, we would have to introduce rules for their syntax (how they form sentences with other words, namely with predicate symbols, names, and variables) and for their semantics (what they contribute to the meaning, that is, the truth value, of the sentences they are in). This would lead us afield here, and we will not introduce these rules. To handle the problems that arise in giving the semantics of English sentences, we would have to complicate SPL much beyond what we have done here. In fact, even PC will not handle all of the aspects of English semantics. In particular, it will not handle any sentences that talk about possible worlds.

In any case, I will point out that an English sentence like 'All humans are mortal' translates into PC as follows: '(ALL x) (if x is HUMAN then x is MORTAL)'. We can read this as 'for all x in the universe of discourse, that is, all the things we can talk about, if x is human then x *is mortal'*. 'Some humans are male' translates as '(SOMEx) (x is HUMAN and x is MALE)'. We can read this as 'for some x, one or more, in the universe of discourse, x is human and x is male'.

2.7. LOGICAL PROPERTIES OF ENGLISH SENTENCES

Translating English sentences into SPL and then into the language of thought can expose **logical properties** of these sentences. Logical properties are properties sentences have because of the *form* of their meanings, and not because of the way the world is. For example, a sentence like 'John is tall' is true simply because John happens to be tall in the world we are talking about, but we could easily imagine the world being different. But a sentence like 'Bachelors are unmarried' is true not because of the way the world is, but because of the meaning it has ('bachelor' means *unmarried male,* so the sentence could not fail to be true). We could not imagine a world in which it was false. The truth of 'Bachelors are unmarried' is a logical property of the sentence, due to the language and not to the world.

To see how translation into SPL and then into the language of thought uncovers such logical properties, consider the English sentence in 18a, with its SPL translation in 18b, and its translation into the language of thought in 18c:

18a. John is a male bachelor

18b. MALEj and BACHELORj

18c. MALEj and NOT MARRIEDj and MALEj

The translation 18c shows that the English sentence in 18a is REDUNDANT since it repeats a piece of information in its meaning (18c), namely MALEj.

There are a number of other such logical properties that sentences can have. Consider, for example, the following:

19a. John is a female bachelor

19b. FEMALEj and BACHELORj

19c. NOT MALEj and NOT MARRIEDj and MALEj

The English sentence in 19a is shown by its translation into the language of thought (19c) to be a CONTRADICTION, since it claims that something is both true (MALEj) and not true (NOT MALEj).

A sentence like 'Bachelors are unmarried' is ANALYTICALLY TRUE because an *analysis* of its meaning (and not the world) shows that it could not conceivably fail to be true. Though we need the resources of PC to represent its meaning fully, an inspection of this meaning readily shows that the sentence could not be false (in fact, its final translation in 18c constitutes a logically valid argument, since any argument of the form 'PREMISE: x is Y; CONCLUSION: x is Y' is valid):

20a. Bachelors are unmarried

20b. (ALL*x)* (if *x* is a BACHELOR then *x* is UNMARRIED)

20c. (ALL*x)* (if *x* is NOT MARRIED and *x* is MALE then *x* is NOT MARRIED)

Sometimes the SPL or PC translation of an English sentence already makes clear that it has some logical property, without having to consider the translation of the sentence into the language of thought. This is the case with a sentence like 'Unmarried males are unmarried':

21a. Unmarried males are unmarried

21b. (ALL*x*) (if *x* is UNMARRIED and *x* is MALE then *x* is UNMARRIED)

21c. The translation into the language of thought is not significantly different than the PC translation in 21b.

Sentence 21b, the PC translation of 21a, already makes clear that the English sentence 21a could never fail to be true in any possible world. When the PC or SPL translation makes clear that a sentence must be true (could never be false under any circumstances), the sentence is said to be LOGICALLY TRUE. A sentence like 'Unmarried males are not males' is said to be LOGICALLY FALSE since its PC translation ((ALL*x*) (if *x* is UNMARRIED and *x* is MALE then *x* is NOT MALE)) already makes clear that it could in no circumstances be true.

─────────────── E X E R C I S E ───────────────

Exercise M. For each of the sentences below, say whether it has any logical properties. If it does, say whether the sentence is redundant, a contradiction, analytically true, or logically true, or more than one of these. (NOTE: A sentence can be redundant and also a contradiction, analytically true, logically true, or have no additional logical properties. All logically true sentences are also analytically true. Treat 'female' as translating into the language of thought as NOT MALE, or treat it as translating as FEMALE and 'male' as translating as NOT FEMALE. It doesn't matter which way you do it.)

1. Max is a young kitten.
2. Max is a cat.
3. Women are females.
4. Young boys are males.
5. Young kittens are kittens.

2.8. SEMANTIC ROLES

In the previous section, we saw that sentences are composed of predicates whose places are filled by nominals. In the following sentences, the *main predicate* is printed in italics and explained below each sentence.

22a. Mary *kissed* John
>(*kiss* is predicated of, said to be true of, John and Mary)

22b. Mary *is tall*
>(*being tall* is predicated of, said to be true of, Mary)

22c. Mary *is in Africa*
>(*being in Africa* is predicated of, said to be true of, Mary)

To give a more detailed picture of the meanings of sentences, we will now add a new and important element to our representations of meaning. The main predicate in a sentence can be looked at as if it names a particular *drama*. And the nominals in the sentence can be looked at as if they name *players* in the drama. Thus, we can see the main verb in a sentence like 'Mary *gave* the book to John' as designating a drama of *giving*. In this drama, Mary plays the role of the *giver*, the book plays the role of the *"givee"* (the thing given), and John plays the role of the *recipient* or person given to. These roles that nominals play in the drama designated by a predicate are called **semantic roles** (**roles** for short).

There is a sense in which, in a sentence like 'Mary sent a book to John', *Mary, the book,* and *John* are playing the same sorts of roles they were playing in 'Mary gave a book to John', though the drama is somewhat different—now it is a drama of *sending,* rather than of *giving.* If we want to capture this similarity between the role *Mary* is playing in the two sentences, we have to view roles somewhat more generally or abstractly than 'giver' or 'sender'. To do this, we will say that in both these sentences, Mary is an ACTOR, that is, one who initiates the action named by the verb. She is also a SOURCE, that is, the *beginning point* of the action of giving or sending, where the action *starts.* John is a RECIPIENT, that is, one who gets or receives something. He is also a GOAL, the place where the action *ends* or *terminates,* the *end point* of the action. Linguists have a special name for the ROLE that the book is playing in these two sentences. They call anything that is *transferred,* or that *moves* from one place to another, as the book does in these actions of giving and sending, the **theme** of the action. 'Theme' is a poor word because it has so many other meanings (like the "theme" of an essay, book, or movie), meanings that are not related to our use of the term here. But since the word is in wide use in linguistics, I will use it here. Treat it merely as a technical term, having only the meaning I give it here.

We can label each nominal in a sentence in terms of the role it plays in the drama designated by the predicate. Thus, our two example sentences can be represented as follows, where the nominals associated with the verbs are labeled with their roles:

23a. Mary (ACTOR/SOURCE) gave the book (THEME) to John (RECIPIENT/GOAL)

23b. Mary (ACTOR/SOURCE) sent the book (THEME) to John (RECIPIENT/GOAL)

Classes of Predicates: States Versus Events

Equipped with semantic roles, we will survey the semantics of predicates in English. The most important semantic distinction in regard to predicates is that between predicates that denote (name) *states* and those that denote (name) *events.* We will assume that STATE and EVENT are basic concepts in the language of thought. To say that something is in a certain state is to say that it is *in a certain condition* or has *a certain property* (like being smart, tall, old, sick, happy, or dizzy), or that it is *in a certain location* (like being in New York, at home, or in Africa). Events, on the other hand, are *happenings* in the world, either *processes* that just occur over time (like a river flowing) or *actions* (like Mary kissing John).

Most adjectives (like 'sick' or 'happy') name states. For verbs, there are several tests to determine whether a verb names a state or an event. One of these is the following: With verbs that name states, the simple present tense can be used to express present time, as in 'Max loves Mary', which says Max, at this present moment, loves Mary. Thus, 'loves' names a state. With verbs that name events, the simple present tense expresses not present time, but habitual or future events, as in 'Max kisses Mary', which doesn't mean he is doing it this moment, but that he often does it or will do it in the future (as in 'Next, Max kisses Mary'). To locate Max's kissing at the present moment, we have to use the present progressive, as in 'Max is kissing Mary'. Thus, 'kiss' names an event, not a state.

─────────────────────── **E X E R C I S E** ───────────────────────

Exercise N. Classify the verbs in the following list into states or events using the test discussed in the preceding section.

Example Answer. Take the verb 'see'. This verb can be used in the simple present tense to express present time ('What do you see? I *see* a robin'). Thus, 'see' names a state. Take the verb 'eat'. This verb cannot be used in the simple present tense to express present time. A sentence like 'John eats rice' does not mean he is eating it now, but rather that he often or usually eats it, or that he is willing to eat it. Thus, 'eat' names an event.

believe
ask
wash

hate
sit
listen
hear

States—Type 1: Physical Locations.   All states involve something having a certain property (like 'being sick' or 'being tall') or being in a certain place (like 'being in Africa' or 'staying in London'). The semantic role of the thing that is in the state (sick, tall, in Africa, in London) is called the THEME (extending this term from the use we made of it above). Thus, for a sentence like 'Mary is tall', which says that Mary has the property of being tall (that she is in the state of tallness), we will say that Mary is playing the semantic role of the THEME. THEME will mean then

> THEME = the semantic role of something that is in a particular state or that changes from one state to another.

The simplest and most fundamental state things can be in is a LOCATION, as in 'John is in Africa', which says that John is located in the location 'Africa'. John is the thing placed in this LOCATION, so John is labeled the THEME. We will label 'in Africa' with the role LOCATION. Example 24a shows the sentence 'John is in Africa', labeling its nominals with their semantic roles, and then shows the translation of this sentence into the language of thought:

24a. John (THEME) is in Africa (LOCATION) =
John (THEME) BE LOCATED IN Africa (LOCATION)

States—Type 2: Properties.   There are three types of states other than locations. However, all of them can be thought of as types of *figurative* (metaphorical) locations. Take a sentence like 'John is sick'. Obviously, sickness is not a physical place, not a location in the literal sense. Nonetheless, we tend to talk about properties such as sickness *as if* they were locations; we tend to think of them *as if* they were places where people could be, or places where they could move into or out of.

Thus, note the following different ways we can talk about John being sick, all of which bring out the way in which we tend to treat properties as if they were locations. We can say 'John is *in ill health',* where we use a locative phrase 'is in', just as in 'John is in Africa'. We can say 'John came to be sick', or 'John got sick', as if he moved from being not sick to being in the figurative location of sickness (compare 'John came to be in Africa', 'John got to Africa'). We can even say 'John quickly went from being quite sick to being quite well again', where we speak as if John moves from one place (being quite sick), figuratively speaking, to another (being quite well). Finally, note 'John is out of danger now', where we speak as if he has moved out of a place (compare 'John is out of Africa now').

Thus, we will treat a state like 'John is sick' as meaning that John is located in the figurative location of sickness. We will treat properties like 'sick' and 'tall' as 'property locations', figurative places in which things can be placed. Thus, we will translate a sentence like 'John is sick' into the language of thought as in 24b:

24b. John (THEME) is sick (LOCATION) =
John (THEME) BE (FIGURATIVELY) LOCATED AT SICKNESS (PROPERTY LOCATION)

States—Type 3: Possession. There are two other types of figurative locations in which things can be placed. One is POSSESSION. A sentence like 'The book belongs to John' essentially says that the book (THEME) is located or placed in the possession of John. Of course, he need not be physically holding the book. Nonetheless, people are treated as locations (POSSESSORS) where things can be "held" in possession. Each of us, in a sense, is treated as a "place" where our possessions are located, figuratively speaking. Thus, we can analyze this sentence into the language of thought as follows:

24c. The book (THEME) belongs to John (LOCATION) =
The book (THEME) BE LOCATED AT John (POSSESSOR LOCATION)

English often reverses the positions of the THEME and LOCATION in possession sentences, especially when it uses its possession verb 'have':

25. John (POSSESSOR LOCATION) has the book (THEME)

This is still understood as meaning that the book is located at John as a possessor. In many languages, such sentences translate literally into English as something like 'The book is at John' (meaning John owns the book, not that he need be holding it at the moment). This way of saying it overtly shows how we humans think of possession as a type of figurative location.

States—Type 4: Mental States. The final type of state is MENTAL EXPERIENCE, cases where people (or animals) experience something in their minds or with their emotions. A sentence like 'The painting pleases Mary' means that the painting is experienced by Mary in a pleasing way. The painting is located in Mary's mental experience. It is, so to speak, inside Mary's head in such a way that it brings her pleasure. The painting is part of Mary's experience of the world. Thus, we can treat people's minds (or their mental experience) as a type of figurative location, where things can be placed.

In fact, we often talk about our minds as if they were places into which and out of which things went: 'John couldn't get the idea *into his head*', 'John *grasped* the point', 'John *lost* the point', 'John couldn't get the scene *out of his mind*', 'John had the idea firmly *in his head*', and so on through many more examples.

We will label people and animals when they are playing the role of *mental locations* as EXPERIENCERS, in addition to LOCATIONS. And we can translate the sentence 'The painting pleased Mary' into the language of thought as follows:

24d. The painting (THEME) pleases Mary (LOCATION/EXPERIENCER) =
The painting (THEME) BE LOCATED AT Mary's MIND (EXPERIENCER/LOCATION)

Of course, more would have to be added to 24d to bring out its full meaning (something like 'The painting (THEME) BE LOCATED AT Mary (EXPERIENCER LOCATION) IN A PLEASING MANNER).

Just as with possession, English often reverses the order of the THEME and EXPERIENCER LOCATION in its sentences from what we saw in 'The painting pleases Mary'. Thus, consider the following examples:

26a. John (EXPERIENCER LOCATION) knows the answer (THEME)
[The answer is in John's head]
26b. John (EXPERIENCER LOCATION) loves Mary (THEME)
[Mary is located in John's emotions]

All of the types of states we have discussed fundamentally amount to the same basic pattern in terms of their meaning: The THEME is placed or located (either literally or figuratively) in a certain LOCATION, either literal ones, like Africa (in 24a), or in various figurative locations, such as the PROPERTY LOCATION in 24b, the POSSESSOR LOCATION in 24c, or the EXPERIENCER LOCATION in 24d.

_____ E X E R C I S E _____

Exercise O. Categorize the following states as physical locations (like 'is in Africa'), properties (like 'is sick'), possession (like 'belongs to John'), or mental states (like 'pleases Mary'). In each sentence, identify the THEME and LOCATION (literal or figurative):

stand: The statue stands in the park.

believe: John believes the story.

have: John has a book.

dizzy: John is dizzy.

see: John saw a vision.

own: John owns the house.

old: John is old.

sit: John sat on the bench.

Events—Go Type. Now we turn from states to events. We can easily understand the *go* type of event once we have understood the states we just discussed. These events are just movements into and out of those states. Many English verbs mean that something (which we will label the THEME) goes from *not* being in a certain state to being in that state—that is, *something changes state.* A sentence like 'The vase fell to the ground' can be analyzed as meaning that the vase (THEME) went from *not* being in the state (LOCATION) of being on the ground to the state (LOCATION) of being on the ground. A sentence like 'The vase broke' can be analyzed as meaning that the vase (THEME) went from the state (PROPERTY LOCATION) of *not* being broken to the state (PROPERTY LOCATION) of being broken.

We saw above that there were four types of states, each of which involved the meaning BE LOCATED. The four types were differentiated in terms of four types of locations: physical locations (in Africa), property locations (sick), possessor locations (John's possession), and experiencer locations (Mary's mind). To each one of these types of state verbs corresponds a type of event verb that means to GO from not being in that state to being in that state. For example,

27a. The vase (THEME) fell to the ground =
The vase GOES FROM NOT BEING LOCATED ON THE GROUND TO BEING LOCATED ON THE GROUND

27b. The vase (THEME) broke =
The vase GOES FROM NOT BEING LOCATED AT THE PROPERTY LOCATION BROKEN TO BEING LOCATED AT THE PROPERTY LOCATION BROKEN

27c. John (POSSESSOR LOCATION) got/received the vase (THEME) =
The vase GOES FROM NOT BEING LOCATED AT THE POSSESSOR LOCATION John TO BEING LOCATED AT THE POSSESSOR LOCATION John

27d. John (EXPERIENCER LOCATION) learned French (THEME) =
French GOES FROM NOT BEING LOCATED AT JOHN'S MIND TO BEING LOCATED AT JOHN'S MIND

Notice that a sentence like 'John learned French' may be used to stress John's efforts in learning French (he did it on purpose or worked at it = John tried to learn French), in which case John can also be marked as an ACTOR. Or it can be used just to stress that the learning took place (John came to know French, for example, in his sleep, or simply by being exposed to it), in which case John can be marked simply as an EXPERIENCER LOCATION.

Events—Simple Actions. ACTIONS are events that involve ACTORS. Actions themselves come in two types. The first is simply the case where an ACTOR performs, initiates, or effects a simple action. For example,

28a. John (ACTOR) is singing
28b. The wind (ACTOR) was whistling through the trees (PATH)

28c. The boy (ACTOR) yelled at his sister (GOAL)

28d. Mary (ACTOR) lied to her brother (GOAL)

28e. The puppy (ACTOR) was playing

28f. The horn (ACTOR) honked

28g. The tea kettle (ACTOR) whistled

Note that I have labeled 'through the trees' as PATH in 28b, since it names the PATH along which the whistle went. I have labeled 'at his sister' in 28c and 'to her brother' in 28d as GOALS, since they both name the location at which the action of the verb is directed and where it terminates.

We could, if we wished, distinguish between different types of ACTORS. For example, an intentional act could be seen as the act of an AGENT, so that 'John' in 28a, 'the boy' in 28c, and 'Mary' in 28d could be said to express the role AGENT. Depending on your view of animals (whether or not you think they can have intentions), you may or may not want to mark 'the puppy' in 28e as an AGENT. 'The wind' in 28b could be marked as a NATURAL FORCE, and 'the horn' and 'tea kettle' in 28f and 28g could be marked as DEVICES. But this is not really necessary, at least for the level of analysis we are engaged in here. Whether or not an ACTOR has acted intentionally follows partly from whether or not it is human (or a higher animal) and partly from how one interprets the verb.

Events—Directed Actions. The second type of action is the case where an ACTOR directs the action of the verb at, on, or toward another participant to directly affect that participant, or where the action of the ACTOR results in the existence of another participant. I will call the participant that is affected by the action of the verb, or that results from the action of the verb, the PATIENT. I will call this class of verbs DIRECTED ACTIONS. In these cases, English places the PATIENT in the object position after the verb, with no preposition in front of it. For example,

29a. The girl (ACTOR) beat the boy (PATIENT)

29b. The puppy (ACTOR) bit the man (PATIENT)

29c. The man (ACTOR) built the house (PATIENT)

29d. The horse (ACTOR) kicked the man (PATIENT)

29e. The girl (ACTOR) hit the boy (PATIENT)

29f. The wind (ACTOR) hit the boy's face (PATIENT)

29g. The girl (ACTOR) sang a rock song (PATIENT)

Some verbs expressing DIRECTED ACTIONS can take either the ACTOR as their subject or what I will call an INSTRUMENT/THEME, a ROLE that labels an object that is used by an ACTOR to carry out an action or that by accident or natural force carries out the sort of action an ACTOR could accomplish:

30a. Mary (ACTOR) hit John (PATIENT) with a stone (INSTRUMENT/THEME)

30b. A stone (INSTRUMENT/THEME) hit John (PATIENT)

31a. Mary (ACTOR) kicked John (PATIENT) with her left foot (INSTRUMENT/THEME)

31b. Mary's left foot (INSTRUMENT/THEME) kicked John (PATIENT)

Events—Causatives.   Just as the language of thought includes a type of GO verb corresponding to each type of STATE verb, so also there is a type of CAUSATIVE verb corresponding to each type of GO verb. These causative verbs mean that an ACTOR CAUSES the THEME to GO FROM NOT BEING LOCATED AT ONE LOCATION TO BEING LOCATED AT THAT LOCATION. Since the THEME here is often affected by the ACTOR who does the CAUSING, it could also be marked as a PATIENT/THEME.

Next, I give an example of the four types of CAUSATIVE verbs. Each type has a particular type of GO in its meaning: GOING through physical locations, property locations, possessor locations, or experiencer locations:

32a. John (ACTOR) put the flowers (THEME) in the vase (LOCATION) =
John CAUSED the flowers to GO FROM NOT BEING LOCATED IN the vase TO BEING LOCATED IN the vase

32b. John (ACTOR) broke the vase (THEME) =
John CAUSED the vase TO GO FROM NOT BEING LOCATED AT THE PROPERTY LOCATION BROKEN TO BEING LOCATED AT THE PROPERTY LOCATION BROKEN

32c. John (ACTOR) gave the book (THEME) to Mary (GOAL) =
John CAUSED the book TO GO FROM NOT BEING LOCATED AT THE POSSESSOR LOCATION Mary TO BEING LOCATED AT THE POSSESSOR LOCATION Mary

32d. Mary (ACTOR) taught French (THEME) to John (GOAL) =
Mary CAUSED French TO GO FROM NOT BEING LOCATED AT John's MIND TO BEING LOCATED AT John's MIND

Many adjectives and verbs in English that name properties (like 'be sick' or 'be broken') enter into systematic patterns in terms of which they vary meanings among STATES, GOINGS, and CAUSATION. For example, notice the following patterns, into which many adjectives and verbs enter:

33a. The soup (THEME) is *thick* = STATE =
The soup (THEME) BE LOCATED AT PROPERTY LOCATION OF THICKNESS

33b. The soup (THEME) *thickened* = GO =
The soup (THEME) GO FROM NOT BEING AT THE PROPERTY LOCATION OF THICKNESS TO BEING AT THE PROPERTY LOCATION OF THICKNESS

33c. The chef (ACTOR) *thicken* the soup (THEME) = CAUSE GO =
The chef (ACTOR) CAUSE the soup (THEME) GO FROM NOT BEING AT THE PROPERTY LOCATION OF THICKNESS TO BEING AT THE PROPERTY LOCATION OF THICKNESS

34a. The vase (THEME) is broken = STATE =
The vase (THEME) BE LOCATED AT PROPERTY LOCATION BROKEN

34b. The vase (THEME) broke = GO =
The vase (THEME) GO FROM NOT BEING AT THE PROPERTY LOCATION BROKEN TO
BEING AT THE PROPERTY LOCATION BROKEN

34c. John (ACTOR) broke the vase (THEME) = CAUSE GO =
John (ACTOR) CAUSE the vase (THEME) GO FROM NOT BEING AT THE PROPERTY
LOCATION BROKEN TO BEING AT THE PROPERTY LOCATION OF BROKEN

    Though CAUSATIVE verbs tend to have the THEME as their objects (of course, the ACTOR is always the subject), many CAUSATIVE verbs have an option of having their LOCATIONS or GOALS or SOURCES as objects, rather than the THEME, while certain verbs prefer one or the other (sentences with an asterisk are unacceptable —see Chapter 6 below):

35a. John gave a book (THEME) to Mary (GOAL)

35b. John gave Mary (GOAL) a book (THEME)

36a. Mary planted the flowers (THEME) in the garden (LOCATION)

36b. Mary planted the garden (LOCATION) with flowers (THEME)

37a. *Mary filled flowers (THEME) in the vase (LOCATION)

37b. Mary filled the vase (LOCATION) with flowers (THEME)

38a. *John robbed 10 dollars (THEME) from Mary (SOURCE)

38b. John robbed Mary (SOURCE) of 10 dollars (THEME)

39a. John stole 10 dollars (THEME) from Mary (SOURCE)

39b. *John stole Mary (SOURCE) of 10 dollars (THEME)

40a. John sold a book (THEME) to Mary (GOAL)

40b. John sold Mary (GOAL) a book (THEME)

41a. John bought a book (THEME) from Sue (SOURCE) for Mary (GOAL)

41b. John bought Mary (GOAL) a book (THEME) from Mary (SOURCE)

Summary of Predicate Types

We have covered a tremendous amount of ground in short compass, surveying a large number of types of English sentences. It is important not to get lost in the trees and miss the beauty of the forest. The system here is actually quite elegant and fairly simple. It is also very unlikely to be anything but universal, since it represents the basic ways in which we humans perceive and think about the world (it is a part of our common human "metaphysics"). Of course, each different

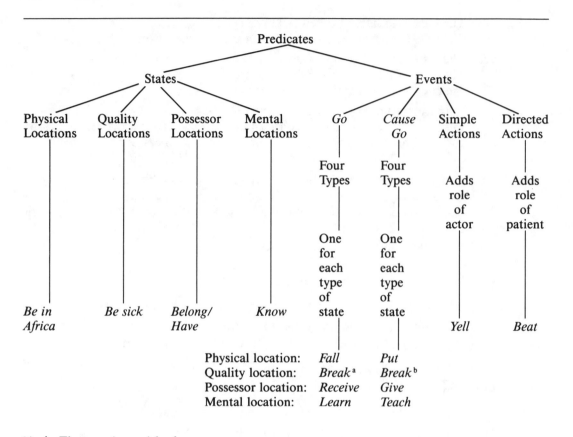

^aAs in The vase (THEME) broke
^bAs in John (ACTOR) broke the vase (THEME)

FIGURE 2-1. Types of Predicates

language expands on and varies this basic system in different ways, reflecting in turn its own way of looking at reality.

Figure 2-1 summarizes the basic system of predicate types in English (and in all likelihood most other languages).

────────────── **E X E R C I S E** ──────────────

Exercise P. For each of the sentences, label each nominal with its semantic role, and explicate the predicate in terms of the categories discussed in this chapter and summarized in Figure 2-1.

Example Answer. Consider sentence 3: 'John knows the answer'. The predicate in this sentence ('knows') names a (figurative) STATE, and this STATE is the state of something being located in the mind. In this sentence, 'the answer' is the THEME and is said to be located in the mind of John, and so 'John' is the LOCATION. This type of LOCATION we have also called an EXPERIENCER. The sentence means 'The THEME ('the answer') BE LOCATED AT John's mind'. Of course, to capture the full meaning of the particular verb 'know', we would have to add other information. For example, both 'John knows the answer' and 'John believes the claim' locate something (the answer, the claim) at John's mind, but these things are "in the mind" in different ways, or these verbs say somewhat different things about the mind and the way information in it relates to the world. These latter, more specific differences among predicates, are not relevant to the sort of information summarized in Figure 2-1 and may be ignored in answering this question.

1. John owns a car.
2. John is in the car.
3. John knows the answer.
4. John is tall.
5. John is certain of the answer.
6. John dropped the ball.
7. John went to the park.
8. John sang to Mary.
9. John kicked the puppy.
10. The ice melted.
11. John melted the ice.

Analytic Versus Lexical Causatives

The causative verbs we have looked at in the previous section are called LEXICAL CAUSATIVES because the verb itself ('put' or 'break', for example) involves as part of its meaning (sense)—that is, as part of its translation into the language of thought—the concept of causation. This concept CAUSATION in the language of thought means *to directly or immediately cause.* Thus, a verb like 'break' in 'John broke the vase' means something like *to immediately cause to break* where we see that the verb 'break' incorporates into its meaning the concepts CAUSE and BREAK.

There is another way to signal causation in English, and that is with so-called causative verbs like 'make' and 'have', as in sentence 42b. These are called ANALYTICAL CAUSATIVES, because the causative meaning is carried by a separate word ('have' or 'make') and not incorporated into the meaning of another word (like 'break' above):

42a. The magician broke the cup = LEXICAL CAUSATIVE

42b. The magician made the cup broke = ANALYTICAL CAUSATIVE

Sentence 42a usually implies that the magician broke the cup by directly interacting with it, but 42b implies that he used some less direct route, like a trick or a spell.

Summary of the Semantic Roles in English

ACTOR = Participant who initiates the action of a simple action, a directed action, or a causative. If there is an ACTOR in a sentence, it is always in subject position in an active (a nonpassive) sentence.

PATIENT = Participant directly affected by the action of the ACTOR in a directed action or the product produced by the action of the ACTOR in a directed action. If there is a PATIENT in a sentence, it is always in object position in an active sentence.

THEME = Participant that is in a state (BE LOCATED) or that moves or changes from state to state (GO FROM NOT BEING LOCATED AT A LOCATION TO BEING LOCATED AT THAT LOCATION). The THEME is often in the subject position if there is no object, and otherwise in the object position. At times it appears in a prepositional phrase headed by 'of' or 'with'.

LOCATION = Participant that serves as the physical location, property location, possessor location, or experiencer location in verbs with BE or GO in their meanings. LOCATIONS are often marked by prepositions like 'in', 'on', 'at', 'under', and other locative prepositions.

SOURCE = The beginning LOCATION, location where an action starts, usually marked by the directional preposition 'from' when the SOURCE is not also an ACTOR (in which case the ACTOR is in subject position).

GOAL = The ending or terminal LOCATION, location where an action terminates or is directed, usually marked by the directional prepositions 'to' or 'toward', sometimes marked by 'at'.

PATH = The route along which something is directed or travels, usually marked by the prepositions 'through', 'along', 'across', and others.

EXPERIENCER = The participant who mentally or emotionally experiences a state or change of state, that is, mental LOCATIONS. Usually in the subject position.

POSSESSOR = The participant that serves as a POSSESSOR LOCATION. Can be in almost any position and marked by a variety of prepositions.

RECIPIENT = A POSSESSOR LOCATION that is also a GOAL. Can be in subject or object position; otherwise it is usually marked by the prepositions 'for' or 'to'.

INSTRUMENT/THEME = Participant that is used to carry out an action by an ACTOR, or that, though it carries out the action by accident or through some natural force, is the sort of thing that could have been used by an actor.

————————————— E X E R C I S E —————————————

Exercise Q. Label each nominal in these sentences with its semantic role, using the summary given above.

1. The ball rolled across the lawn into the swimming pool.
2. John rolled the ball across the lawn into the swimming pool.
3. John hit Bill with a club.
4. John gave a book to Bill.
5. John inherited a million dollars from his uncle.
6. John went from New Jersey to New York.
7. John sold the books to Mary.
8. John died.
9. John killed Bill.
10. John loves Mary.

Buy and Sell: Meaning as a Perspective on the World

English has a number of verbs that essentially name the same activity, but that differ in which semantic role is in subject position. Thus, consider the following sentences:

43a. John (ACTOR, SOURCE) sold the bike (THEME) to Mary (GOAL)

43b. Mary (ACTOR, GOAL) bought the bike (THEME) from John (SOURCE)

Sentences 43a and 43b could be used about one and the same action in the real world. The *a* version places the SOURCE (the seller) in the subject position and treats it as the ACTOR. The *b* version places the GOAL (the buyer) in the subject position and treats it as the ACTOR.

These two sentences are simply different PERSPECTIVES on the same event, two different ways to view one and the same event. Both sentences mean something like 'John CAUSE the bike to GO to Mary for some price and Mary CAUSE the price to GO to John for the bike'. One sentence focuses on the seller as the main initiator of the action; the other focuses on the buyer as the main initiator of the action. In fact, there can be no such transaction unless both parties are initiators—one of a transference of the bike and the other of the price for the bike.

These sentences constitute a good example of how language is not just *about* the world; rather we *actively construct* what counts as reality by the perspective or view we take on the world. And language gives us the resources to carry out this constructional work. Ultimately, language is always about our perspective on or view of the world, not the world itself.

RECOMMENDED FURTHER READING

ALLAN, KEITH (1986). *Linguistic Meaning.* Vols. 1 and 2. London & New York: Routledge & Kegan Paul. (A detailed, accessible, and up-to-date survey of linguistic semantics.)

ALLWOOD, JENS, ANDERSSON, LARS-GUNNAR & DAHL, OSTEN (1977). *Logic in Linguistics.* New York: Cambridge University Press. (A remarkably clear, helpful, and relatively short book.)

CHIERCHIA, GENNARO & McCONNELL-GINET, SALLY (1990). *Meaning and Grammar: An Introduction to Semantics.* Cambridge, Mass.: MIT Press. (A solid introduction to semantic theory in formal linguistics. Requires basic knowledge of syntactic theory.)

CLARK, HERB H. & CLARK, EVE (1977). *Psychology and Language.* New York: Harcourt Brace Jovanovich. (Much of this well-written and helpful book deals with meaning as it functions in language use and language acquisition.)

JACKENDOFF, RAY (1983). *Semantics and Cognition.* Cambridge, Mass.: M.I.T. Press. (A fairly technical but important book; deals with semantic roles, types of verbs, and the figurative extension of locative meanings.)

KEMPSON, RUTH (1977). *Semantic Theory.* New York: Cambridge University Press. (A clear introduction to some of the more philosophical and technical issues in the theory of meaning.)

LYONS, JOHN (1977). *Semantics.* Vols. 1 and 2. New York: Cambridge University Press. (Masterful survey; use for browsing or as a reference work.)

McCAWLEY, JAMES D. (1981). *Everything That Linguists Have Always Wanted to Know About Logic, But Were Ashamed to Ask.* University of Chicago Press. (Entertaining introduction to logic and language.)

WIERZBICKA, ANNA (1985). *Lexicography and Conceptual Analysis.* Ann Arbor, Mich.: Karoma. (An idiosyncratic and fascinating theory of the meanings of words.)

CHAPTER 3

Phonology
The Sound
of Language

3.1. HUMAN-LIKE COMMUNICATION SYSTEMS

Suppose you were to invent a medium of communication for creatures much like human beings. However, these creatures cannot use sounds (as in a language like English) or sign with the hands (as in a language like American Sign Language). Their communication system must therefore be graphic. You first need to select a set of *symbols* and then assign each symbol a meaning. It does not really matter what the symbols are made of or look like, as long as the creatures that are going to use them can clearly tell one symbol from the other.

Suppose you have the following graphic symbols, among others, to use: 'X', 'Y', '&', ')', '}', 'V', and '/'. We will assume that the creatures will paint them on rocks with little brushes. Now you need to assign each symbol a meaning. How this can be done turns out to be a deep philosophical question, but let's just assume that you manage it (either by pointing and other types of instruction, or by using translations in terms of another symbol system the creatures know). Ultimately, you assign the following meanings to the symbols (where the words in small capital letters, like DOG, stand for concepts or ideas in the minds of the creatures):

X means DOG

Y means ROCK

& means LOVE

) means STAR

} means HAPPY

/ means RED

etc. (through a list of all the symbols you have available)

This is obviously not going to get you very far in creating a communication system, because if there are 10,000 things our creatures want to communicate about, they are going to have to have 10,000 discrete symbols. This will overtax both their memories and the perceptual abilities. They will have to remember 10,000 separate symbols and, worse still, will have to be able to perceive a clear difference between each one and its 9,999 mates. It will also overtax our ability to create new symbols for them. Even if we could do it, and our creatures could handle it, it is not a very efficient use of our effort or theirs.

So how are we going to allow our creatures to communicate about lots of things but not have to use lots of different symbols? That is, how are we going to design lots of symbols without overtaxing the memory and perceptual skills of our creatures as well as our own creative energy? The trick is this: Treat *combinations* of our original symbols as themselves *single* simple symbols. That is, 'X' can count as a single symbol and mean DOG, and 'Y' can count as a single symbol and mean ROCK, but we can also let the combination of 'X' and 'Y' together—that is, 'XY'—count as a single symbol and mean something else, say CHAIR. We are treating 'XY' just as if it were a single, simple symbol, like 'X' or 'Y' alone. We ignore the fact that it is made up of two things ('X' and 'Y') and treat it as if it were only one thing.

This trick is the basis of all human languages. No animal communication system has hit on it. Each piece of an animal communication system is meaningful—but in 'XY' meaning CHAIR, 'X' means nothing, nor does 'Y', only the combination 'XY' means CHAIR. It is rather like a magician's trick: now you see it ('X' and 'Y' are two things) and now you don't ('XY' is only one thing—the symbol for CHAIR).

This trick eases the burden on perception: If our creatures' perceptual systems can tell 'X' from 'Y', they can certainly tell 'XY' from 'X' alone or 'Y' alone. It means we can create new symbols out of our old ones, so we only need a relatively small stock of original symbols. We can go yet further if we want and treat a sequence of three of our original symbols as a single symbol and assign it a meaning—for example, let 'XY&' mean CAT. We can do the same for sequences of four and five symbols, and so on, up to the limit where we will overtax our creatures' memories and perceptual abilities.

Obviously, now we are going to get a lot more mileage out of our original symbols, and will be able to name many more things. We might have a list of symbols and meanings like the following:

X means DOG

Y means ROCK

& means LOVE

) means STAR

} means HAPPY

/ means RED

XY means CHAIR

XY& means CAT

X/ means BLUE

YX/ means EARTH

etc. (We can make up many more sequences and assign them meanings.)

Notice that the symbol 'X' alone means DOG, but in combination with other symbols, as in 'XY', it means nothing; only 'XY' as a whole has meaning, namely CHAIR. If we had a symbol (for example, '/') that only occurred in sequences (for example, say 'X/' means SAD), then it would never have any meaning by itself. Only the combinations it was in would have meaning. Furthermore, notice that 'X' in the system above really has no constant meaning: Alone it means DOG, but in combinations with other symbols it means nothing (rather, the whole combination has meaning).

This type of communication system has three very interesting properties. First, it has a certain *arbitrariness:* It does not really matter what the symbols are made of, or even what they look like at all. It is a completely arbitrary fact that we have chosen 'X' to mean DOG and 'XY&' to mean CAT. If we replaced each of our original symbols with a completely different one, and thus also replaced them in all the combinations they entered into, nothing important would change. As long as these new symbols were clearly separate from each other, the exact same things could be communicated. If '?' replaced 'X', then DOG would be '?' and CHAIR would be '?Y'. But these would work as well as 'X' and 'XY', and nothing important would have changed. Call this property the *arbitrariness property.*

Second, in most of their uses, our original symbols have no meaning themselves (for example, 'X' means nothing in 'XY&' or 'XY'). The pieces of our composite symbols (like 'X' and 'Y' in 'XY' and 'X', 'Y', and '&' in 'XY&') mean nothing at all. Call this the *meaninglessness property.*

Third, the symbols have to be *produced* somehow to be used for communication (written, spoken, cut out of paper, painted on flags, or brushed on rocks, as we have assumed for our creatures). This act of production can affect the symbols in various ways (mistakes can be made, individuals can perversely refuse to brush them right, the rocks can affect them in various ways). Our nice, pristine symbols will fall prey to time, chance, the people who use them, and the conditions under which they use them. Call this the *production property.*

These three properties (arbitrariness, meaninglessness, and production) each separately and all together seem trivial and mundane. This is misleading, however, because in fact they are crucial to any understanding of language, or of communication generally. Don't be fooled: Remember that a magician has played a trick here, and the trick is the heart of human language. People say that the thing with magicians is to watch their hands carefully and don't take your eyes off them, but skillful magicians are good at getting our eyes off their hands. Likewise, we are tempted to ignore the properties of language that are the subject of this chapter, but if we do, we miss the key trick altogether.

So back to our symbol system. The three properties—arbitrariness, meaninglessness, and production—give our symbols a life of their own. When we aren't watching, they come alive and live a life all their own, quite apart from their assigned job to communicate meaning.

Consider the situation we would be in if something like the following happened (and with creatures that are anything like human beings, we are guaranteed it will). Say our creatures want to produce 'XY' to communicate CHAIR. But sometimes they get sloppy and start to produce the symbols very quickly. So they sometimes draw 'XX' instead of the intended 'XY', since 'Y' looks something like 'X', and it is easier to produce (brush on the rock) an 'X' after an 'X' rather than a 'Y' after an 'X'. That is, in production, they sometimes *assimilate* the symbol 'Y' to a preceding 'X' and make it look like that 'X'. So sometimes we get 'XY' for CHAIR, and sometimes we get 'XX'.

More generally, we might notice that sometimes when a 'Y' follows an 'X' we see it brushed as an 'X' and not 'Y'. So not only do we sometimes see 'XX' for CHAIR instead of 'XY', but we sometimes see 'XX&' for CAT instead of 'XY&', and so on for many other cases where we would expect to see a 'Y' following an 'X' (but instead see an 'X' following an 'X').

So now what will happen? People are producing 'XY' when they are being careful and formal, and 'XX' when they are being quick and casual. This can lead the communication system to have two properties it did not have originally. That is, quite magically, two new things grow up—one a *new type of meaning* and one a *new structural property.*

First, the new type of meaning: The creatures can use the formal and careful form ('XY') to signal that they are being careful and formal and thus treating the addressee as important and worthy of special care, perhaps because the addressee is of higher status or because the addressee is a stranger or outsider. They can use the casual and quick form ('XX') to signal that they are being quick and causal, thus treating the addressee as one with whom one can be comfortable and more carefree, perhaps because the addressee is not of higher status or because the addressee is a peer or a friend.

These are *social* meanings. The original system had no symbols for them, but now all of a sudden it does: It signals deference and respect by *careful* productions, and comradeship and insiderhood by quick and *casual* productions. And further, a whole host of pedantic members of our creatures' community can band together to condemn 'XX' productions as "sloppy," "degenerate," and "bad communication" when they are used by others, unaware that they are also used from time to time by themselves.

And now the new structural property: Anyone who can understand the symbols that our creatures use must now realize that sometimes CHAIR is produced as 'XY' and sometimes as 'XX', and that CAT is sometimes produced as 'XY&' and sometimes as 'XX&', and so on for all cases where a 'Y' follows an 'X' in any of our composite symbols. Furthermore, one could predict that if a new symbol came into use, like 'XXY' to mean SKY, this would sometimes be produced as 'XXY' and sometimes as 'XXX'.

This knowledge of our creatures' communication system can be stated as a general rule: A 'Y' can show up as an 'X' when it is preceded by an 'X' in casual communication. This general knowledge allows us to realize that 'XX' and 'XY' can both mean CHAIR. But such a rule must be known also by the creatures producing (and not just understanding) the communication system, both because they produce 'XY' and 'XX' for CHAIR, and because they can all understand the communication system (they are all both producers and understanders).

Thus, this rule is *neutral* with respect to production and understanding; it really tells us something that such creatures *know* about their communication system. They do not have to know this *consciously,* they may know it only *unconsciously.* Knowledge is in people's (and our creatures') heads, and so the rule, like the rest of the symbol system, is in our creatures' heads. So our communication system is made up not just of the list of symbols and meanings, but of a rule as well. In addition to growing a new type of meaning (social meanings), the system has grown a new structural property: *rules.*

Of course, we have no idea how this rule is encoded in the brains of our creatures. As linguists, we can write it in several different ways, all of which amount to the same thing:

Rule 1

1a. 'Y' changes to 'X' when it is preceded by 'X' (in casual communication)

[Here we write the rule in English and take it to mean any Y can change to X when, in any string of symbols, it is preceded by X.]

1b. . . . XY . . . → . . . XX . . . (in casual communication)

[Here we use a new symbol system to write our rule in. ' . . . ' stands for any symbols that might be to the left or right of 'XY', and the arrow means *changes to,* so the whole thing means 'XY', when either by itself or with any other symbols to the right or left, can change to 'XX', with whatever is to the left or right, if anything, held constant'.]

1c. Y → X / XY (in casual communication)

[Here we use a different symbol system to write the rule in. This one means 'any Y changes to X when (the slash, /, means *when*) the Y is preceded by X'. The material after the slash (here 'XY') states the conditions under which the change before the slash (here 'Y → X') happens; it does not matter to the rule if any other symbols are to the right or left of 'XY'.]

What has happened so far—the way our communication system has grown both social meanings and rules—is due to the three properties of arbitrariness, meaninglessness, and production. Since it is quite arbitrary that 'XY' means CHAIR, and any other symbol or symbol communication could have done as well, then 'XX' carries out the job just fine. The 'X' in 'XY' means nothing, neither does either 'X' in 'XX'; rather, 'XY' (or 'XX') as a whole means CHAIR. Finally, in being produced, the symbols are prey to whatever hazards may come upon them, given their arbitrary nature and the meaninglessness of their parts.

You might wonder what would happen if our creatures sometimes produce 'XX' for 'XY' (meaning CHAIR), as we are hypothesizing they do, but the communication system already happens to have a composite symbol 'XX' meaning something other than CHAIR (for example, WATER). Will this stop them? Probably not, because in the context of real communication it would rarely be the case that understanders of the language could not readily figure out whether the producer meant by 'XX' CHAIR or WATER. If one of our creature's houses is on fire and he rushes out and paints the symbol for FIRE (whatever it is) and then follows up with 'XX', those standing by are unlikely to hand him a chair; instead they will run for water.

As time goes on, we may notice that something else begins to happen to our communication system. We see that our creatures, in quick and casual communication, are not only producing, 'X's' where we would expect 'Y's' when these 'Y's' follow 'X's'. They are also changing the symbol '/' to an 'X' when it follows an 'X'. Thus, for 'X/' meaning BLUE they sometimes produce 'X/' and sometimes 'XX', and for 'YX/' meaning EARTH they sometimes produce 'YX/' and sometimes 'YXX'—and so on for all cases where the symbol '/' follows 'X'. They begin to treat '/' just as they have been treating 'Y'. This means that in addition to Rule 1, we have a second rule:

Rule 2. '/' changes to 'X' when it is preceded by an 'X'.

There is something very peculiar about Rules 1 and 2. Why are our creatures doing this to 'Y' and '/' (when they follow an 'X') and not to other symbols, like '&' or ')' or '}'? What's so special about 'Y' and '/'? For one thing, they both look more like—bear more perceptual similarity to—'X' than do any of the other symbols. The symbol '/' just looks like half an 'X', and a 'Y' looks like an 'X' that didn't continue all the way down. The other symbols are all made out of curves and not lines the way 'X', 'Y', and '/' are.

But this suggests that Rules 1 and 2 are really part of one bigger rule that says that figures made out of *lines* and not *curves* change to resemble 'X' when they follow 'X'. But how can we state this rule and capture the similarity of 'X', 'Y', and '/', a similarity that we hypothesize is causing Rules 1 and 2 to operate?

To see how to do this, reconsider our list of symbols and meanings:

X means DOG

Y means ROCK

& means LOVE

) means STAR

} means HAPPY

/ means RED

XY means CHAIR

XY& means CAT

X/ means BLUE

YX/ means EARTH

etc. (We can make up many more sequences and assign them meanings.)

Looking at our symbols, we can see that some ('X', 'Y', and '/') are made out of lines, and others ('&', ')', and '}') are made out of curves. Let's refer to all the ones made out of lines as [+line] and the ones made out of curves as [−line]. [+line] and [−line] are called VALUES (+ or −) of the FEATURE [line]. It is just as if we were to say that men and boys are [+male] and women and girls are [−male]. In the previous case, we could have used [−curve] and [+curve] just as easily, just as we could have used [+female] and [−female] for women and men, respectively.

The only point is that features allow us to see things as having different values (+ or −) on the same scale or property. So the symbols made out of lines have the value '+' on the feature [line] and the symbols made out of curves have the value '−', just as men have the value '+' on the feature [male] and women have the value '−'. The feature names we use are arbitrary (but remember, being arbitrary is nothing to look down on when we are talking about symbols—that's precisely what gives them a life of their own, which is the point of this section).

A feature like [line] allows us to state Rules 1 and 2 as one rule and thus capture what these two rules have in common. It allows us to capture the fact that these two rules are really one process (making things that look like 'X' resemble 'X' even more). We can state the single rule replacing Rules 1 and 2 as follows (we will call the rule "the X assimilation rule," because it causes symbols to "assimilate" to 'X'):

THE X ASSIMILATION RULE (which collapses Rules 1 and 2 into one rule):

Any [+line] symbol changes to 'X' when it is preceded by 'X'.

Since the symbols '/', 'Y', and 'X' are marked as [+line], this rule will change these symbols to 'X' (vacuously for 'X' itself) when they follow an 'X'.

Rules like the X assimilation rule, which have now become part of our creatures' communication system, introduce yet another new structural property into their system: *features and their values*. Feature values are aspects or properties of symbols (for example, [+line] is a property that 'X', 'Y', and '/' share, and the others don't; the others share the feature [−line]). Features and their values have no meaning, they are not even symbols, and yet they are part of the system—things in the minds of our creatures.

Notice how our communication system keeps growing things that have no direct tie to meaning, things that are themselves meaningless (like 'X' in 'XY', or our rules, or the features and their values). Yet they are part of the system and in the minds of the creatures. This is indeed the way that our symbol system takes on a whole life of its own, apart from meaning. This is precisely the sort of thing we bought into when we played our trick of letting our original, arbitrary symbols (like 'X' and 'Y') enter into combinations that were treated as single symbols (like 'XY') with a single meaning (like CHAIR), a meaning that had nothing to do with the parts of the composite symbol. Our creatures are beginning to have to store in their heads all sorts of *structural knowledge* (symbol combinations, rules, features, and values).

In fact, since all human languages have just the properties we are studying here (as we will see later), human languages require brains capable of storing this sort of structural knowledge (and, since human languages are much more complex, they require much more of it). Thus, unless human evolution had given rise to such brains, there would have been no languages, at least not of the type we know.

More can happen to our communication system. Suppose that over time the quick and casual version ('XX' instead of 'XY') is used more and more—so often, in fact, that it is almost always the form used. Two things will happen: First, 'XX' will lose its ability to signal social meaning, since it will be used so often that in many cases 'XX' will occur instead of 'XY', even in formal and deferential contexts (communicating to important people).

Second, the new generation of children who are learning the communication system will "mistakenly" think that the only way to say CHAIR, for instance, is 'XX' (not 'XY'), or the only way to say CAT is 'XX&' (not 'XY&'). Once the new generation grows up, this "mistake" will no longer be a mistake, since it will now constitute the real system (everyone who knew—unconsciously, of course—that 'XX' came from 'XY' by the X assimilation rule will be dead or dying). This means that the rule changing 'X' or '/' (anything [+line]) to 'X' is lost; children have failed to realize it was part of the system. The children have changed the system (dropping the X assimilation rule).

Of course, on the other hand, these children are producers as well as understanders, and so nothing stops them from introducing new quick and casual productions, thereby eventually introducing new social meanings and new rules to make up for those that have been lost. After a number of generations have done this (lost and gained rules), if our original creatures were to return from the grave, they would not recognize (or know) their communication system any more. The symbol system lives a life that is quite independent of any of our creatures' intentions to communicate meanings like CHAIR and CAT.

─────────────────── E X E R C I S E ───────────────────

Exercise A.   Imagine the creatures we discussed in the previous section did not do what we said there, but only the following: They sometimes (when being careful) brushed 'XY' for CHAIR and sometimes (when being less careful) 'YY' for CHAIR. Indeed, they do this same sort of thing in all words where an 'X' precedes a 'Y'. Write the rule they unconsciously know in this case. Now, assume that later in the history of this language we find that all words with '/Y' in them sometimes show up with '/Y' in them (when the brushers are being careful) and sometimes with 'YY' (when the brushers are being less careful), in addition to all words with 'XY' in them continuing to sometimes show up as 'XY' (careful) and sometimes as 'YY' (less careful). Write the rule (using a feature) for what they now unconsciously know.

3.2. INDIVIDUAL SOUNDS AND THEIR RULES

The Sound Symbols of Human Language

All human spoken languages work like the symbol system we have designed for our creatures (and so do various signed languages, like American Sign Language, but their symbols are visual, not auditory as in spoken languages). The symbols of spoken languages are produced not by being brushed on rocks but by being formed by the mouth and projected to the hearer through the air.

These spoken symbols are also arbitrary, have parts that are not meaningful, and are subject to the vagaries of production. Think of a word like 'cost' as a sound symbol; it is *not* a visual image (like 'XY' brushed on a rock), but a "sound image" in our heads. It is arbitrary that we use the sound image 'cost' for the concept COST and not some other one (other languages use different-sounding words for this concept). We could just as easily have used some other sound image (and indeed 'cost' was pronounced differently in earlier stages of the language).

The sound image 'cost' is composed of four sound parts: It starts with the sound /k/, which is followed by the sound /a/ (this is the symbol linguists use for the vowel sound 'ah'), and it ends with the sounds /s/ and /t/. These sounds are completely meaningless; they only have meaning in combination with other sounds. Furthermore, when 'cost' is actually produced (pronounced), very often, in casual speech, people say it as [kas] ('cos′'), leaving off the final /t/ sound.

It is important to remember for the rest of this chapter that we are talking about *sounds,* not the way words are spelled. Many of the world's languages have never been written, and people learn to speak their language before they can write it. Spelling is a symbol system that is parasitic on sound, and it is sound systems that we want to understand here.

The English spelling system can be very misleading if we want to think about the way things are said and heard, not the way they are seen on a page. For example, the word 'cost' is spelled with a 'c' and the word 'kitten' is spelled with a 'k', but they both begin with the same sound, a sound we will represent as /k/. In the word 'citizen', the 'c' at the beginning is said as an /s/, not a /k/. Words like 'bear' and 'bare' are spelled differently, but said the same; a word like 'read' is spelled one way, but said in two different ways (compare 'Every night these days, I read', 'Yesterday, I read'). The sound /f/ is spelled as 'f' in 'fun', as 'ph' in 'phrase', and as 'gh' in 'rough'. But 'gh' in 'bough' (as in the 'bough of a tree'—rhymes with the exclamation 'Wow!') is not pronounced at all. The 'ou' in 'bough' rhymes with 'wow', in 'rough' it rhymes with 'stuff', in 'dough' it rhymes with 'oh', and in 'cough' it rhymes with 'off'.

Obviously, the English spelling system is no way to represent sound—and I will ask you to forget about spelling for the rest of this chapter. We will gradually introduce and use a system for representing sounds that is used widely by many linguists and that stems from the International Phonetic Alphabet (see Chapter 4). As we proceed, you will sometimes see sound segments and words enclosed between slashes (as in /kast/ for 'cost') and sometimes between brackets (as in [kas] for 'cos'', that is, 'cost' said without its /t/). It will gradually become clear why I do this, but for the time being ignore it.

Chapter 4 discusses how sounds are physically produced and the ways in which linguists classify them. It also lists the entire set of symbols we will use for representing individual sounds. You may choose either to read Chapter 3 first, where such matters will be introduced gradually and only as needed, or to read Chapter 4 and return to this chapter afterward.

If you are wondering why words are spelled so oddly in English, the reason is in part related to the sorts of things we saw happening in the communication system we designed in the previous section. At one time, the spelling of a word like 'knight' (which now has no /k/ sound in it, but begins with /n/) did reflect the way the word was said, but as the language changed the spelling system did not always keep pace with the change. Old pronunciations are often "frozen" into the spelling system.

Thus, the word /kast/ ('cost') is a symbol, like the symbol 'XY&' in our creatures' communication system. It is composed of meaningless parts: /k/, /a/, /s/, and /t/. I will call these meaningless parts "sound segments" of the symbol /kast/ ('cost'), or just "segments" for short. Now what are these segments and what exactly does it mean to say that a word like 'cost' has four segments in it? This question is trickier than you might think: We are so accustomed to print with its nice separate letter symbols and neat spaces that we may think this a trivial question. But in fact it is a difficult and intriguing one, once we get our minds thinking about sound and not spelling.

When we speak, we push air out of our lungs and through our throat and mouth. The organs of speech (the vocal chords, lips, teeth, and tongue, operating in the mouth cavity) disturb this flow of air, causing small variations in air pressure that occur rapidly one after another. These disturbances (variations in air pressure) are communicated to the molecules of the surrounding air and propagated in the form of sound waves through the air, somewhat like the ripples on a pond hit by a stone. When the sound waves reach the ear of a listener, they cause the eardrum to vibrate. A graph of a sound wave is very similar to a graph of the movements of the eardrum.

There are no clear boundaries in the sound wave, and furthermore we know from research on speech perception that information relevant to the identity of any segment in a word (the vowel /a/ in 'cost', for instance) is spread out throughout the whole sound wave, not concentrated just in its middle. It has been shown that in a word like 'tip' (/tɪp/), English speakers can tell what the vowel is (here /ɪ/) even if it is cut out of the word by recording the word and deleting its vowel from the tape. They can make this judgment based on the effect that the vowel /ɪ/ has had on the initial /t/ and the final /p/ (or, in other words, by the information contained in the beginning and end of the sound wave about what is in its middle). In fact, for most of us, speech in a language we do not know sounds like a more or less continuous "mush" in which we can pick out few discrete sounds.

A word like 'arm' (/arm/) ends in a *nasal* sound, that is, a sound in which air is allowed to come out of the nose. The first two sounds of /arm/, that is, /a/ and /r/, normally do not have any nasal air (they are said to be *oral* sounds, with air coming out of the mouth only). But in the word 'arm', speakers usually "anticipate" the upcoming /m/ and allow air to flow through the nose from the beginning of the word, so that /a/ and /r/ are *nasalized*. The nasal feature that belongs to the /m/ is in actuality spread throughout the word. Equally, the /r/ sound affects the /a/ vowel in such a way that /a/ is said rather differently than it is in the word 'cost' (/kast/). Thus, individual segments "bleed" their features throughout the sounds around them. Thus, the question is, how does the hearer unravel this mushed-up mess to get to discrete segments?

To make matters worse, factors like the age and gender of the speaker, whether the speaker has a cold, and the emotional state of the speaker (for example, anger), as well as the rate at which the speaker is talking, affect the shape of the sound waves the speaker produces. The word 'cost' said by a four-year-old and by a forty-year-old with a voice hoarse from smoking sounds very different indeed. Yet hearers can recognize that both the child and the adult have said the "same" word with the same segments.

It is something of a miracle, then, that we recognize the segments /k/, /a/, /s/, and /t/ in 'cost', and this miracle is performed by the human brain. Indeed, unless the human brain had evolved to pull off this miracle, there could be no communication of the sort we discussed at the beginning of this chapter, at least none using sound. How the brain actually does this job is part of the study of speech perception in psychology, and we do not fully understand the phenomena as of yet. The point is, however, that the segments are not "out there" in the world. All that is "out there" in the world are continuously changing sound waves, with no clear segmental boundaries, waves that carry some information that has nothing to do with what word was said (for example, age, gender, emotional state, health, and rate of speaking).

This means that segments like /k/, /a/, /s/, and /t/ in 'cost' are *not* physical entities but operations that have been performed on the sound wave by the human mind and "images" of that operation that are stored in the minds of speakers. A segment like /k/ is something in the mind, a piece of linguistic knowledge; there are no /k/'s in the physical world. Humans must use their mouths to produce this segment and the words it is in (like /kast/, 'cost'), but their physical production of it should never be confused with the segment, or the words, which are mental entities.

Just as we saw with 'Y' in 'XY' in our earlier communication system, lots of things can happen to /k/ when it gets put into production. When mental entities get dragged into the physical world, they go kicking and screaming, as we will see.

—————————— **E X E R C I S E S** ——————————

Exercise B. In Section 3.2, I say that

> As we proceed, you will sometimes see sound segments and words enclosed between slashes (as in /kast/ for 'cost') and sometimes between brackets (as in [kas] for 'cos″, that is, 'cost' said without its /t/). It will gradually become clear why I do this, but for the time being ignore it. (Here is a hint: In talking about our creatures' communication system in the first section of this chapter, I said, "The symbol /XY/ meaning DOG is sometimes produced— brushed—as [XY] and sometimes as [XX]").

Using the hint in the parentheses above, speculate on what the difference is between placing symbols in slashes (/XY/) and placing them in brackets ([XY] and [XX]).
In the statement

> The word <u>kast</u> ('cost') is sometimes said as <u>kast</u> (in slow, careful speech) and sometimes said as <u>kas</u> (in fast, informal speech)

place 'kast', 'kast', and 'kas' in slashes or brackets as you think appropriate, given what you take slashes and brackets to mean.

Exercise C. In Section 3.2, I said that a word like /kast/ ('cost'), and even a segment in this word, like /k/, are not physical entities, but mental ones (entities in the mind, though, of course, they are ultimately stored somehow in the brain, which is a physical thing). Think of visual perception: When I claim to see the color red in the world, is the red I claim to see a physical or a mental entity? Discuss the matter (there is no right answer here, though there are thoughtful ways to approach the problem). What about when I claim to see a cat—is the cat I claim to see a physical or a mental entity?

Phonological Rules

We are not going to be concerned here with how people actually produce sounds; that is not the linguist's job (see Chapter 4 for an overview of the matter, however). The linguist is concerned rather with *what people know (unconsciously) about how things conventionally get produced in a language.* This may seem only subtly different from studying what people actually do, but it is not: A person could lose the capacity to speak, and thus lose the capacity to produce sounds. But such a person would not have lost her *linguistic knowledge* about the way the language is pronounced.

Even if one of our creatures had lost the ability to brush symbols on rocks, she would still know that there are two ways to brush 'XY' (either 'XY' or 'XX') and thus would still know the *rule:* 'XY' is changed to 'XX' in casual communication. Indeed, understanders (as opposed to producers) don't produce anything, but they still must know this rule to decode the symbols they see. So we are interested in *knowledge* (what I called "competence" in Chapter 1), in *representations* (like 'XY' or /kast/), and *rules,* all of which are in the mind.

Let's take a concrete example of a rule native speakers of English unconsciously know about the pronunciation of their language, one that matches closely the sort of rule we saw in our creatures' communication system. The English word 'cost' is represented in people's heads as /kast/. When it is spoken slowly, these are the segments that their ears and brains tell them are there (though, of course, what they actually produce are muscle movements in their mouths, which give rise to sound waves that other people's ears decode). However, in quick and casual speech, the word 'cost' is often said as [kas] ('cos' '), that is, the final /t/ is dropped.

This is not true just of a word like 'cost'; in fact, it is true of words that resemble 'cost' in a certain way. Thus, 'desk' is said in formal speech as [dɛsk], but in casual speech as [dɛs], and 'kept' is said in formal speech as [kɛpt], but in casual speech as [kɛp]. In fact, any word ending in two consonants can be said in fast speech with the last consonant dropped.

The discussion of our creatures' communication system has taught us to expect two things in a case like this. First, the two variants of each word should carry *social* meaning. The formal pronunciation should be used to signal respect, deference, or distance, the casual one to signal comradeship, in-group standing, or equality of footing. Second, the people who use this system know a rule that tells them that sometimes words like 'cost', 'mist', and 'desk' are said one way and sometimes another way. Furthermore, since this rule is true not just of one word like 'cost', it must be stated in terms of *features* (like [+line] and [−line]). Features allow us to capture what the segments that the rule applies to have in common. Thus, we do not have to mention them all separately or pretend there is a separate rule for each one.

Let's make a distinction between sound segments that are VOWELS and those that are CONSONANTS. Vowels are produced with an open vocal tract, and the air from the lungs flows out relatively unimpeded. Consonants have some type and degree of restriction in the mouth that causes the air to be briefly stopped or to become turbulent as it flows past an obstruction that does not stop the air, but impedes its flow.

Let's call consonants "[+consonantal] segments" and vowels "[−consonantal] segments". Just as we saw in the case of [+line] and [−line], we could have used other feature names (for example, [−vocalic] and [+vocalic] respectively), just as we can use [+male] and [−male] for men and women, or [−female] and [+female]. The important thing is the distinction between two classes (vowels and consonants, men and women) that we are trying to make.

We can now state the rule that English speakers (unconsciously) know, which tells them that sometimes 'cost' is said as [kast] and sometimes as [kas], and equally for many other similar sorts of words. The rule is as follows:

CONSONANT DELETION RULE

A [+consonantal] segment can be deleted if it follows another [+consonantal] segment at the end of a word, in quick and casual speech.

More formally, this rule can be written as follows:

CONSONANT DELETION RULE (Formal Version)

[+consonantal] → zero / [+consonantal] __ #

This means that: a [+consonantal] segment changes to zero (becomes nothing, is deleted) when (the slash, /, means *when* or *in the environment of*) it is preceded by a [+consonantal] segment and followed by the end of the word (we use the symbol # for a word boundary, to mark the end of a word). In the rule, the blank between "[+consonantal]" and the word boundary symbol "#" is a placeholder for the thing that is changing (going from being a consonant to being deleted). To see more clearly how this blank is used, imagine I wanted to state a rule that said that John disappears whenever he stands between Sue and Mary, just as the consonant deletion rule says that a consonant is deleted (disappears) when it stands between another consonant and the end of the word (#). This could be written as:

John → zero / Sue ___ Mary

The blank here stands for John who takes on the property of disappearing whenever he is placed between Sue and Mary. This rule is exactly equivalent to writing the more unwieldy formula below:

Sue John Mary → Sue zero Mary

Just as we could have written for our consonant deletion rule:

[+consonantal][+consonantal] # → [+consonantal] zero #

Thus, in the word /kast/ ('cost'), a /t/, which is [+consonantal], follows, at the end of the word, another [+consonantal] segment (namely /s/), and therefore can be deleted, to give us [kas]. The same is true of /dɛsk/ ('desk'), which can become [dɛs]; or /lɪft/ ('lift'), which can become [lɪf]; or /lɪmp/ ('limp'), which can become [lɪm].

This rule tells us not that people actually delete consonants in their heads as they speak, but rather that they know that there are two ways to say 'cost'—[kast] and [kas]. Whether they say [kast] or [kas], what happens in their mouths is muscle movements and what comes out of their mouths are mushed-up sound waves. What comes to the listener's ear are the mushed-up sound waves. The nice clean sound segments are *mental entities* in any case. To give a full account of actual pronunciation, we would have to spell out rules of how the segments in either [kast] or [kas] are turned into muscle movements and sound waves. These are not linguistic rules and belong to another science (speech science).

Furthermore, while we have defined the features [+consonantal] and [−consonantal] in terms of aspects of sound production (whether the vocal tract is relatively wide open or not), this is not really relevant. We could have defined lots of other features based on aspects of production (or sound waves, or audition, for that matter). We choose our features *because* they give us the right classes of sounds to account for the rules that native speaker–hearers of the language unconsciously know (and that they show us they know by how they behave).

The feature [consonantal] divides the sounds in the right way to state the consonant deletion rule, and that rule seems to be the correct one for English. In the end, we must settle on a whole set of features based on the whole set of rules in the language. But this choice is based on research as to what is the best set of features to use to account not only for the rules of English, but of all other languages as well.

The consonant deletion rule is an example of a **phonological rule.** Such rules state relationships between sound forms (like [kast] and [kas]) that native speaker–hearers (unconsciously) know to hold in their language. When we find such an alternation, we pick one form as **basic** or **canonical** (/kast/, /dɛsk/, /mɪst/, and so forth in the case of the consonant deletion rule). The other form ([kas], [dɛs], [mɪs]) is said to be derived from this basic or canonical form by the phonological rule. The basic or canonical form is always on the left side of the rule, and the derived form on the right.

We have picked the forms of the words with both consonants at the end (/kast/, /dɛsk/, /mɪst/, etc.) as basic forms because it is easier to state the rule that way. It is certainly easier to say of words ending in two consonants that the last consonant can be deleted than to say of forms like /kas/, /dɛs/, and /mɪs/ that a consonant is added to the end in more formal speech (how would we know what consonant to add!). Furthermore, speakers' behavior in slow and formal speech shows that they know that the word 'cost', for example, ends in a /t/, even if they drop this /t/ in fast speech.

We will assume that all speaker–hearers of a language have a mental dictionary in their heads, which we call the **mental lexicon.** This lexicon lists all the words in the language that that speaker–hearer knows. With each word is listed all the speaker–hearer's linguistic knowledge about that word—for example, its part of speech (whether it is a noun, verb, adjective, or adverb), its phonological representation, and its meaning. Of course, we have no idea how such information is stored in the brain. We simply represent it by our linguistic notation—things like /kast/ for 'cost'.

We will *not* assume that for a word like 'cost' both the form /kast/ and the form /kas/ are each listed as words, and likewise for all other words ending in two consonants. This would be silly, since it misses the fact that the native speaker–hearer (unconsciously) knows that these two forms are *related* to each other by the consonant deletion rule.

Instead, we will only list the basic or canonical form of the word in the lexicon. Thus, we will only list for 'cost' the form /kast/; and for 'desk' the form /dɛsk/; and for 'mist' the form /mɪst/. These basic or canonical forms are also called the **lexical forms** of the words, precisely because they are the forms listed in the mental lexicon. The derived forms ([kas], [dɛs] and [mɪs], for instance) are derived by the consonant deletion rule—it is this rule that tells the speaker–hearer of English that such forms exist (and where they can be used). They need not be listed in the lexicon.

Let me give another example of a phonological rule. Notice that in slow speech the word 'bet' is said as /bɛt/, as in the phrase 'I will bet you $10' said slowly. However, if we say this phrase fast, we get 'I'll *betch* ya $10', where 'bet' is said as /bɛč/ (/č/ is the symbol of the sound often spelled 'ch' or 'tch'—it is a single sound in English). Thus, there are two ways to say 'bet', either as /bɛt/ or /bɛč/.

The /t/ in 'bet' changes to /č/ in fast speech because of the following /y/

sound in the word 'you' (or 'ya'). The segment /t/ is made by stopping the air from the lungs with the tip of the tongue placed at the alveolar region of the mouth (the bony ridge right behind the front teeth). And /y/ is made by thrusting the tongue toward the palate (the roof of the mouth), which is somewhat behind the alveolar ridge. Thus, in [beč], the /t/ is moving back from the alveolar region to the palatal region (/č/ is made at the palate) to 'agree with' the /y/ sound, making the pronunciation of 'bet' easier in this environment (that is, in front of /y/).

This same change happens to a small set of other sounds that are also made at the alveolar ridge and that move to be made near the palate when they occur before /y/ in fast speech: When preceding /y/, the sound /d/ becomes /ǰ/, the sound beginning 'joy'; /s/ becomes /š/, the sound beginning 'shoe'; and /z/ becomes /ž/, the sound spelled as 's' in the middle of 'pleasure'.

Thus, it would not be enough simply to say that /t/ changes to /č/ when it precedes a /y/ in fast speech. Rather, we need to find a feature or small set of them that characterize just /t/, /d/, /s/, and /z/ (something they all have in common, and that no other segments do) and write the rule in terms of this feature or this small set of features. For example, since all of them are made at the alveolar ridge, we could have something like the following rule: A [+alveolar] segment changes to become [+palatal] when it precedes a [+palatal] segment. We will not actually use these features below (there is a better set for wider purposes), but they make the point.

Finally, our basic point is, to know English, one cannot simply know words and what they mean. One has to know what sound segments (meaningless parts of words) English uses and what rules the native speaker knows about these segments, as well as the features that are used in these rules to characterize groups or classes of sound segments. And all this knowledge has nothing directly to do with meaning.

———————————————— **E X E R C I S E** ————————————————

Exercise D. The data below is from a nonstandard dialect (version) of English that you probably do not speak. Nonstandard dialects are perfectly normal and rule governed; they are just different than the "standard" (the standard is the dialect normally used in the news media and in schools—see Chapter 9). Below, I write out a set of standard English words and then the fast-speech and slow-speech versions of these words in the nonstandard dialect. I represent these words in English spellings or "pseudo-English" spellings that attempt to make clear to you how the word is pronounced. These spellings are followed in parentheses by the phonetic spelling of the pronunciations, that is, the pronunciations as they would be represented by linguists using the system we use in this chapter and that we explicate in Chapter 4.

Propose one or more phonological rules to account for the data in the nonstandard dialect. You can state your rule or rules in English, but be as clear and explicit as you can. Assume that the phenomena you observe here happens after all vowels, and not just the ones here—that is, refer to "vowels" (or a feature [−consonantal] or [+vocalic], as you wish) in your rule or rules. HINT: The sound /d/ is a consonant made by momentarily stopping the air with the tongue at the alveolar ridge (the bony ridge behind the front teeth). It is said to be a *voiced* ([+voice]) sound because the vocal chords in the throat are vibrating when it is made. The sound /t/ is just like /d/, but it is *voiceless* ([−voice]); the vocal chords are not vibrating. The sounds /t/ and /d/ are said to be *stops;* /t/ is a voiceless stop and /d/ is a voiced stop. The phenomenon you observe in this exercise is exemplified for /t/ and /d/ only, but the same thing happens for all voiced and voiceless stops (thus, also for /p/ and /b/, and /k/ and /g/). State your rules in terms of "voiceless stop" and "voiced stop" (that is, your rule or rules should read "Voiceless (or [−voice]) stops become . . . when they are . . ." or "Voiced (or [+voice]) stops become . . . when they are . . .").

STANDARD ENGLISH	FAST SPEECH	SLOW SPEECH
boot	boo ([bu])	boot ([but])
wood	woot ([wʊt])	wood ([wʊd])
lot	la ([la])	lot ([lat])
load	loat ([lot])	load ([lod])
boat	boa ([bo])	boat ([bot])
sit	si ([sɪ])	sit ([sɪt])
lid	lit ([lɪt])	lid ([lɪd])

After stating your rule or rules, give the *basic forms* for the nonstandard dialect of each of the words. Place each of these forms between slashes (for example, /boot/ using English spelling or /but/ using phonetic spelling). Clearly specify whether you are using English spellings or phonetic spellings.

Optional Versus Obligatory Phonological Rules

The consonant deletion rule tells us that in the case of words like 'cost', two different forms alternate, namely [kast] and [kas]. We have chosen /kast/ as the basic, or canonical, or the lexical form—all mean the same thing here—listed in the mental lexicon. The form [kas] is a *derived* form, accounted for by the consonant deletion rule. These two different forms of the word 'cost' occur in different contexts (slow and fast speech, respectively) and in different styles (formal and informal styles, respectively), and they communicate different social meanings (deference and comradeship, respectively).

It is also clear why the rule came to exist in the first place. In fast speech, it is easier to pronounce a single consonant following a vowel ('cos″ [kas]) than it is to pronounce two of them ('cost', [kast]). There are many phonological rules that take place in fast speech, rules like the consonant deletion rule or the rule that changes /bɛt/ ('bet') to [bɛč] ('betch') in front of /y/. Operating together they can alter the pronunciation of words dramatically.

For example, consider the phrase 'do you want to'. In slow and formal speech this could be said as [du yu want tu] ('do you want to'). However, even in fairly careful speech, the unstressed vowels in /du/ and /yu/ would be reduced to the brief central vowel [ə], which is called "the schwa vowel" (we will discuss *stress* below). This vowel occurs pervasively in English, since almost all un-stressed vowels are reduced to this vowel regardless of how they would have been said if they had been stressed. Thus, 'do you want to' would, even in fairly formal speech, normally be said as [də yə want tu].

As one's speech gets more quick and casual, more fast-speech phonological rules apply. For example, 'want to' can be contracted to [wantə] (spelled 'wanta'—note that here English spelling spells the schwa vowel with 'a'), giving 'da ya wanta'. And, going further, the /t/ of 'wanta' can be deleted, giving 'da ya wana'; or 'do you' can be contracted together to give 'dya wana'. Finally, the whole phrase can be said as one word, 'jawana', where the /d/ of 'do' and the /y/ of 'you' have been fused into a [ǰ], a "soft g sound." Thus, we get a series of possible forms, ranging from the most formal 'do you want to' to the least 'jawana', through several other versions, each one of which is created by the application of more and more phonological rules that apply in fast speech and casual styles. Each such adjustment makes the phrase easier to say in ever-faster speech.

Each of these different forms is used in a slightly different style, and the use of each signals a slightly different social meaning on the scale from highly formal and deferential communication to highly informal and peer-oriented communi-cation. There is not really a dichotomy here, but rather a whole scale of styles and social meanings, each appropriate to different occasions of use.

However, not all phonological rules are fast-speech rules. There are phonological adjustments that also make pronunciation easier but that are made *in all styles.* These can be said to be **obligatory** processes. Since they always occur, they cannot give rise to two different forms of one word.

For example, when any vowel in English precedes one of the consonants /m/, /n/, or /ŋ/, it is pronounced a little bit differently than when it occurs anywhere else. When in front of these consonants, vowels are said with air coming out of the nose as well as out of the mouth (they are said to be *nasalized* or *nasal vowels*). When vowels are said anywhere else (in front of any other consonants, or when ending a word), they are said with air coming out of the mouth only, but not out of the nose (they are said then to be *oral vowels*). Thus, the vowel /ɪ/ in the word 'sit' is said as an oral vowel with no nasal air, and in the word 'sin' it is said as a nasal vowel, with nasal as well as oral air.

The consonants /m/, /n/, and /ŋ/ are the only consonants in English that are themselves produced with air coming out of the nose—that is, they themselves are nasalized. They all involve momentarily stopping the airstream from the lungs in the mouth while letting air out the nose (eventually, letting go the obstruction in the mouth and letting air out of the mouth also). An /m/ is just like a /b/, except that /m/ has air coming out of the nose and /b/ does not (say 'mop' and 'bop'). An /n/ is just like a /d/, except that /n/ has air coming out of the nose and /d/ does not (say 'not' and 'dot'). An /ŋ/ is just like a /g/, except that /ŋ/ has air coming out of the nose and /g/ does not (say 'sang' and 'sag'). Thus, vowels add the feature [+nasal] (that is, they nasalize—add nasal air) when they precede consonants that have the feature [+nasal] (nasalized consonants); the vowel's nasalization anticipates the nasalization of the consonant and makes the words easier to pronounce.

Given the fact that vowels nasalize in front of nasal consonants, we find the sort of data in English that is given in the list below. In this list, the tilde (~) over the vowel sounds in some words means that air is let out of the nose (they are nasalized, have the feature [+nasal]) as well as the mouth. If a vowel has no tilde, then no air is let out of the nose (only out of the mouth) and they are said to be oral vowels.

sit	/sɪt/	sin	/sĩn/
peg	/pɛg/	pen	/pɛ̃n/
at	/æt/	am	/æ̃m/
road	/rod/	roam	/rõm/
log	/lag/	long	/lãŋ/
see	/si/	seem	/sĩm/

The data shows clearly that vowels are always nasalized in front of nasal consonants (/m/, /n/, and /ŋ/). It is not that human beings cannot produce a pronunciation of an oral vowel (a vowel with air only coming out of the mouth) in front of a nasal consonant. It is just that English speakers in general do not do it.

Perhaps at one time English speakers did produce oral vowels in front of nasal consonants and only occasionally changed these oral vowels to nasal vowels because it was easier. Indeed, there is a tendency in all languages occasionally to nasalize vowels in front of nasal consonants, even if speakers do not always do this or do not nasalize the vowels to any great degree. It *does* make pronunciation easier, given how the human vocal tract works (it's easier to open the nasal passage, by lowering the velum, a little bit before forming the obstruction for the nasal consonant). Eventually, however, in English and some other languages, it became obligatory to pronounce all vowels with nasalization when they are before nasal consonants.

Thus, a physical tendency (which can be overridden) became an obligatory convention. This obligatory convention constitutes a *rule*. While this rule had its origins in a physical tendency due to the way the human vocal tract is constituted, like all rules it is a mental phenomena, not a physical one. The language need not have made this tendency into a rule in the first place. Whether or not the English vowel nasalization rule arose this way (and it probably did), many phonological rules certainly did (and continue to do so in the world's languages).

Looking at the above list, one can easily formulate the rule that is at work to produce this configuration of data, a rule we have stated informally already: When a vowel (any vowel) precedes a nasal consonant (/m/, /n/, and /ŋ/), it is nasalized (adds the feature [+nasal]). When a vowel precedes any other sound or ends a word, it is not nasalized (said with no air coming out of the nose, it is just an oral vowel). The rule is stated below, first informally, but using features, and then more formally. Remember that we are using the feature [−consonantal] to pick out vowels and the feature [+consonantal] to be pick out consonants. The feature [+nasal] picks out nasalized sounds, while [−nasal] picks out sounds with no nasalization (oral sounds).

VOWEL NASALIZATION RULE

[−consonantal] segments add the feature [+nasal] when they precede sounds that have both the features [+nasal] and [+consonantal] (that is, vowels add the feature [+nasal] when they precede nasal consonants).

VOWEL NASALIZATION RULE (Formal Version)

$$[-\text{consonantal}] \rightarrow [+\text{nasal}] \ / \ \_\!\!\_ \begin{bmatrix} +\text{consonantal} \\ +\text{nasal} \end{bmatrix}$$

This more formal notation says the following: Any segment that has the feature [−consonantal] changes to add the feature [+nasal] when (the slash, '/', means *when*) that sound (the blank, or underline, signals the place or location of the sound that we are concerned with) is followed by any segment that has both the features [+consonantal] and [+nasal] (that is, consonants that are nasalized, thus /n/, /m/, and /ŋ/, the only such in English).

Basic Segments Versus Derived Segments

In the last section we saw that, thanks to the vowel nasalization rule, each vowel segment in English has two forms, an oral form ([ɪ] in [sɪt], for instance) and a nasal form ([ĩ] in [sĩn], for instance). Now let's compare this rule to the consonant deletion rule. The consonant deletion rule, since it was optional and applied in different styles, gave us two forms of a single word ([kast] and [kas] for 'cost'). We chose one of them as the *basic* or *canonical* form, the form to be listed in the lexicon (for example, /kast/), and we derived the other form (for example, [kas]) by rule. In the case of the vowel nasalization rule, we get not two different forms of a single word but two different forms of a single segment: two forms of each vowel segment—an oral form (for example, [ɪ] in 'sit') and a nasal form (for example, [ĩ] in 'sin').

Here too we want to make a distinction between a basic or canonical form and a *derived* form, a form derived by a rule from the basic form. But in this case, it will be a distinction between *basic* and *derived* segments (for example, oral vowels versus nasal vowels), not different forms of the same word (as in [kast] and [kas] as forms of 'cost').

We will pick the *oral* vowel forms as basic or canonical, in part because they occur in more places than the nasal vowel forms (have a wider distribution in the language). But our main reason is that it is easier to write the rule relating oral and nasal vowels if we pick the oral vowels as basic and derive the nasal ones from them. It is clearly the following nasal consonants that are causing the oral vowels to take on an additional feature (that is, [+nasal]) so that they more closely resemble these nasal consonants.

We assume that speaker–hearers store in their heads not only a mental lexicon but also a list of the *basic systematic sounds* of their language. This list is part of the PHONOLOGICAL COMPONENT or PHONOLOGICAL MODULE of their mental grammar. The oral vowels of English are part of this list of basic systematic sounds. The nasal vowels are not. Speakers derive the nasal vowels (that is, know about them—that they constitute part of the language) through the vowel nasalization rule. They are *derived* sounds.

Thus, we are proposing that a speaker–hearer of English knows (unconsciously) what sounds there are in English by knowing, first, the list of the basic systematic sounds (for the basic sounds) and, second, knowing rules, like the vowel nasalization rule. These rules derive nonbasic segments (derived segments) from the list of basic ones, adapting the basic segments to particular environments in which they occur (for example, in front of nasal consonants).

The basic vowels segments of English are the oral ones: /ɪ/ ('sin'), /i/ ('see'), /ɛ/ ('set'), /e/ ('say'), /æ/ ('sat'), /ʊ/ ('soot'), /u/ ('suit'), /o/ ('so'), /ɔ/ ('sought'), /ʌ/ ('gut'), and /a/ ('sod'). We do not need to add the nasal versions of each of these vowels to the list—we know they are in the language thanks to the vowel nasalization rule but that they are special-purpose versions (derived versions) of the basic oral vowels.

A segment is *not* basic if its distribution is predictable by a rule. Thus, as we saw above, nasal vowels are not basic because we can predict where they will occur, namely in front of nasal consonants. A segment is basic if we cannot predict in specific terms where it will occur. If I ask where the nasal vowel [ã] occurs in English, you would say "in front of nasal consonants." If I ask where the oral vowel [a] occurs, all you could say is "everywhere else." Its distribution is not predictable in any more specific terms. Thus, the nasal vowel segment [ã] is not basic, and the oral vowel segment [a] is.

The fact that any derived segment is derived from a basic one by a rule (as the nasal vowel [ã] is derived by the vowel nasalization rule from the oral vowel /a/) leads to an important relationship between a basic segment and the derived segment that is derived from it: Since the derived segment is derived from the basic one by a rule, the derived segment and the basic one can never occur in the same place. The nasal vowel [ã] occurs before nasal consonants, the oral vowel [a] everywhere else. They are said to be in **complementary distribution.** Two segments are in complementary distribution if, given all the positions in words in which they could occur, one occurs in a subset of these places (for example, all the positions before nasal consonants) and the other in a different and distinct subset (for example, everywhere else), and they never occur in the same position.

The fact that two segments never occur in the same place means that they can never directly contrast with each other. That is, it could never happen that you could substitute one of these segments for the other one in a given word and thereby get a different word, a word with a different meaning. If you take a word like 'sin', which contains the nasal vowel [ĩ] ([sĩn]), and you try to substitute the corresponding oral vowel [ɪ], you do not get a different word, but just an odd and foreign-sounding pronunciation of 'sin'—[sɪn], with an oral vowel. Vice versa, if you take a word like 'sit', which contains the oral vowel [ɪ] ([sɪt]), and you try to substitute the nasal vowel [ĩ], you do not get a different word, but just an odd and foreign-sounding pronunciation of 'sit' ([sĩt] with a nasal vowel). This is precisely what it means to say that oral vowels (like [ɪ]) and nasal vowels (like [ĩ]) do not contrast with each other.

On the other hand, basic segments and segments derived from different basic segments *do* contrast with each other. Thus, the vowel segment [a], which is a basic segment, contrasts with all other basic vowel segments. If you substitute [a] for any other vowel ([o], for example) in a particular word, you can get a different word, a word with a different meaning. For example, if you substitute [a] for [o] in the word 'coat' [kot], you get a new word (not an odd un-English pronunciation), namely 'cot' [kat]. Thus, [a] and [o] directly contrast with each other. If you substitute the nasal vowel [ĩ], a segment derived from the oral vowel [ɪ], for the nasal vowel [õ], a segment derived from the oral vowel [o], in the word [fõn] ('phone'), you get a different word, namely [fĩn] ('fin'). In general, all segments—basic or derived—in a language contrast with the other segments in the language, except for basic segments and segments derived from them by rule (for example, [ɪ] and [ĩ]).

Another way we can word all this is to say that the distinction between oral vowels (like [a]) and nasal vowels (like [ã]) is not *distinctive* in English (that is, the two do not distinguish any words in English). Equivalently, we can say that the feature [+nasal] is not distinctive for English vowels because it cannot be the single difference that causes two words to be different words ([sɪt] and [sĩt] are not different words, just different pronunciations of the same word, one of them "odd").

Note that the distinction between nasal consonants (/m/, /n/, and /ŋ/) and oral consonants (such as /b/, /p/, /d/, /t/, /g/, and /k/) *is* distinctive in English. If you substitute an [m], for example, for a [b] in a word—for example, the word 'mit' ([mɪt])—you get a different word, namely 'bit' ([bɪt]). Thus, [m] and [b] directly contrast. Furthermore, no rule can predict in specific terms where [m] will occur or where [b] will occur—indeed, they can occur in the very same position, as in [mɪt] versus [bɪt] (that's what allows them to distinguish meanings). Equivalently, we can say that the feature [+nasal] is distinctive for consonants in English. The only difference between [b] and [m] is that the latter is [+nasal] and the former is [−nasal]; otherwise they are made in exactly the same way. Yet this difference alone can make a difference of meaning in English (again, as in [mɪt] versus [bɪt], which are two different words).

In other languages, the feature [+nasal] may behave differently. For example, in French, the feature [+nasal] is distinctive for vowels. Thus, there are contrasts like [lo] (which means *prize*) versus [lõ] (which means *long*). If we substitute a nasal version of a vowel for an oral version in French, we can change the meaning of a word. Therefore, French has no such rule as the vowel nasalization rule. There is no rule that can predict where the nasal [õ] appears by deriving it from the oral [o]. The nasal [õ] is not derived from the oral one as basic.

Let's look at another example of the distinction between basic segments and derived ones, involving vowels. Consider the following data from English. In this data I use the symbol ':' following a vowel segment to mean that the vowel is *longer* than the same vowel segment without this symbol. The question we will ask is, can we predict where long vowels occur in relation to vowels of regular length?

goat	[got]	goad	[go:d]
bus	[bʌs]	buzz	[bʌ:z]
leaf	[lif]	leave	[li:v]
bat	[bæt]	bad	[bæ:d]
back	[bæk]	bag	[bæ:g]
loose	[lus]	lose	[lu:z]
at	[æt]	add	[æ:d]

If you inspect this data, you will notice that all the words in the left column end in a *voiceless* consonant, and the words in the right column end in a *voiced* consonant. Consider the first pair, 'goat' and 'goad'. 'Goat' ends in a [t], and 'goad' ends in a [d]. These two sounds are made in exactly the same way (the air from the lungs is momentarily stopped by the front of the tongue being placed at the alveolar ridge, the bony ridge behind the front teeth), except that in the case of [d] the vocal chords in the throat are vibrating, and in the case of [t] they are not.

When the chords are vibrating during a segment, the segment is said to be *voiced;* when a segment has no vocal chord vibration, it is said to be *voiceless.* In each pair above, the segment ending the word on the left is a voiceless version of the voiced sound ending the word on the right ([s] is voiceless, [z] voiced; [f] is voiceless, [v] is voiced; [k] is voiceless, [g] voiced). The segments ending these words in each pair differ only by the feature [−voice] versus [+voice].

Once we know that all the words on the left end in a voiceless consonant (a segment with the feature [−voice]) and all the words on the right end in a voiced consonant (a segment with the feature [+voice]), we can see what is causing the vowels to lengthen. Vowels become longer when they precede a voiced consonant. This is yet another phonological rule of English. Since we can predict the distribution of the long vowels in terms of a rule changing the regular vowels to [+long], we are treating the long vowels as derived from the regular ones as basic. Thus, we have the following rule:

VOWEL-LENGTHENING RULE

A [−consonantal] segment adds the feature [+long] when it precedes a segment with both the features [+consonantal] and [+voice].

VOWEL-LENGTHENING RULE (Formal Version)

$$[-\text{consonantal}] \rightarrow [+\text{long}] \ / \ \underline{\quad} \begin{bmatrix} +\text{consonantal} \\ +\text{voice} \end{bmatrix}$$

Now we can ask an interesting question: What about vowels in front of nasal consonants (/m/, /n/, and /ŋ/)? All these nasal consonants are voiced ([+voice]). We know these vowels will nasalize by the vowel nasalization rule. But, since nasal consonants in English are all voiced, we would expect that these vowels would also lengthen (get the feature [+long] by the vowel-lengthening rule). If you compare how 'sit' ([sɪt]) is said to how 'sin' ([sĩn]) is said, you will notice that the vowel in 'sin' is indeed longer than the vowel in 'sit' (besides being nasalized), despite the fact that these are otherwise very similar vowel sounds. Thus, the real representation of 'sin' should be [sĩ:n] with a lengthened vowel, and not [sĩn] as we have been writing it so far.

Thus, we see that two of our phonological rules have applied to the word 'sin': the vowel nasalization rule and the vowel-lengthening rule. We can think of these rules applying one after the other, applying to the basic segment (/ɪ/) in the word 'sin' to transform it progressively to the way it is actually pronounced. Below, I give a graphic representation of the rules applying step by step to the three words 'sin', 'Sid' (a proper name), and 'sit':

BASIC SEGMENTS	/sɪn/	/sɪd/	/sit/
Vowel nasalization rule:	sĩn	—	—
Vowel-lengthening rule:	sĩ:n	sɪ:d	—
OUTPUT	[sĩ:n]	[sɪ:d]	[sɪt]
	sin	Sid	sit

The rules apply to the word in its basic segments and progressively change these segments (for example, by adding features to them that are predictable).

The rule applies only if its conditions for application are met. Thus, the vowel nasalization rule cannot apply to /sɪt/ because here the vowel is not followed by a nasal consonant; and the vowel-lengthening rule cannot apply to /sɪt/ because the vowel is not followed by a voiced ([+voice]) consonant.

The step-by-step progression, moving from a representation in terms of basic segments to a final output via phonological rules, is called a **derivation.** As a matter of convention, we will place the basic segments in slashes ('/') and the final output of a derivation in brackets ('[' and ']'). The intermediary steps will be enclosed by neither slashes or brackets.

The representation that we have labeled "basic segments" and enclosed in slashes (for example, /sɪn/), is sometimes called the **underlying representation,** the **systematic phonemic representation,** or the **lexical representation.** These all amount to the same thing. This underlying representation in terms of basic segments indicates the way the words are stored in the mental lexicon. The output representation, enclosed in brackets (for example, [sĩ:n]), is closer to the way the words are actually pronounced (though we would still have to specify how these symbols are translated by the mind and mouth into actual muscle movements). This output representation is sometimes called the **phonetic representation** or the **surface representation.** It includes information that is predictable by rule and that is added by rule to the basic or underlying representation.

Of course, many more phonological rules can apply to the same underlying representation. For example, consider the derivation below of the fast-speech pronunciation of the word 'mend' as 'men′' (as in the sentence, 'This thing will never men′ right'). This derivation involves most of the rules we have seen so far:

BASIC SEGMENTS (UNDERLYING REPRESENTATION)	/mɛnd/
Vowel nasalization:	mɛ̃nd
Vowel lengthening:	mɛ̃:nd
Final consonant deletion (fast-speech rule):	mɛ̃:n
OUTPUT (PHONETIC REPRESENTATION)	[mɛ̃:n]

You can think of the underlying representation (here /mɛnd/) as what is stored in the mental lexicon, a mental representation that includes all and only the information that is basic and unpredictable about the word. In turn, you can think of the phonetic representation as a mental representation that contains all the information about the word that is needed to pronounce it as it is actually said (and not merely as it is "thought of" in the head), and that can be sent to the muscles of the mouth to be turned into a set of muscle movements (though it need never actually be sent—a person who has lost her speech still knows how the word is pronounced even though she cannot in fact say it; she still knows that /mɛnd/ is actually said as [mɛ:n] in fast speech).

─────────────── E X E R C I S E S ───────────────

Exercise E. The data below is from an imaginary language, which we will call 'Imagine' (in this case, and for exercises below involving imaginary languages, a number of actual languages work in a similar way; the exercises, however, avoid various complications that might obscure the point that I am trying to make). This data is written in phonetic representation (in brackets) followed by a translation of the Imagine word into English:

[roti]	dew	[rol]	sand
[radil]	speak	[tal]	small
[soro]	laugh	[sil]	silly
[irãmi]	shout	[ilkop]	number
[kiri]	cat	[ipalso]	take

The data indicates that [r] and [l] are in complementary distribution, that is, they never occur in the same position in a word. In this language, these two sounds are related to each other by a rule—they are both surface (phonetic) variants of the same underlying representation. Answer the following questions:

1. Show that [r] and [l] are not related by a phonological rule in English, that is, give an example that shows substituting one for the other in a word in English can change the meaning of the word.

2. Consider /r/ the basic segment for Imagine and write a rule that says where /r/ changes to [l] in this language (your rule should begin "In Imagine, /r/ becomes [l] when . . ."). HINT: Be sure you pay attention to the consonants and vowels near the [r] or [l] sound in the data.

3. Consider that /l/ is the basic segment and write a rule that says where /l/ changes to [r] in this language (your rule should begin "In Imagine, /l/ becomes [r] when . . .").

4. Can you think of any reason to prefer one of these rules to the other (that is, for taking /r/ as basic or /l/ as basic), or do you think we would need more data?

Exercise F. The data below is also from Imagine:

[fovo]	love	[boto]	bottle
[savo]	need	[lugbil]	carry
[tiva]	radio	[buru]	hole
[ovu]	ask	[tab]	reply
[togavi]	road	[todbob]	far

The sounds /v/ and /b/ are both basic sounds of English, as the fact that they can be substituted one for the other and cause a change in meaning shows: *vat* versus *bat*. These two sounds are somewhat similar in how they are made, however. The sound /b/ is made by momentarily stopping the air from the lungs by banging the lips together. It is a voiced sound (/p/ is just like /b/, except it is voiceless). Such sounds are called **stops,** because they momentarily stop the air coming from the lungs by a stoppage in the mouth. The sound /v/ is not a stop, but a **fricative.** A fricative creates a constriction in the mouth that lets air pass out, but forces it through the tight constriction, thus causing turbulence or friction. The sound /v/ is made by causing a tight constriction between the top teeth and the bottom lip. It is voiced (/f/ is just like /v/, except it is voiceless). The sounds /b/ and /v/ thus are both made with the lips involved, and both are voiced. Answer the following questions:

1. In Imagine, [v] and [b] are not both basic segments; rather, one segment is derived from the other (that is, you can predict where one will occur based on characteristics of the position in words where it occurs). Choose one segment as basic and state a rule deriving the other segment from this one (state a rule beginning "/b/ becomes [v] when . . ." or "/v/ becomes [b] when . . .").

2. Why did you choose /b/ as the basic segment? (If you didn't, you'd better change your answer to the last question!)

3. Would you expect [p] and [f] in Imagine to be related in the same way as [b] and [v]? Why? State the rule relating [p] and [f] (that is, choose one as basic, place it in slashes, and derive the other one, placed in brackets, from it by a phonological rule).

4. If we say that [p] and [b] share the two features [+stop] and [+labial] and that these features distinguish them from all other sounds in the language, and [f] and [v] share the features [−stop] and [+labial], and these distinguish them from all other sounds in the language, how would you state the relationship between [p], [b], [f], and [v] in Imagine in a single rule? (Your rule will look like, "Sounds with the features . . . change to have the feature or features . . . when they occur . . .") NOTE: In the next section of this chapter, we will use the feature values [−continuant] and [+continuant] instead of [+stop] and [−stop], where [+continuant] means that the air stream continues rather than is stopped.

Phonemes

Our distinction between basic segments and derived ones can be looked at in a slightly different way. We have seen that any basic vowel segment has a number of forms in which it can occur. A vowel like /o/ can occur as a lengthened vowel ([o:]) when it occurs in front of voiced consonants, and it can occur as a nasalized vowel ([õ:]) when it occurs in front of nasal consonants (where it will also be lengthened because nasal consonants, which cause the nasalization of the preceding vowel, are also voiced consonants). In other situations (when not before a voiced consonant or a nasal consonant), the vowel appears in its basic or regular form ([o]). This is true of each basic vowel segment in the language.

Thus, in the case of vowels, we get the following picture in terms of basic segments and the forms they can take. Each basic segment can be produced in its basic form, or in any of its derived forms, depending on where it occurs in the stream of speech. I list each basic vowel segment (leaving out diphthongs—see Chapter 4 for a discussion of them). Underneath each basic vowel, I list all its derived forms (those we have discussed—there are others) and the basic form itself, as this is the form that shows up if no rule applies to change it. The forms created by rule (derived forms) I list on the first line under the basic segments, and the basic form itself (the form that shows up when no rules apply) I list in the next line. We can treat the basic form as a derived form in the sense that it is derived when no rules apply. I include basic segments in slashes and forms that are actually found in speech (the output of the rules) in brackets.

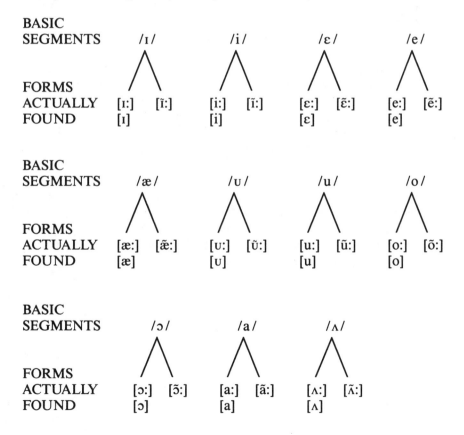

BASIC SEGMENTS	/ɪ/	/i/	/ɛ/	/e/
FORMS ACTUALLY FOUND	[ɪ:] [ɪ̃:] [ɪ]	[i:] [ĩ:] [i]	[ɛ:] [ɛ̃:] [ɛ]	[e:] [ẽ:] [e]

BASIC SEGMENTS	/æ/	/ʊ/	/u/	/o/
FORMS ACTUALLY FOUND	[æ:] [æ̃:] [æ]	[ʊ:] [ʊ̃:] [ʊ]	[u:] [ũ:] [u]	[o:] [õ:] [o]

BASIC SEGMENTS	/ɔ/	/a/	/ʌ/
FORMS ACTUALLY FOUND	[ɔ:] [ɔ̃:] [ɔ]	[a:] [ã:] [a]	[ʌ:] [ʌ̃:] [ʌ]

One traditional way to view the picture given above of phonological segments is as follows: All the forms that are listed under "forms actually found" (segments derived by rule from a basic form or the basic form itself, which surfaces if no rules apply) can be considered a *class* or *set* or *group* (all these terms mean the same thing here) of segments. No segment in the group attached to each basic segment can contrast with any other one in the group—they never occur in the same place, and if you substitute one for the other in a given word, all you will get is an odd pronunciation, not a different word.

Each of these groups of sounds—for example, the group connected with the basic segment /o/ (made up of [o:], [õ:], and [o])—is called a PHONEME. The phoneme is *named* by the basic segment symbol. Thus, the group of segments under the basic segment /o/ is called the /o/-phoneme, or the phoneme /o/. Each of the segments in the group attached to the basic segment—each of them in the group of segments that constitutes the phoneme /o/, for instance—is called an ALLOPHONE of the phoneme (allophones of the phoneme /o/, for example). Allophone means the variant ('allo' means *variant*) sounds ('phone' means *sound*) that represent the phoneme under different conditions. The allophones of the phoneme /o/ are the various forms that /o/ can take ([o:], [õ:], and [o]), depending on the positions in which it occurs in the stream of speech. The allophones of /o/ together constitute the phoneme /o/.

Linguists have argued whether the phoneme (/o/, for example) ought to be viewed as *just* its set of allophones (the group or set <[o:], [õ:], and [o]>: When we want to talk about a set or group of things we enclose them in angled brackets.) or whether the phoneme is itself a separate mental entity above and beyond its various realizations, a mental image that is realized physically in several different ways. I am sympathetic to the latter view.

For example, consider the fact that H_2O (water) has many different manifestations, depending on the conditions in which it is found: water, ice, steam. Humans need not know that water is H_2O to know what water and ice and steam are, or even to know they are related. In normal human conditions (when the temperature is not too cold and not too hot), we say that water (a liquid) is the basic or normal form of water. Water freezes (becomes frozen, adds the feature of being frozen) at 32 degrees Fahrenheit, thus becoming ice. When heated, it turns to steam. Representing water as we have represented phonological relationships, we would get a picture like this:

/water/

[ice]   [steam]
[water]

Humans tend to view water not just as the set of <ice, steam, and water>, but as fundamentally a liquid they call 'water', which manifests itself under certain specifiable conditions as ice or steam, and otherwise as the liquid referred to as 'water'. They have a mental image of water and a set of rules (knowledge of relationships) that tell them what water will look like under certain conditions.

Of course, not just vowels occur in basic segments and derived ones. All segments in a language do. To see this, consider an example of a phonological rule that creates derived segments for some consonants in English. The data we will consider in this regard concerns the distribution of STOP CONSONANTS in English.

The consonants /p/, /b/, /t/, /d/, /k/, and /g/ are made by completely stopping the air from the lungs momentarily by an occlusion in the mouth. The segments /p/ and /b/ are made by closing the upper and lower lips together (they are said to be *bilabial* sounds). /P/ is a voiceless bilabial stop, and /b/ a voiced bilabial stop. The segments /t/ and /d/ are made by placing the front of the tongue against the alveolar ridge. /T/ is a voiceless alveolar stop; /d/ is a voiced alveolar stop. The segments /k/ and /g/ are made by closing off the air from the lungs by placing the back of the tongue against the velum (the soft part of the top of the mouth behind the palate or roof of the mouth). /K/ is a voiceless velar stop; /g/ is a voiced velar stop.

All these stops differ from another large class of consonants in English, namely the FRICATIVES. Stops involve a full stoppage of the air from the lungs, which is then released, while the class of fricatives involves not fully stopping the air from the lungs but blocking it just enough to cause turbulence as the air flows past the obstruction. Segments like /f/, /v/; /s/, /z/; and /š/ ('sh'), /ž/ ('zh') are fricatives. The fricatives all have the feature [+continuant] (the air continues through the mouth), and the stops all have the feature [−continuant] (the air fails to continue and is momentarily stopped).

In the data below, I use a raised 'h' on a stop to signal *aspiration,* an audible puff of air that is released when voiceless stops ([p], [t], and [k]) are released (when the stoppage of air is let go). In a word like 'pit', you can feel this air come off the [p] if you moisten your finger and put it next to your mouth. In a word like 'spin', you will not feel it (though you will hear and feel turbulence from the fricative [s]). The question about the data below is, Where do the aspirated stops occur ([pʰ], [tʰ], and [kʰ]) and where do the nonaspirated ones occur ([p], [t], and [k])? Are either derived from the other, or are both aspirated and nonaspirated stops basic segments?

pit	[pʰɪt]	spin	[spɪn]	tip	[tʰɪp]
pot	[pʰat]	spot	[spat]	top	[tʰap]
pool	[pʰul]	spool	[spul]	soup	[sup]
top	[tʰap]	stop	[stap]	pot	[pʰat]
tell	[tʰɛl]	step	[stɛp]	debt	[dɛt]
told	[tʰold]	stole	[stol]	tote	[tʰot]
kit	[kʰɪt]	skip	[skɪp]	tick	[tʰɪk]
cool	[kʰul]	school	[skul]	nuke	[nuk]
can	[kʰæn]	scan	[skæn]	lack	[læk]

It is clear from this data that aspirated stops occur at the beginning of a word, and nonaspirated ones occur everywhere else (after /s/, for instance, as shown in the second column, and at the end of a word, as shown in the third column). Thus, it is plausible to derive the aspirated ones from the nonaspirated ones by a rule that says that voiceless stops (segments that have the features [−continuant] and [−voice]) add the feature [+aspirated] when they occur at the beginning of a word. More formally, the rule is as follows (where '#' stands for a word boundary):

STOP ASPIRATION RULE

$$\begin{bmatrix} -\text{continuant} \\ -\text{voice} \end{bmatrix} \rightarrow [+\text{aspirated}] \ / \ \# \ \underline{\quad}$$

If we looked at more data, we would learn that this rule would have to be changed slightly (the real rule is that voiceless stops become aspirated when they are at the beginning of a syllable—but we have not discussed syllables yet). But the rule as it stands above makes the point that each voiceless stop comes in two versions: an aspirated version (such as [pʰ]), and the unaspirated form, a basic version that shows up when no rule applies (such as [p]). In terms of our concept of phonemes, we have the following picture:

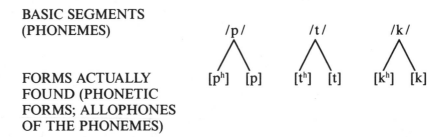

BASIC SEGMENTS
(PHONEMES)   /p/   /t/   /k/

FORMS ACTUALLY   [pʰ] [p]   [tʰ] [t]   [kʰ] [k]
FOUND (PHONETIC
FORMS; ALLOPHONES
OF THE PHONEMES)

Thus, in English, [pʰ] and [p], for instance, are allophones of the same phoneme; they are variant forms or versions of the same basic segment. The version [pʰ] is derived by the stop-aspiration rule, and the version [p] shows up otherwise, when no rules have applied. On the other hand, consider the data from Assamese, a language of northeastern India:

[pat]   leaf
[pʰat] split

This data shows us that [p] and [pʰ] *contrast* in Assamese. If you substitute one for another in a word (like [pat], meaning *leaf*), you get another word (namely [pʰat], meaning *split*). This could never happen in English. The segments [p] and [pʰ] occur in different places and represent the same basic segment. One, namely [pʰ], occurs at the beginnings of words and the other, namely [p], occurs elsewhere. If you tried to substitute one for the other in a word—for example, if you tried to substitute [p] for [pʰ] in the word 'pit' (which is normally pronounced [pʰɪt])—you would not get a new word, just an odd pronunciation of the word 'pit' (namely [pɪt]—try saying 'pit' without aspirating the 'p'; it is very hard for an English speaker to do so). But in Assamese you do get a new word. Thus, in Assamese, /p/ and /pʰ/ belong to different phonemes, they constitute different basic segments, and neither is derived by rule from the other (though each might have their own variants in other contexts).

Another way we can state the contrast between English and Assamese is that in English the feature [+aspiration] is not distinctive: No two words are distinguished solely in that one word has an aspirated segment where the other one has an unaspirated segment. But in Assamese, the feature [+aspiration] is distinctive. The words /pat/ (meaning *leaf*) and /pʰat/ (meaning *split*) are different words and differ solely in that one has a segment with aspiration where the other has a similar segment without it.

————————————— E X E R C I S E S —————————————

Exercise G. The data below is from another imaginary language, called Example:

[dot]	hate	[to:]	run
[lo:ta:]	ready	[o:li:]	oil
[logba:]	express	[ulti:]	save
[ha:pi:]	satisfied	[taffi:]	count
[ti:]	enough	[tift]	diverse

I have used the symbol ':' to mark lengthened (longer) vowels. Are long vowels in Example predictable—that is, are they allophones of phonemes that include both the shorter and longer vowels as allophones? If you think long vowels in Example are predictable, state the rule predicting where they occur (you can simply use ordinary English to state the rule).

Exercise H. The data below is from yet another imaginary language, called Fiction. This data shows the operation of several phonological rules. One rule aspirates certain stops. In addition, in Fiction, vowels are lengthened in two environments. State these rules (you can state two rules, or one collapsed rule, for the lengthening of vowels). Then answer the questions below the data.

[tʰiːd]	love	[vit]	ask
[pʰoːdiː]	puppy	[spaːb]	wonder
[kʰup]	give	[tpiː]	morning
[oːdaː]	see	[otaː]	effect
[skiːg]	leave	[kʰok]	cool
[liːv]	never	[lis]	why
[tʰaf]	candy	[pʰoːv]	fur
[bot]	swim	[giːdiː]	loud
[duːboː]	feel	[khituː]	poet

1. What is the phonemic form (lexical representation, representation in terms of basic segments—they all mean the same thing) of the following words in Fiction:

love

wonder

why

candy

poet

puppy

feel

see

2. What is the phonetic form of the following words from Fiction, which are listed in their phonemic representations (basic segments)?

/tibo/	bone
/spi/	cruise
/lotud/	mouse
/kigo/	kick

Syllables

Individual sound segments (like /p/ or /a/) pattern into larger units called **syllables.** Syllables are very odd entities indeed. Every speaker of a language can readily identify syllables. English speakers can easily tell that the word 'educated' is made up of the syllables 'ed' 'u' 'ca' 'ted'. In fact, people who have not been educated in an alphabetic writing system (like the one used for English, in which individual consonants and vowels are given separate symbols) find it difficult to think of syllables as being made up of individual consonants and vowels. To them, psychologically, the syllable seems like the basic or primary unit of sound. And there are many writing systems across history and across the world today in which there is one written symbol for each syllable. Yet at the same time linguists have had a very hard time defining or understanding exactly what a syllable is or why syllables exist.

Thus, although nearly everyone can identify syllables, almost nobody can define them. If I ask you how many syllables there are in the word 'organization' you can easily count them and tell me. There are five: 'or', 'gan', 'i', 'za', and 'tion'. While it is subjectively clear in most cases what the syllables of a word are, nevertheless it is difficult to state an objective procedure for locating the number of syllables in a word.

Each syllable contains a segment that constitutes the *peak of prominence* in that syllable. This is the segment that is heard as the loudest in the syllable. Whether a sound segment is heard as louder than another one is a matter, in part, of its inherent loudness (this is called the *sonority* of a sound) and, in part, a matter of the actual length, stress, and pitch of the sound as it is actually said in a particular context.

In general, vowels have more prominence than consonants. And the consonants /l/, /r/, /m/, /n/, and /ŋ/ have more prominence than other consonants (enough that in the absence of a vowel in a syllable these consonants can be the most prominent segment in the syllable or constitute a syllable in their own right, as in 'kitten' /kɪt-n/, where /n/ is a syllable by itself).

In any syllable, we will call the segment with the most prominence (usually the vowel) the **nucleus** of the syllable, and say that this segment has the feature [+syllabic]. The other segments in the syllable have the feature [−syllabic]. Vowels, when a syllable has one, are always [+syllabic]. Most consonants are always [−syllabic], and the consonants /r/, /l/, /m/, /n/, and /ŋ/ are sometimes [+syllabic] (when there is no vowel in the syllable) and sometimes [−syllabic] (when there is a vowel). The [+syllabic] segment (usually the vowel) is the most prominent part of the syllable, and the "heart" of the syllable, so to speak.

Syllables, in English, vary in the amount of **stress** they are heard as having. Stress in a very important property in a variety of respects in English. It is important to realize that stress is a *psychological* property to English speakers. Various combinations of length, loudness, and *pitch* (rising or lowering the pitch of the voice) can cause a syllable to be heard as stressed. Furthermore, these physical factors can often "trade off" with each other: More loudness can make up for less length, or greater pitch make up for less loudness, and so on. But, of the three physical properties, pitch is the most important for recognizing stress differences.

Some words in English are differentiated for the most part solely by which of their syllables are stressed. For example, say 'he is a *convict*' (where 'convict' is a noun); now say 'they always *convict* criminals here' (where 'convict' is a verb). These two words differ mainly by which of their syllables is stressed (and this is usually marked by a complex combination of lengthening stressed syllables, saying them somewhat more loudly, and varying the pitch of the voice on these syllables). In the noun 'convict', the first syllable is stressed: CONvict. In the verb 'convict', the second syllable is stressed: convICT (when I am concerned only with stress in a word, I will use the convention of writing the word in its spelled form with the stressed syllable in small capitals). There are many other pairs of nouns and verbs that are differentiated this way—for example, 'object' (compare the noun 'an OBject' to the verb 'to obJECT'), 'permit' (compare the noun 'a PERmit' to the verb 'to perMIT'), 'pervert' (compare the noun 'a PERvert' to the verb 'to perVERT').

Syllables, thus, constitute important boundaries within words: A word is composed of syllables, and these syllables in turn are composed of sound segments (vowels and consonants). Thus, the word 'computerize' has the following composition in terms of syllables: com-pu-ter-ize. It is important to notice that the syllables in a word have nothing to do with the word's meaning. The word 'computerize' is made up of several meaningful parts: the word 'compute' (the verb 'to compute'), the ending 'er' (which is added to verbs to yield a noun meaning *a person or thing that does the action of that verb,* as in 'computer', 'baker', 'lover', etc.), and the ending 'ize' (which is added to nouns to yield verbs, as in 'organize' from 'organ', or 'criticize' from 'critic', or 'idolize' from 'idol', etc.). Thus, in terms of meaning, the word 'computerize' has the parts comput-er-ize. Each of these meaningful parts of a word are called **morphemes.** Compare, then, the syllables and morphemes in 'computerize' (they are obviously not the same):

computerize
SYLLABLES: com-pu-ter-ize
MORPHEMES: comput-er-ize

The example above constitutes a clear demonstration of the independence of sound structure (syllables and their segments) and meaning (words and their morphemes). As we have seen throughout this chapter, sound follows its own principles of organization. Somewhat miraculously, out of these principles, which are independent of meaning, all meaning in language ultimately flows.

When I say that every native speaker can readily identify the syllables in a word, I do not mean to imply that there are no complexities in this area. Here, in fact, is one: A word like 'happy' is spelled with two 'p's', but in fact has only one /p/ in its pronunciation. The word has two syllables, but each syllable shares the single /p/ segment. That is, its syllable structure is 'hap-py', where the single /p/ segment ends the first syllable (by the closing of the lips) and begins the second (by the opening of the lips). This is presumably why it, and so many words like it, are spelled with two consonants ('p' in this case), where only one is said. Speakers also psychologically feel that the /p/ belongs to both syllables and will have difficulty assigning it to just one of them if they are forced to do so. We could write the syllable structure of 'happy' as follows (where 's1' stands for the first syllable in the word and 's2' stands for the second syllable in the word):

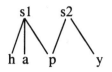

————————————— E X E R C I S E S —————————————

Exercise I.   The data below is from the imaginary language Example. This time I have shown you the syllables in the words (I place a hyphen ('-') between syllables; if a word has no hyphen, then it is just one syllable long). Can you restate the rule for where vowels are lengthened (become [+long]) in Example in terms of syllable structure? HINT: In any language, a syllable that ends in a vowel is called an **open** syllable, and a syllable that ends in one or more consonants is called a **closed** syllable.

[dot]	hate	[to:]	run
[lo:-ta:]	ready	[o:-li:]	oil
[log-ba:]	express	[ul-ti:]	save
[ha:-pi:]	satisfied	[taf-fi:]	count
[ti:]	enough	[tift]	diverse

Exercise J.   Give the organization in terms of morphemes and in terms of syllables of the following English words:

organization

baker

happy

lover

satisfied

Exercise K.   Why do you think /p/, in English, shows up as aspirated ([pʰ]) in the words in the left column and nonaspirated ([p]) in the words in the right column? (Remember that in a word like 'happy', there is only one /p/, which is shared by both syllables; it closes the first syllable and begins the second. Thus we have hap-py, where I underline the /p/ to make clear it is one sound splitting itself between two syllables.) NOTE: In the words below, 'y' in the spelling stands for a vowel sound in the pronunciation.

ha<u>pp</u>y	hapless
hypo	dampness
sa<u>pp</u>y	tipsy
di<u>pp</u>ing	stripling
repo	ripeness

3.3. THE RHYTHM OF SENTENCES

Stress, Pitch, and Intonation

We saw above that words are composed of syllables and that some syllables are stressed. In long words, often more than one syllable is stressed. Thus, in the word 'photograph', both the first and the third syllables are stressed: PHO-to-GRAPH. In such cases, one syllable is said to bear the **primary stress,** and the other stressed syllable or syllables bear nonprimary stresses. In 'photograph', the first syllable bears the primary stress (is heard as more prominent than the third syllable). I will underline the primary stressed syllable: <u>PHO</u>-to-GRAPH (I should point out that some people hear stress differences *consciously* better than others, though all native speakers *unconsciously* hear them, because they pronounce the words properly and understand them properly).

In English, lack of stress leads to the phenomenon of **vowel reduction.** In most cases, if a syllable is not stressed, then the vowel of that syllable is reduced to the neutral, unstressed vowel [ə], called the *schwa* vowel (it sounds like a very weak 'uh'). Thus, when said at the normal rather rapid rate of conversation, the vowel in the second syllable of 'photograph' (<u>PHO</u>-to-GRAPH)—the syllable spelled 'to'—is a schwa. So are the vowels in the second and last syllables of 'inclination': IN-cli-<u>NA</u>-tion. So is the last vowel in 'sofa' (<u>SO</u>-fa) and the first vowels in 'reduce' (re-<u>DUCE</u>) and the verb 'produce' (pro-<u>DUCE</u>). Any vowel can be reduced to schwa if it has no stress. Note that English spells schwa ([ə]) in many different ways.

This process of vowel reduction in unstressed syllables is part of what gives English its special "sound." This process does not happen in Spanish, for instance. Often, when English speakers speak Spanish they reduce unstressed vowels to schwa, rather than giving them their full value, and thus have an "English accent" (and sound "mushy" to Spanish speakers). In turn, Spanish speakers often fail to reduce unstressed vowels in English to schwa and thus sound like they are overarticulating (they say something like [fo-to-græf] instead of [fo-tə-græf]).

Sometimes in English we vary the pattern of stressed and unstressed syllables in a word as we vary its grammatical form. Note the example below, where in each case the primary stressed syllable is in a different place, and different syllables are unstressed and thus reduced to schwa:

photograph	PHO-to-GRAPH	Primary stress on PHO
	[fo-tə-græf]	Schwa in second syllable
		Nonprimary stress on GRAPH
photography	pho-TO-gra-PHY	Primary stress on TO
	[fə-ta-grə-fi]	Schwa vowels in first and third syllables
		Nonprimary stress on PHY
photographic	PHO-to-GRAPH-ic	Primary stress on GRAPH
	[fo-tə-græf-ək]	Schwa vowels in second and last syllables (in this word, for some speakers, the reduced vowel in the last syllable is a bit different than the reduced vowel in the second syllable)
		Nonprimary stress on PHO

Stress also plays a role in the distinction between LEXICAL (CONTENT) words and GRAMMATICAL (FUNCTION) words in English. Lexical words (also called 'content' words) are those words whose meanings carry specific content (like 'dog', 'love', and 'beauty'); they fall into the classes of noun, verb, and adjective. Grammatical words (also called "function" words) are those words whose meanings have to do with the grammar and structure of the sentence, or that carry less specific content (like 'the', 'can', 'of', and 'that').

In English, grammatical words are usually said with no stress (or, rather, no appreciable stress—they must have some minimal degree of stress to get out of the mouth at all) and thus their vowels are reduced to schwa. Thus, listen to the sentence 'The cat has ran to Bill' said very slowly, one word at a time:

[θi kæt hæz ræn tu bɪl]

and to the same sentence said rapidly and normally:

[θə kæt həz ræn tə bɪl].

In the latter case, only the content words are stressed and have full vowels ('cat', 'ran', and 'Bill'), and the grammatical words ('the', 'has', and 'to') have no stress and have reduced vowels (schwas).

This process of reducing grammatical words is what, together with the stress and syllable patterns of the words in a sentence, gives English sentences their characteristic rhythm, with alternating weak and strong syllables (for example, the CAT has RAN to BILL).

When words enter into phrases or sentences, the grammatical words have little or no stress, and each content word brings to the sentence its stressed syllable or syllables. However, not all these stressed syllables are given equal prominence in the phrase or sentence—some are somewhat downplayed or subordinated in regard to others. If you take the adjective 'red' and the noun 'coat' and combine them into the phrase 'a red coat', the stress on 'red' is subordinated somewhat to the stress on 'coat', which is the most prominent stress in the phrase (in American English).

In fact, it is typical in English phrases that the last stressed syllable in the phrase is the most prominent one and the other stressed syllables in the phrase are all downgraded a bit—their stress is lowered a bit. So in a phrase like 'lost the battle', the stressed syllable of 'battle' (BATtle) would often be the most prominent stress in the phrase, and the stress on 'lost' would be downplayed a bit. Of course, 'the', being a grammatical word, normally has little or no stress and has a reduced vowel.

On the other hand, in a compound noun made up of 'red' and 'coat' as in 'redcoat' (a British soldier in the American Revolution), the stress on 'coat' is subordinated to the stress on 'red', which is the most prominent. This is typical of most compound words in English. Thus, we get a RED COAT' (a phrase meaning a coat that is red) versus 'a REDcoat' (a compound noun naming a type of soldier), with the most prominent syllable underlined.

This process of words accommodating or adjusting their stressed syllables to the stressed syllables of the other words in phrases or compounds is carried further in full sentences. In a short sentence, each grammatical word carries little or no stress, while each content word carries more stress. But one word is chosen as the **intonational focus** of the sentence, and this word receives the most prominent degree of stress in the sentence. All the rest of the stressed syllables in the sentence are downgraded (made less prominent, sound somewhat less stressed, though they are still stressed to a certain degree).

Often, in English, the intonational focus is the stressed syllable of the last content word in the sentence. Thus, in a sentence like 'The redcoats lost the battle', the word 'battle' would often be the FOCUS and we would also have a whole set of additional stress adjustments made. For example, in the compound 'redcoats', 'coats' would be downgraded in relation to 'red' (as we saw above), while in the phrase 'lost the battle', 'lost' would be downgraded in relation to 'battle' (as we also saw above). Finally, 'battle' as the FOCUS would get the most prominent stress, and all the other stressed syllables would be downgraded in relation to it. Thus, the sentence is composed of ever-varying hills and valleys of stress:

1. The REDcoats LOST the BATtle
   (with BAT, the intonational focus, the most prominent syllable, RED the second most prominent, and LOST the third most prominent. 'Coats' is less prominent than any other lexical word, but more prominent than the function word 'the')

For the rest of this chapter I will ignore some of these degrees of stress and just distinguish between the intonational focus (underlined and in small capitals), stressed syllables (of whatever degree; these will just be in small capitals), and unstressed (often reduced) syllables (which will be left in small letters).

The choice of intonational focus is connected directly to what the speaker thinks and intends to signal is the most important information in the sentence. It is also the key to the **intonation pattern** or **intonation contour** of the sentence, that is, the characteristic patterns of pitch changes across English sentences. Intonational patterns are crucial to the meanings of English sentences, to the way speakers package information, to the interaction between speaker and hearer, and to the rhythm and sound of English sentences. We will study them, and their relation to stress, in the next section.

Intonation Contours

Listen to just the pitch of the voice (its rise and fall) while someone says a sentence. You will find that it is changing continuously. In singing, you change pitch all the time also, but you hold a given note for a noticeable length of time and then jump to the pitch of the next note. But in speaking, as against singing, there are no steady-state pitches (you don't hold the same pitch for any length of time, but continuously move up or down). Throughout every syllable in a normal conversational utterance the pitch is going up or down. (Try talking with steady-state pitches and notice how odd it sounds.)

The intonation contour of a string of words (a phrase or sentence, for instance) is the pattern of pitch changes that occurs. The part of a sentence over which a particular intonational contour extends is called a **tone group.** A short sentence often forms a single tone group, while longer ones are made up of two or more. I will show the major pitch changes in a tone group by lines placed above the sentence (thus showing the intonational contour graphically but leaving out many intricacies in actual contours), as in the sentence below.[1]

2. The GIRL GAVE the MONey to her FAther

Each stressed syllable is capitalized; the intonational focus is underlined as well. The pitch of the voice moves downward throughout sentence 2, with a little perturbation in this downward trend for each stressed syllable. I have not shown these little perturbations (which in fact help mark each stressed syllable as stressed), since what is most important is the overall downward trend.

The overall pitch pattern of a tone group (in this example, a slight downward trend) must change on the intonational focus. On this syllable, the pitch will change somewhat dramatically (for example, either quickly rising or falling). In the sentence above, the pitch on the stressed syllable of 'father' rises just a bit from the general downward trend of the sentence and then falls quickly.

[1]The examples in this section are from Pete Ladefoged's *A Course in Phonetics* (New York: Harcourt Brace Jovanovich, 1975, pp. 93–101), and my discussion is based on Ladefoged's work.

This pitch change marks this syllable (and the word it is in) as the intonational focus of the intonation contour.

Thus, within a tone group there is usually a single syllable that stands out because it carries the major pitch change in the intonation contour defining the tone group. I have called this syllable the intonational focus (it is also called the *tonic* syllable). This syllable is the most stressed syllable in the tone group, and all other stressed syllables in the tone group are subordinated to it. In many sentences, including sentence 2 above, the primary stressed syllable of the last lexical word in the tone group is the intonational focus (here, the first syllable of 'father'). But it may occur earlier, as in the example below:

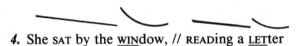

3. He WANTed to GO to GERmany on MONday

Here the intonational focus is on GERmany (the pitch falls quickly). Notice also how the pitch change that starts on the intonational focus (and that defines it as such) continues on the following syllables. In the examples given above, the fall in pitch starting on the intonational focus continues (but at a slower rate) until the end of the sentence.

Sometimes there are two or more tone groups within a sentence:

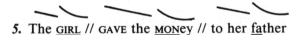

4. She SAT by the WINdow, // READing a LETter

I use double slashes ('//') for the boundary between two tone groups. There is no syntactic unit that corresponds exactly with the tone group (for example, not all tone groups are sentences and not all sentences are tone groups). When speaking slowly in a formal style, a speaker may choose to break a sentence up into a large number of tone groups, so that it becomes

5. The GIRL // GAVE the MONey // to her father

The way in which a speaker breaks up a sentence into tone groups depends largely on what that person considers to be the important information points in the sentence. A tone group is a unit of information rather than a syntactically or structurally defined unit. It is only in rapid conversational style that there is likely to be one tone group per sentence.

The choice of what will be the intonational focus is also not predictable by any rule. Again, this is a matter of how the speaker views the information he or she is communicating. The choice of intonational focus depends on what the speaker considers to be the most important information in the tone group. In general, new information is more likely to be the intonational focus than material that has already been mentioned. Also, the *topic* of a sentence is less likely to be the intonational focus than the *comment* that is made on the topic. Thus, if I were discussing the properties of water, I might say

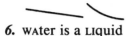

6. wᴀter is a ʟɪquid

Here the intonational focus is 'liquid'. In this case, the topic of the sentence is *water,* and the comment on that topic is that it is a liquid (I am saying "about the topic water, it's a liquid"). But if I were discussing liquids and considering that as the topic, I might say

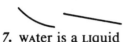

7. wᴀter is a ʟɪquid

Here the intonational focus is 'water', and I am saying, about the topic of liquids, water is one of them.

For simplicity's sake, in all our examples so far the intonational focus has been marked by a fall in pitch. Various other pitch changes are possible on the intonational focus.

The intonational focus can be the start of an upward glide in pitch, rather than a fall. This kind of pitch change, which we will simply refer to as *rising,* is typical of questions requiring a yes or no answer, such as

8. Do you wᴀɴᴛ some ᴄᴏғfee?

As with falling pitch changes, an intonational focus that is marked with a rising pitch change is not necessarily the last stressed syllable in the tone group. It occurs earlier in the next example:

9. Do you ᴛᴀᴋᴇ ᴄʀᴇᴀᴍ in your ᴄᴏғfee?

Questions that cannot be answered with yes or no, such as the following, often have a falling intonational focus, not a rising one:

10. wʜᴇʀᴇ did you ᴘᴜᴛ the ᴘᴀper?

A rising pitch change on the intonational focus often occurs in the middle of sentences, a typical circumstance being at the end of a clause, as in example 11.

Here we have two tone groups in a single sentence. Such a rising intonation in the middle of a sentence often means "I'm not finished, there's more to come":

11. The MAN who TOOK the COFfee // was my FAther

The intonational focus of an intonation contour can also be *both* rising and then falling (we will call this rising-falling) or falling and then rising (we will call this falling-rising). Intonational contours that have a falling-rising pitch change on the intonational focus commonly convey doubt. If you tell me someone's name and I do not believe you, I might well say

12. His NAME is PEter?

This is different from the straightforward statement (which would have a simple fall) or a genuine yes/no question (which would have a simple rise). The opposite possibility, a rising-falling pitch change on the intonational focus, is somewhat less common. Among other things, it can signal certainty as opposed to doubt.

To summarize, all the intonation patterns we have discussed so far involve a significant pitch change starting on the primary stressed syllable of the intonational focus and continuing until the end of the tone group. However, you should keep in mind that matters of intonation are quite complicated and we have only touched on the basics here. The sorts of changes in pitch we have briefly looked at here are the basis in English for pervasive and subtle signals about mood, attitude, and the "slant" (perspective) the speaker takes on the information being communicated.

——————————————— **EXERCISE** ———————————————

Exercise L. Using the sorts of graphic devices we have been using in the preceding section, give the intonational contours for the following sentences, using their most natural pronunciations (in two cases, I have included a context in brackets—just represent the sentence that is not in brackets).

1. The redcoats lost the war.
2. Did the redcoats lose the war?
3. The girl gave the money to him.
4. [Who's the leader?] John is the leader.
5. [What is John?] John is the leader.

RECOMMENDED FURTHER READING

ANDERSEN, STEPHEN R. (1985). *Phonology in the Twentieth Century: Theories of Rules and Theories of Representations.* University of Chicago Press. (A demanding, sometimes dry, but brilliant book.)

EDWARDS, MARY L. & SHRIBERG, LAWRENCE D. (1983). *Phonology: Applications in Communicative Disorders.* San Diego: College Hill Press. (A good descriptive overview for people interested in language disorders.)

GOLDSMITH, JOHN (1991). *Autosegmental and Metrical Phonology.* Oxford: Basil Blackwell. (A clearly written, detailed, but technical, introduction to aspects of current phonological theory.)

HOGG, RICHARD & McCULLY, C. B. (1987). *Metrical Phonology: A Coursebook.* New York: Cambridge University Press. (An up-to-date and accessible introduction to some aspects of current work in phonological theory.)

HYMAN, LARRY (1975). *Phonology: Theory and Analysis.* New York: Holt, Rinehart and Winston. (Still the best-written introduction to phonological theory, though now dated—still well worth reading.)

KATAMBA, FRANCIS (1989). *An Introduction to Phonology.* London & New York: Longman. (An accessible, hands-on, and up-to-date introduction to phonological theory for the beginner.)

KENSTOWICZ, MICHAEL & KISSEBERTH, CHARLES (1979). *Generative Phonology: Description and Theory.* New York: Academic Press. (A standard textbook in phonological theory, though now dated.)

LADD, D. ROBERT (1980). *The Structure of Intonational Meaning: Evidence from English.* Bloomington, Ind.: Indiana University Press. (A very informative and readable book.)

LASS, ROGER (1984). *Phonology.* New York: Cambridge University Press. (Wide in coverage, basically descriptive.)

SCHANE, SANFORD (1973). *Generative Phonology.* Englewood Cliffs, N.J.: Prentice-Hall. (A small and very readable book, though now dated.)

WOLFRAM, WALT & JOHNSON, ROBERT (1982). *Phonological Analysis: Focus on American English.* Washington, D.C.: Center for Applied Linguistics and Harcourt Brace Jovanovich. (Good description of some central facts of English phonology.)

CHAPTER 4

Phonetics

Description and Notation of Language Sounds

4.1. SYMBOLIZING SOUNDS

When we want to talk about the sounds of English or any other language, we are faced with several problems. First, the English spelling system is not very consistent. It often spells the same sound differently in different words. Thus, the letter 's' spells many different sounds. For example, 's' in 'sit' is the sound /s/, but in 'sure' it is the sound often otherwise spelled 'sh' (as in 'shoe'), and in 'cards' the spelled 's' represents the sound /z/ as in the word 'zen'. On the other hand, the sound /s/ is not always spelled with an 's'. For example, in the word 'citizen', the initial 'c' spells the sound /s/. Or, to take an example from how we spell vowels, the sound of the vowel in 'she' ('ee') is spelled in many different ways: bel<u>ie</u>ve, s<u>ee</u>, p<u>eo</u>ple, s<u>ei</u>ze, s<u>ea</u>, sill<u>y</u>, k<u>ey</u>, mach<u>i</u>ne. Notice that in some of these words the vowel is spelled with two letters (though it is a single sound) and in others with one letter.

Second, we want to symbolize sounds in such a way that we can represent the words of any language, not just English. However, different languages use different sorts of writing systems, and even when they use the same sort of writing system, they often spell the same sounds with different letters.

In 1888, the International Phonetic Association (IPA) developed a phonetic alphabet that could be used to symbolize the sounds found in all languages. Because many languages use a Roman alphabet like that used in English writing, the IPA system is based on Roman letters. The IPA system represents each sound with one and only one symbol, and each symbol represents one and only one sound, unlike the English alphabet. The IPA effort was based on a variety of earlier "universal" phonetic alphabets, developed by a number of scholars.

We will use a version of the IPA alphabet to symbolize sounds. Unfortunately, linguists have not always used the IPA exactly, but have varied a few symbols

TABLE 4-1. Symbols for the Sounds of English

CONSONANTS				VOWELS			
p	pit	θ	thigh	i	beet	ɪ	bit
b	bit	ð	thy	e	late	ɛ	let
m	mit	š	shoe	u	boot	ʊ	foot
t	to	ž	azure	o	boat	ɔ	caught
d	do	č	chill	æ	bat	a	pot
n	no	ǰ	joke	ʌ	but	ə	sofa
k	kill	l	low	aɪ	bite	aʊ	out
g	gill	r	row	ɔɪ	boy		
ŋ	sing	y	yes				
f	fan	w	win				
v	van						
s	seal						
z	zeal						

here and there. This has led to different linguists using slightly different systems to describe sounds. Table 4-1 lists the symbols we will use here, giving an example of the sound in a common word. However, keep in mind that, particularly with vowel sounds, there is dialect variation. Your pronunciation for the word I use as an example may not be the same as the dialect I describe here.

Before I list the symbols we will use for sounds, let me point out two things about the material in this chapter. First, **phonetics** (the physical description of sound in terms of how sounds are heard and produced in languages) is not part of linguistics. Linguists use descriptions from phonetics so they can go on to talk about sound systems and phonological rules in the world's languages (see Chapter 3). Phonetics is thus a useful tool to do another job. We will use only a small part of phonetics here, just enough to have a way to talk about sounds in English.

Second, there is a good bit of simple descriptive detail in this chapter, much like in a manual that comes with a new product. In my opinion, it is better to familiarize oneself with the basic ways in which the sounds of English are described and then look up details when needed, as in a reference book, rather than to memorize everything. Most of the material is given both in the text and in separate figures, tables, and lists.

EXERCISE

Exercise A. The English spelling system is often criticized as being "inconsistent," and, indeed, in many cases it is. A word like 'knight' is spelled with an initial /k/ because it once used to be pronounced with one. However, the pronunciation of the word changed, but the spelling did not. Thus, linguists can sometimes use the spelling systems of some languages as clues to how words used to be pronounced and the sorts of changes that may have occurred. In other instances of mismatches between spelling and pronunciation, there is a deeper logic to why English spells things the way it does. Considering the two cases below, say why you think English spells different sounds with the same symbol in these cases:

1. cat<u>s</u>   's' = /s/
   lad<u>s</u>   's' = /z/
2. electri<u>c</u>   final 'c' = /k/
   electri<u>c</u>ity second 'c' = /s/

4.2. VOICED AND VOICELESS SOUNDS (IN FEATURE TERMS [+VOICE] AND [−VOICE])

When we speak, air is pumped from the lungs up through the throat and into the mouth. As this **airstream** from the lungs is on this route, several things can happen to it. Each thing that can happen defines a different type of speech sound.

One of the first things that can happen gets its chance to occur as the air passes through the **glottis** (see Figure 4-1). The glottis is an opening between two chords in the lower part of the throat. These chords—called the **vocal chords**—are like thick rubber bands. If the vocal chords are held apart, the air from the lungs passes through them without anything happening. But if they are held together, the airstream forces its way through them and causes them to *vibrate*. When a sound is made this way, with the vocal chords vibrating, the sound is said to be a **voiced** sound. When a sound is made with the vocal chords apart, and therefore not vibrating, the sound is said to be **voiceless.**

The sound /z/ is voiced and the sound /s/ is just like it except that it is voiceless. If you say /z/ continuously (z-z-z-z) and press gently on your "Adam's apple" (the middle of your throat—despite what you have heard, females have "Adam's apples" too), you will feel the vibrations of the vocal chords. If you say /s/ continuously (s-s-s-s) and press gently on your throat, you will not feel the vibration (though you will hear hissing coming from the mouth, as you do also with the sound /z/).

So we can classify all speech sounds as to whether they are voiced or voiceless. We will treat this distinction in terms of a **feature**. A feature is a property that one thing has and another thing lacks, and that thus distinguishes the two things. The thing that has the property has the value '+' (plus) on the feature, and the thing that lacks the property has the value '−' (minus) on the feature.

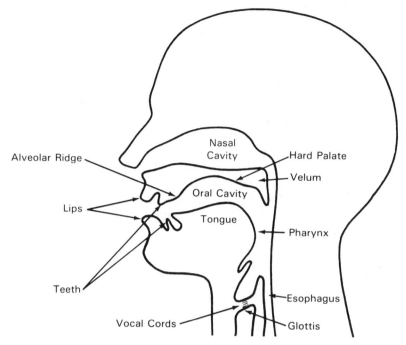

FIGURE 4-1. The Human Vocal Track.

So, for example, if you were comparing a tall and a short person, you could just say that one was TALL and one was SHORT. But this fails to capture that tall and short are related—you cannot be both at the same time. Being tall implies you are not short, and being short implies you are not tall. To capture the relationship between tallness and shortness, we could set up a feature TALL and assign a tall person the value [+tall] and the short person the value [−tall] on the feature [tall]. Of course, we could as easily have called the feature SHORT and assigned the tall person the value [−short] and the short person the value [+short]. But the point is that, either way, we treat the two people as related by the fact that one has what the other lacks.

Notice that the feature approach is something of a conceptual trick. When we say that some people are [+tall] and others [−tall], we are treating height as if it came in only two degrees (tall = [+tall] and short = [−tall]). This is not true of the real world, where there are many degrees of height and some people are in the middle, neither tall nor short. The feature approach ignores this multiplicity of heights and treats height as a dichotomy—you are either tall or short. This may or may not be a good approach to height, but linguists have long argued that it is a good approach to the properties of speech sounds.

So we can treat the distinction between voiced and voiceless sounds in terms of a feature. Voiced sounds, sounds where the vocal chords are vibrating, have the value [+voice] on the feature [voice]. On the other hand, sounds that are voiceless, where the vocal chords are not vibrating, have the value [−voice] on the feature [voice]. Another way to look at this feature is as follows: You can ask of any sound the question, "Do the vocal chords vibrate when this sound is said?" If the answer to this question is yes, then the sound is [+voice]; if the answer is no, the sound is [−voice].

Just as with height, there are actually many degrees of voicing, with the vocal chords vibrating a lot, not at all, or many degrees in between (both in terms of how fast they vibrate and how long they vibrate through the duration of the speech sound—the chords often vibrate only a part of the time in which a single sound is produced). But the feature approach says (correctly, I believe) that in speech this does not matter. All that matters, in the way humans perceive and produce speech, is that a sound either counts as voiced ([+voice]) or not voiced ([−voice]). A certain amount and duration of vocal chord vibration makes humans hear a sound as voiced. Below this degree, the sound counts as voiceless. That is, it is a key property of sound as used in language that a continuum made up of many possible degrees (here various amounts and durations of vibration) is treated as a simple two-way distinction ([+voice] versus [−voice]).

———————————————— **E X E R C I S E** ————————————————

Exercise B.   Rewrite the words below and circle the voiced sounds. (HINT: All vowels are voiced sounds.)

      cats   sin   bob   talk   kill
      lads   zen   pop   doll   gill

4.3.   NASAL AND ORAL SOUNDS
(IN FEATURE TERMS [+NASAL] AND [−NASAL])

One of the next things that can happen to the airstream as it moves from the lungs through the throat to the mouth is that the air can be allowed to go out of the mouth and nose, or just out of the mouth alone, with the nose closed up.

If you look at Figure 4-1, you will see a thing called the **velum** at the very back of the mouth. The velum is a soft piece of flesh that can move up and down. When it is down—as shown in Figure 4-1—air is allowed to enter the nasal cavity and go out of the nose (of course, it also goes into the mouth as well). When the velum is raised up, it closes off the nasal cavity, and therefore the air from the lungs cannot go into the nasal cavity and out the nose. All the air goes into the mouth and eventually out of the mouth.

Sounds in which air is allowed to go into the nasal cavity and out of the nose are called **nasal** sounds. Sounds in which air is not allowed into the nasal cavity, and all the air goes into and out of the mouth, are called **oral** sounds. The sound /b/ is an oral sound, where air goes into the mouth, is momentarily stopped or blocked by the lips, until it builds up a bit and is then released out of the mouth. The sound /m/ is just like /b/, except that the air is allowed to go in and out of the nose as it also goes into, gets blocked, and is released from the mouth.

We can treat the distinction between oral and nasal sounds in terms of a feature. A nasal sound, like /m/, has the value [+nasal] on the feature [nasal], and an oral sound like /b/ has the value [−nasal] on the feature [nasal].

English has three nasal consonants: the sounds /m/, /n/, and /ŋ/ (the sound often spelled 'ng', as in 'sing', but it is a single sound). The sound /m/ is just like /b/ except that /m/ is a nasal ([+nasal]) sound and /b/ is an oral one ([−nasal]). The sound /p/ is just like these, except that it is [−voice] and they (/b/ and /m/) are [+voice]. All three of these sounds are made by momentarily stopping the air from the lungs by placing the lips together. Thus, they are **bilabial** ("two lips") **stops.**

The three sounds /n/, /d/, and /t/ are related in the same way. The sound /n/ is just like /d/, except that /n/ is nasal and /d/ is oral. The sound /t/ is just like both of them except that it is voiceless ([−voice]) and they (/d/ and /n/) are voiced ([+voice]). All three of these sounds are made by momentarily stopping the air from the lungs by placing the front of the tongue on the **alveolar ridge** (see Figure 4-1), the bony ridge behind the front teeth. Thus, they are **alveolar stops.**

The three sounds /ŋ/ (often spelled 'ng' as in 'sing', but it is a single sound), /g/, and /k/ are related in the same way. The sound /ŋ/ is just like /g/, except that /ŋ/ is nasal and /g/ is oral. The sound /k/ is just like both of them except it is voiceless ([−voice]) and they (/g/ and /ŋ/) are voiced ([+voice]). All three of these sounds are made by momentarily stopping the air from the lungs by placing the back of the tongue against the **velum** (see Figure 4-1). Thus, they are **velar stops.**

——————————— E X E R C I S E ———————————

Exercise C. There is one position in English words where the sound /ŋ/ cannot occur, but the other nasal consonants (/m/ and /n/) can. Where is it?

4.4. VOWELS AND CONSONANTS

Every language in the world makes a distinction between vowels and consonants. Vowels are made with a relatively open mouth (for example, say /a/, the sound 'ah' that the doctor asks you to make when using a tongue depressor). Consonants are made with a relatively more closed mouth (for example, /s/ or /f/ or /p/). We can distinguish vowels and consonants in terms of a feature [consonantal]. Consonants have the value [+consonantal] on the feature [consonantal], and vowels have the value [−consonantal] on this feature. Of course, we could have used the feature name [vocalic] (and reversed the values, so that vowels were [+vocalic] and consonants were [−vocalic]), but we will stick with the feature name [consonantal].

There is another important distinction between vowels and consonants. Speech is produced in *syllables,* small combinations of consonants and vowels that are pronounced together as a tight cluster or unit. So, the word 'poetry' has the following three syllables: 'po', 'e', and 'try'. And the word 'wonder' is made up of the two syllables 'won' and 'der'. English speakers can usually recognize the syllables in a word if they say the word slowly. A syllable is usually built around a vowel as its center, core, or **nucleus** (they all mean the same thing). Thus, in 'poetry', the first syllable ('po') is built around the vowel /o/, the second ('e') around the vowel /ɛ/, and the last ('try') around the vowel /i/.

A syllable can be made up of a single vowel, or of a vowel with some accompanying consonants, but usually a syllable cannot have just a consonant with no vowel sound. Thus, the word 'open' has two syllables, 'o' and 'pen', with the first syllable made up of just the single vowel /o/. So, in general, syllables must have vowels, but they need not have consonants (though, of course, they can). This is another sense in which vowels are the heart of the syllable.

Since vowels are the nucleus around which syllables are built, they are sometimes called **syllabic** sounds. Consonants are said to be **nonsyllabic** sounds. We can treat this property as a feature also. Vowels have the value [+syllabic] on the feature [syllabic] and consonants have the value [−syllabic] on the feature [syllabic].

However, this picture of a clear distinction between vowels and consonants is disturbed by the presence of two types of sounds that are intermediary between vowels and consonants. These sounds share properties with both vowels and consonants. The first such type are the sounds /r/ and /l/, which are **liquids.** The second such type are the sounds /w/ and /y/, which are **glides.**

Let's take the glides first. Glides are produced with a more closed mouth than vowels, but more open than with any other consonants. Furthermore, they often occur with vowels and, so to speak, *lengthen* the vowel, creating what are called **diphthongs,** as in 'boy', which has the vowel /o/, followed by the glide /y/ (/boy/), or 'how', which has the vowel /a/ (the sound 'ah') followed by the glide /w/ (/haw/). The glide /y/ draws the vowel sound out by moving the tongue upward and to the front of the mouth, and the glide /w/ draws the vowel sound out by moving the tongue upward and to the back of the mouth. However, these sounds can also occur at the beginning of a word (as in 'yes' and 'win').

The sounds /r/ and /l/, called liquids, have an even more closed mouth than the glides and are usually just treated as consonants. But they have an odd property that makes them in some ways like vowels. They can occur in syllables with no vowel present. When they do, they function as the nucleus of the syllable, and are thus [+syllabic] sounds (like vowels) in these situations.

Thus, in the word 'medal', there are two syllables: 'med' (with the vowel /ɛ/) and just the sound /l/ ('med-l'). Since the second syllable has only an /l/, the /l/ is *syllabic* here, playing the sort of role a vowel usually does. By the way, to have only an /l/ in the second syllable, you have to say the word fast; if you say it more slowly and stick in a vowel before the /l/, as in the pronunciation /mɛd-əl/, with a vowel that sounds like 'uh' in the second syllable, then this vowel is the syllabic sound and /l/ is no longer syllabic. This is true of all the cases discussed below as well.

This can happen with /r/ as well, as in 'feather', which has the syllables 'feath' (built around the vowel /ɛ/) and the single sound /r/. Thus, in the last syllable, /r/ is syllabic, since there is no vowel to play this role. So we see that the liquids (/r/ and /l/) can be syllabic if there is no vowel in the syllable. If there is a vowel, then /r/ and /l/ are, of course, nonsyllabic, as in 'hill', where the center of the single syllable that makes up this word is the vowel /ɪ/, not the liquid /l/.

The only other sounds that can sometimes be syllabic, other than vowels and the liquids, are the nasal consonants /m/, /n/, and /ŋ/. Thus, in 'mitten', there are two syllables, 'mit' (with the vowel 'ɪ') and the single sound /n/, which is syllabic in this case, since there is no vowel. We can conclude that vowels are always syllabic when they are present, that liquids and nasals can be syllabic if no vowel is present; otherwise they are not syllabic. Glides and consonants (other than liquids and nasals) are never syllabic but always occur with vowels.

So we need to describe not just regular, mundane vowels (like /a/) and regular, mundane consonants (like /s/, /f/, or /p/), but these special cases—liquids, glides, and the nasals when they are syllabic—as well. We will do so as follows. Vowels will be [−consonantal] and [+syllabic]. Glides (/y/ and /w/) will also be listed as [−consonantal], capturing their similarity to vowels, but [−syllabic], capturing their difference as well (they can never be syllabic, but must occur in a syllable with a vowel). Liquids (/l/ and /r/) and nasals (/m, n, n/) will be listed as [+consonantal] and treated as simple consonants. However, when there is no vowel in their syllable, they will be said to be [+syllabic]; when there is a vowel, it will be syllabic, and they will be given the feature [−syllabic]. All other consonants (like /s/, /f/, and /p/) will be both [+consonantal] and [−syllabic] (since they are never syllabic). This nicely captures the similarities and differences all around. Table 4-2 summarizes our results.

In Table 4-2 we see something typical of any scientific description. The terms 'vowel' and 'consonant' are, in many ways, terms from common-sense descriptions of language. They capture an important insight. But when we try to apply this insight to the actual workings of language, we find a certain degree of complexity. It turns out that the common-sense insight about the distinction between vowels and consonants covers over two different properties. Vowels are syllabic sounds, and they share this with liquids and nasals (when the latter occur in syllables with no vowel) in contrast to glides and the remaining consonants. On

TABLE 4-2. Types of Sounds

	Vowels e.g., /a/	Glides /w/ & /y/	Liquids /r/ & /l/, & Nasals /m, n, ŋ/	Consonants e.g., /s/, /f/, & /p/
Features:				
Consonantal	−	−	+	+
Syllabic	+	−	+/−	−

Types of sounds, with features capturing the way in which glides and liquids are intermediary between true vowels and true consonants. (The value +/− for liquids and nasals means that these sounds are [+syllabic] when they occur in a syllable with no true vowel, and they are [−syllabic] when they occur in a syllable with a vowel; all other sounds marked as [−syllabic] can never occur in a syllable without a true vowel.)

the other hand, vowels are sounds made with an open mouth, and they share this with the glides in contrast to liquids and the remaining consonants.

───────────────── E X E R C I S E ─────────────────

Exercise D.   Write the following words in phonetic notation and place the words into their syllables, if the word contains more than one syllable. Feel free to use Table 4-1 as a guide to the sound a phonetic symbol stands for.

Example Answer.   The word 'expert' is represented in the phonetic symbols given in Table 4-1 as /ɛks-pɛrt/, where I have separated the two syllables of the word by a hyphen.

sing	notice	monsoon	roll	knight
kitten	why	hippo	yes	know

4.5. STOPS (IN FEATURE TERMS [+CONTINUANT] AND [−CONTINUANT])

We saw that the three sounds /p/, /b/, and /m/ are similar sounds. They are all made in the same way (by momentarily blocking the air from the lungs by placing the lips together). They are differentiated by the fact that /p/ is [−voice] and /b/ and /m/ are [+voice], while /b/ and /p/ are [−nasal] and /m/ is [+nasal].

Sounds like /p/, /b/, and /m/ are called *stops* because they momentarily stop the air in the mouth (they stop it until the airstream behind the blockage has built up a bit; then the blockage is released and the air rushes out). Since, as we have just seen, these three stops are made by stopping the air with the two lips, they are called *bilabial stops* ('bilabial' means *two lips*). We name the three sounds in terms of *where* in the mouth they are made.

Where a sound is made in the mouth is called its **place of articulation** (thus, 'bilabial', which names where the stops are made in the mouth, names a place of articulation). All sounds have a place of articulation and can be given a name designating this place of articulation. We can also spell out places of articulation in terms of features, though we will leave that until later.

How, or the manner in which, a sound is made (for example, by stopping the airstream momentarily, or letting it flow without any blockage) is called its **manner of articulation.** Thus, the term 'stop' names a manner of articulation. Manners of articulation can also be spelled out in terms of features, and we will turn to this matter in a moment.

There are other stops in English that come in a voiceless, voiced, and nasal version as well, just like /p/, /b/, and /m/. Thus, /t/ is voiceless, /d/ is voiced, and /n/ is nasal (and voiced). Otherwise, these three sounds are the same. They momentarily stop the air from the lungs by blocking it with the front of the tongue placed at the alveolar ridge (the bony ridge behind the front teeth—often burned while eating pizza). Thus, they are called *alveolar stops* ('alveolar' names the place of articulation and 'stop' the manner of articulation).

/k/ is voiceless, /g/ is voiced, and /ŋ/ (the sound usually spelled as 'ng' as in 'sing', but it is a single sound) is nasal (and voiced). Otherwise, these three sounds are the same. They momentarily stop the air from the lungs by blocking it with the back of the tongue placed at the velum. Thus, they are called *velar stops* ('velar' names the place of articulation and 'stop' the manner of articulation).

All these stop sounds (/p, b, m/; /t, d, n/; /k, g, ŋ/) can be distinguished from all other sounds by the fact that they momentarily block the air *in the mouth* (the nasal stops do let it out the nose, however; the oral stops don't). Other sounds let the air flow out of the mouth without blocking it, though they may disturb it in other ways. Thus, compare /p/ as in 'pan', which stops the air in the mouth, with /f/ as in 'fan', which lets the air out of the mouth (though it constricts the airstream and makes it "fizz" or "hiss" a bit). Thus, we are distinguishing the stops from other sounds on the basis of their manner of articulation (how they are produced).

Sounds that do not completely stop the air from going out of the mouth will be said to have the value [+continuant] on the feature [continuant] (meaning that the air is allowed to *continue* out of the mouth). Sounds that momentarily stop the air from coming out of the mouth (though they may let some out of the nose), that is, the stops, will be said to have the value [−continuant] on the feature [continuant] (the air does not continue out of the mouth unstopped). Thus, the sound /p/ has the value [−continuant] and the sound /f/ has the value [+continuant].

Remember that the feature [continuant] has to do only with whether the airstream is stopped or continues out of the mouth. It says nothing about air coming out of the nose. Since the nasal stops (/m, n, ŋ/) stop the air coming out of the mouth, though they do let it out of the nose, they have the value [−continuant] on the feature [continuant].

4.6. SONORANTS AND OBSTRUENTS
(IN FEATURE TERMS [+SONORANT] AND [−SONORANT])

In the last section we saw that one way to classify sounds is in terms of whether the airstream is stopped in the mouth ([−continuant]) or allowed to flow out of the mouth ([+continuant]). We can also classify sounds as to whether the airstream is *obstructed* (through complete blockage or through being constricted and bothered, but not totally stopped) or is allowed to pass through the *nose or mouth* relatively freely.

Let's look first at sounds that allow the air to pass relatively freely through the mouth or nose. We will call such sounds **sonorants.** They have the value [+sonorant] on the feature [sonorant] (such sounds are called sonorants because they sound sonorous or have a resonating quality to them—they are the heart of any singing). Clearly all vowels (like /a/, the sound the doctor asks you to make when holding your tongue down with a tongue depressor) allow the air to flow freely out of the mouth. So vowels are [+sonorant] sounds. Now consider the nasal stops (/m, n, ŋ/). While these sounds block the air coming out of the mouth (thus they are stops, sounds with the feature [−continuant]), they allow air to flow freely out of the nose (because they are [+nasal]). So they also count as [+sonorant] sounds. The sounds /r/ and /l/, which are called liquids (see above), are also [+sonorant] sounds. So also are the sounds /w/ and /y/—called glides (see above).

Now let's look at sounds that obstruct the airstream in some serious fashion, not allowing it to flow freely out of the mouth or nose. The oral stops (/p, b; t, d; k, g/) stop the air completely in the mouth and nose. So they are given the value [−sonorant]. But there is also a class of sounds traditionally called **fricatives,** which do not completely stop the air coming from the lungs but seriously obstruct it by making a tight (but not complete) constriction in the mouth. The air is restricted by this constriction, and the air particles bang into the constriction and each other, creating turbulence (a fizzing or hissing sound).

These fricative sounds—like /f/ or /v/—are, then, also [−sonorant]. The [−sonorant] sounds (the oral stops and fricatives together) are called **obstruents.**

Oral stops and fricatives, then, are both [−sonorant] sounds, because they do not allow the air to flow freely out of the mouth or nose. Stops and fricatives are distinguished by the fact that stops (oral and nasal) are [−continuant] (air does not flow out of the mouth), and fricatives are all [+continuant] (air, however constricted, does flow out of the mouth).

Like the stops, fricative sounds (sounds that constrict the airstream and thus cause friction) can be named by the places in the mouth where they are made (their places of articulation). Like the stops, they come in voiced and voiceless versions (though there are no nasal fricatives in English).

The fricative sounds /f/ (voiceless) and /v/ (voiced) are made by creating a constriction with the lower lip placed against the top teeth; thus they are called **labio-dental fricatives.** The fricative sound /θ/ (voiceless), usually spelled 'th' as in the word 'thigh', and the sound /ð/ (voiced), usually also spelled 'th' as in the word 'thy', are made by creating a constriction with the tip of the tongue placed between the teeth. Thus, they are called **interdental fricatives.** The fricative sounds /s/ (voiceless) and /z/ (voiced) are made by creating a constriction with the front of the tongue placed near the alveolar ridge. Thus, they are **alveolar fricatives.** The sound /š/ (voiceless), usually spelled 'sh' as in 'shoe', and the sound /ž/ (voiced), spelled as 's' as in 'pleasure', are made by creating a constriction with the body (middle) of the tongue placed near the palate (the high bony ceiling of the mouth; see Figure 4-1). Thus, they are called **palatal fricatives.**

There are also sounds that very quickly combine a stop and a fricative; the two sounds are said so fast that they sound like (and count as) a single sound. Thus, the sound spelled 'ch' in 'church' is really a /t/ followed by a /š/ ('sh'). This sound is voiceless and symbolized as /č/. The sound spelled 'j' at the beginning of 'judge' and 'dg' at the end is really a /d/ followed quickly by a /ž/ (the sound spelled 's' in 'pleasure'). This sound is voiced and symbolized as /ǰ/. These sounds—/č/ (voiceless) and /ǰ/ (voiced)—are called **affricates.** The affricates are counted as [−continuant] and [−sonorant] sounds.

Table 4-3 shows the stops, fricatives, and affricates of English.

If you look at Table 4-3, you will see that there are "gaps" in the English system. For instance, we have bilabial stops (/p, b, m/), but no bilabial fricatives (though we could have them; Spanish does). And we have no interdental or palatal stops to go with our interdental and palatal fricatives. We also have no velar fricatives to go with our velar stops. All these sounds are possible and exist in other languages. In a sense, places and manners of articulation give a space within which a large number of sounds are possible. Each language picks just some of these possibilities from this space. Thus, in any language, there are always gaps like there are in English. The gaps are places where historical change can operate, places where sounds can be added to the language.

TABLE 4-3. **The Stops, Fricatives, and Affricates of English, Classified by Mannner and Place of Articulation**

Stops:	Bilabial	Alveolar	Velar	
Voiceless	p	t	k	
Voiced	b	d	g	
Nasal	m	n	ŋ	

Fricatives:	Labio-dental	Inter-dental	Alveolar	Palatal
Voiceless	f	θ	s	š
Voiced	v	ð	z	ž

Affricates:	Alveolar stop moving quickly to palatal fricative
Voiceless	č
Voiced	ǰ

Manner of articulation: *stop* versus *fricative* versus *affricate*. Place of articulation: *bilabial/labial* versus *interdental* versus *alveolar* versus *palatal* versus *velar*. The places of articulation have been arranged from the front of the mouth (bilabial) to the back (velar). Stops and affricates have the feature value [−continuant], while fricatives are [+continuant]. The nasal stops are [+sonorant] sounds; all other stops and affricates and fricatives are [−sonorant]. We have not yet used features to classify places of articulation. We are simply using names (like 'bilabial' or 'alveolar'). Since the fricatives /s/ and /z/ are made by many people just a little back from the alveolar ridge, between the alveolar ridge and the palate, they are sometimes called **alveo-palatal** sounds.

_____ E X E R C I S E _____

Exercise E. Write the following words in phonetic notation and place the words into their syllables, if the word contains more than one syllable. Feel free to use Table 4-1 as a guide to the sound a phonetic symbol stands for.

fish	church	joy	vine	pleasure
shoe	this	them	think	theme
love	chicken	children	thing	fizz

4.7. THE FEATURE [+STRIDENT] AND [−STRIDENT]

Another feature that is used to distinguish speech sounds in English is the feature [+strident] and [−strident]. The friction created in the production of the fricatives in the words 'fail' (/f/) and 'veil' (/v/); 'sit' (/s/) and 'zip' (/z/); and 'shoe' (/š/) and 'pleasure' (/ž/), as well as the friction created by the ending parts of the affricates in 'church' (/č/) and 'judge' (/ǰ/) causes a hissing sound. The airstream coming against the teeth or the hard bone of the alveolar ridge produces even more noise or stridency than is produced during the articulation of the interdental fricatives, /θ/ (as in 'throw') and /ð/ (as in 'thy'). The harsh hissing sounds are said to have the value [+strident] on the feature [strident], while the softer interdental fricatives and all other sounds (which are less noisy) are said to have the value [−strident] on the feature [strident].

4.8. PLACES OF ARTICULATION (THE FEATURES [+ANTERIOR], [−ANTERIOR] AND [+CORONAL], [−CORONAL])

We still have to discuss a set of features for vowels. But as far as all other sounds go, we are finished, except for the need to introduce features to deal with places of articulation. For example, we want to capture the fact that the stops /p/ and /d/ are similar in that they are made in the front of the mouth, in contrast with the stop /k/, which is made at the back of the mouth. At the same time, we want to capture the fact that /p/ and /d/ differ in that /p/ is made with the lips and /d/ is made with the tongue.

We will introduce two new features to deal with places of articulation. First, sounds that are articulated at or in front of the alveolar ridge will be called [+anterior] sounds. Sounds made behind the alveolar ridge will be called [−anterior] (posterior) sounds. Thus, /p/ (made by the lips) and /d/ (made at the alveolar ridge with the tongue) are [+anterior], and /k/ (made at the velum with the tongue) is [−anterior].

Second, sounds that are made by raising the blade of the tongue (the front of the tongue, including the tip of the tongue) up from its neutral position at the bottom of the mouth toward the top of the mouth are called [+coronal] sounds. All other sounds are said to be [−coronal] sounds. This seems like a funny feature, but it is basically meant to designate sounds made near the middle of the mouth (at the alveolar ridge or at the palate, which are marked as [+coronal]) in contrast to sounds made either in the very front (at the lips or teeth) or very back of the mouth (at the velum or further back), which are all marked as [−coronal]). Thus, the sound /d/, which is made toward the middle of the mouth (not at the very front or back), is [+coronal] and the sounds /p/ (made at the very front) and /k/ (made at the very back) are [−coronal] sounds.

TABLE 4-4. The Stop and Fricative Consonants of English, Showing How the Features [Anterior] and [Coronal] Are Assigned

[+ANTERIOR] SOUNDS				[−ANTERIOR] SOUNDS	
Bilabial sounds	Labio-dental sounds	Inter-dental sounds	Alveolar sounds	Palatal sounds	Velar sounds
p	f	θ	t	š	k
b	v	ð	d	ž	g
m			n		ŋ
			s		
			z		
[−coronal]		[+coronal] sounds			[−coronal]

The stops (/p,b,m; t,d,n; k,g,ŋ /) and fricatives (/f,v; θ,ð; s,z; š,ž /) are arranged in the table from the front of the mouth on the left (bilabial) to the back on the right (velar). Note that sounds made toward the front are [+anterior] and those toward the back are [−anterior]. Sounds made toward the middle are [+coronal], and those made toward the very front or very back are [−coronal].

Table 4-4 shows how the consonants of English are distributed in terms of the features [anterior] and [coronal].

―――――――――――――――――― **E X E R C I S E** ――――――――――――――――――

Exercise F. Classify the following sounds in terms of the features [+coronal] and [−coronal], and [+anterior] and [−anterior]. I have supplied a set of values for /p/. Complete the chart, adding the appropriate feature values.

	p	k	t	n	s	m	f
Anterior	+						
Coronal	−						

4.9. FEATURES AND THE CLASSIFICATION OF SOUNDS

We can view a speech sound as the set of all the feature values that distinguish it from every other sound in the language. Thus, a sound is a set of features and their + and − values. Therefore, the sound /p/ can be seen as the set of feature values: [+consonantal, −syllabic, −sonorant, −continuant, −strident, −nasal, +anterior, −coronal, −voice], and these features distinguish it from every other sound in English. The sound /m/ can be seen as the set of feature values [+consonantal, + or −syllabic, +sonorant, −continuant, −strident, +nasal, +anterior, −coronal, +voice] (remember, nasal consonants can be syllabic if no vowel is in their syllable, otherwise they are nonsyllabic). The order in which we list the features within the sound is of no significance.

We can also compare sounds in terms of how similar or different they are in terms of features and feature values. Thus, compare the feature values of the four sounds in Table 4-5 (/p, b, m, s/).

Each sound /p, b, m, s/ can be viewed as the set of feature values listed underneath it in Table 4-5. At a glance, we can see where each sound is similar or different from each other sound. Thus, /p/ and /b/ are exactly alike except on the feature [voice], where /p/ is [−voice] and /b/ is [+voice]. The sounds /b/ and /m/ are identical except on the features [nasal] and [syllabic]. The sound /m/ differs from /p/ on three features: [voice], [nasal], and [syllabic], but from /b/ on only two: [nasal], [syllabic]. Thus, /m/ is closer to /b/ than it is to /p/. On the other hand, /m/ is closer to both /p/ and /b/ than it is to /s/. The sound /s/ differs on seven features from /m/: [syllabic], [sonorant], [continuant], [strident], [nasal], [voice], and [coronal]. Thus, /m/ resembles /p/ and /b/ more than it resembles /s/.

The more similar sounds are (the more feature values they share), the more they pattern together in both the processes of historical change and in the phonological rules of the language. Thus, it would not be at all surprising to find /p/ and /b/ functioning together in a sound change in the language (undergoing the same change) and even for /p/, /b/, and /m/ to pattern together. And the same would be true of a phonological rule in a language (they might all cause or

TABLE 4-5. Four Sounds of English Listed in Terms of Their Feature Values

	p	b	m	s
Consonantal	+	+	+	+
Syllabic	−	−	+/−	−
Sonorant	−	−	+	−
Continuant	−	−	−	+
Strident	−	−	−	+
Nasal	−	−	+	−
Anterior	+	+	+	+
Coronal	−	−	−	+
Voice	−	+	+	−

undergo the same phonological rule). But it would be quite surprising to see /s/ pattern with any of these sounds (/p, b, m/). It is too different from them.

EXERCISE

Exercise G. Give the full set of features for /s/, /š/, /f/, and /z/, as I have done in Table 4-5. Which two sounds are closest to each other? Which of the two sounds /š/ or /f/ is closer to the pair of sounds /s/ and /z/?

4.10. DISTINCTIVE AND NONDISTINCTIVE FEATURES

We need to make two important points clear. First, we have introduced only features that are needed to distinguish every *English* language sound from every other one. We would need either more or less features to describe the sounds of another language, depending on which sounds and how many that language had.

Second, we have dealt only with the *distinctive features* of English sounds. Each feature we have introduced can make a word differ in meaning if it is changed. Thus, the feature [voice] distinguishes sound pairs like /p/ and /b/, or /f/ and /v/, or /s/ and /z/ from each other. These pairs of sounds (and many others in English) differ only by this feature. If the feature value of this feature is changed in a word, it can change the meaning of the word. Thus, if I take the word 'pit' and change the feature value for the feature [voice] in the sound /p/, which is [−voice], to its opposite, that is, [+voice], I will get the word 'bit', which is a different word. I get /b/ instead of /p/ because /b/ is identical to /p/ except that it has the value [+voice] instead of [−voice]; otherwise /p/ and /b/ share all the same values on the features we have used. When a feature can do this (that is, change the meaning of a word), it is called a **distinctive feature.** So the feature [voice] in English is a distinctive feature. Of course, it need not be distinctive in other languages.

On the other hand, there are features of sound that are not distinctive in English (though they may be so in another language). Each sound adjusts to the sounds around it in the words and sentences in which it occurs. These adjustments are described by nondistinctive features. For example, when the sound /p/ occurs at the beginning of a word (or syllable) before a stressed vowel, it is said with an audible puff of air once the momentary closure of the lips is released. This is called **aspiration.** The /p/ sound is aspirated. However, when a /p/ occurs after the sound /s/, as in 'spin', it is pronounced without the puff of air. In this case it is not aspirated (**unaspirated**). In feature terms, the /p/ sound in 'pit' is [+aspirated] and the /p/ sound in 'spin' is [−aspirated].

But this feature ([aspiration]) is not distinctive in English. When you change the value of a **nondistinctive feature** like [aspiration] in a word, you will not change the meaning of the word, you will just make its pronunciation sound odd and foreign. So if you take the word 'pit' and change the feature value [+aspirated] in the initial /p/ to [−aspirated], you will still get 'pit', but now without any puff of air from /p/ (you will be saying the /p/ in 'pit' just like you normally say the /p/ in 'spin', where it follows an /s/ and is not aspirated). This will simply sound odd. It will not constitute a different word of English, just an odd pronunciation of 'pit'. This is exactly what it means to say that the feature [aspirated] is not distinctive (is nondistinctive) in English.

In some other languages the feature [aspiration] is distinctive. If you change the value of the feature, you would get a different word (that is, 'pit' with aspirated /p/ and 'pit' with unaspirated /p/ would be different words, both correctly pronounced in that language, just like 'pit' and 'bit' are in English).

When we list a sound with only its distinctive features and their values present in the list, this sound is called a **phoneme** (a basic sound of the language). When we add in the nondistinctive features, like [+aspiration] for the /p/ in 'pit' or [−aspiration] for the /p/ in 'spin', we are talking about variant versions of the basic sound /p/ (the phoneme /p/), versions that show up in different contexts. These variant versions are called the **allophones** of the phoneme /p/. When we want to be explicit about the distinction between phonemes (basic sounds) and allophones (variants of the basic sound that show up in different contexts), and do not want to write out the whole feature list, we write the phoneme in slashes, as in '/p/'. We write the allophones in brackets, as '[pʰ]' for aspirated /p/ (the raised 'h' stands for aspiration) and '[p]' for unaspirated /p/. The two variant pronunciations, [pʰ] and [p], are alternate ways to say the basic sound, the phoneme /p/. These alternates are determined by where in a word the /p/ occurs.

In our discussion, we have listed the distinctive features of English, not the nondistinctive ones. There are many nondistinctive variations of the phonemes of English, variations determined by where in a word or sentence they occur. A full description of English would require a discussion of these, and some are discussed in the preceding chapter. But we will not discuss them further here.

─────────────── **E X E R C I S E S** ───────────────

Exercise H. Show that the feature [nasal] is distinctive for consonants in English. Vowels can be *nasalized,* said with air coming out the nose; thus vowels can have the feature [+nasal] in certain contexts. Where does this happen? Is the feature [nasal] distinctive for vowels in English? Say why you believe it is or is not distinctive for vowels.

Exercise I. In some dialects of English, a voiceless stop (/p, t, k/) at the end of a word can be said as unaspirated (for example, [tʰɪp], 'tip') or as aspirated (for example, [tʰɪpʰ], 'tip'). This phenomenon is called *free variation,* because the two variants of the phoneme /p/ occur in the same place but do not cause any difference in meaning. Does this make [aspiration] a distinctive feature in these dialects? Why not? Why would you expect free variation to be a fairly rare phenomenon in languages?

4.11.   VOWELS

Vowels are central to the sound structure of any language. They are the nucleus of syllables, and, as syllabic sounds, the basic carriers of stress and intonation in words and sentences. It is because they are the carriers of stress and intonation that they are the basis of any singing.

Stress stands for the degree of perceptual salience a syllable has in a word or sentence. Humans hear stress by paying attention to a complex combination of cues involving loudness differences (how loud the syllable is, in comparison to others around it), pitch differences (the rise and fall of the tone of the voice), and duration differences (how long the syllable is, in comparison to others around it). Thus, in the word 'important', the middle syllable has more stress, is more salient, than the first and last syllables: im-POR-tant.

Intonation stands for the complex changing patterns of stress and, particularly, pitch across a sentence. Thus, the sentence 'John is happy' said with a slow fall in pitch across the sentence and an accelerated fall at the end constitutes a claim or statement. Said with a rising intonation, accelerating the rise at the end, it constitutes a question. Other patterns of pitch changes can make it sound surprised, incredulous, ironic, threatening or challenging, and many other things. In the case of both word stress and the overall intonation contours of sentences, it is the vowels that carry most of the information necessary for hearers to identify degrees of stress or intonation.

Unfortunately, there is a great deal of dialect variation across the U.S. and the English-speaking world in the pronunciation of the vowels of English. The pronunciation of vowels is much more variable across dialects than that of consonants. In this section, when I list a word as an example of how a particular vowel symbol is pronounced, I will use a particularly common dialect—for example, the vowel symbol /ae/ is for the vowel in 'cat'. But you may very well pronounce the vowel in this word somewhat differently than others (and, thus, a different phonetic symbol would be appropriate for you). If you know your dialect is somewhat different from others around you, you may want to check the pronunciation of various words used here against your own pronunciation.

For example, I pronounce the vowels in the words 'pin' and 'pen' exactly the same. But many other people pronounce the vowel in the first word as /ɪ/, like the vowel in 'pit', and the vowel in the second word as /ɛ/, like the vowel in 'pet'. My vowel in 'pin' and 'pen' is made in a position in the mouth between where /ɪ/ and /ɛ/ are made. Or, to take another example, I do not make any distinction between the vowel in 'cot' (a thing to sleep on) and 'caught', but many others use the vowel

/a / (the vowel in 'father') in the word 'cot' and the vowel /ɔ / (the vowel in 'awful' where the 'aw' is said at the back of the mouth) in the word 'caught'. I use the vowel /a / in both 'cot' and 'caught', and, in fact, do not use the vowel /ɔ / very much, while this latter vowel is very common in many other people's speech.

In the description in this section, I do *not* use my dialect, but one that makes the distinctions (as in 'pen' and 'pin' or in 'cot' and 'caught') that I do not make. The dialect I describe is somewhat more "standard" than the one I speak (for example, the dialect I am describing, not the one I speak, is used on the national TV news).

One other thing that makes matters tricky is that certain sounds, especially /r /, tend to "warp" or change the sound of vowels that precede them. Thus, notice how the vowel /o / sounds in the word 'no' (/no /), and compare this to how it sounds in the word 'nor' (/nor /), where it is followed by /r /.

─────────────── **E X E R C I S E** ───────────────

Exercise J.   Underline the syllable in each of the words below that has the most stress. Transcribe the vowel in this syllable.

Example Answer.   Consider 'important'. The stressed syllable is 'por', thus: im-**por**-tant. The vowel in this syllable is /o /.

important	rerun	photography	photograph
photographer	wonder	sensible	different
never	discussion	redcoat	photo
knowledge	yesterday	tomorrow	blackboard

4.12.   DESCRIBING VOWELS (THE FEATURES [+HIGH], [−HIGH], [+LOW], [−LOW], AND [+FRONT], [−FRONT])

It is not easy to describe what physically happens when one produces a vowel. Vowels are made with a relatively open mouth, which allows the airstream to pass through and out of the mouth in a completely unobstructed way. Because vowels are produced without any articulators (lips, teeth, and tongue) touching or even coming close together, it is often difficult to feel or say what is happening in the mouth when they are produced.

Vowels are usually described in terms of how high or low in the mouth the tongue is held in the production of the vowel, and how far forward or back in the mouth the tongue is held in the production of the vowel. These different positions of the tongue change the shape of the mouth cavity, and thus the air in the mouth cavity resonates differently for different vowels, producing the different vowel sounds.

Thus, imagine the mouth as a space. Within this space, the tongue can be high or low, front or back. For vowels, 'front' means basically near the palate and 'back' means behind this point. 'High' means up toward the top of the mouth, and 'low' down toward the bottom. Given this scheme, we can describe any vowel as high or low, front or back. We will, however, treat these terms in terms of features (for example, [+high] and [−high]).

One thing needs to be kept in mind here. These terms, 'high' and 'low', 'front' and 'back', are rather impressionistic. What actually goes on in the mouth with vowels is rather complicated. But it turns out that the impressionistic terms 'high–low' and 'front–back' work well in describing the vowels that show up in English and other languages.

Three are three types of vowel sounds in English. These are **tense vowels, diphthongs,** and **regular vowels.** Let's start with the regular vowels. The regular vowels in the dialect of English I am describing here are listed below, with their symbols:

/ɪ/   pit, lip, pill
/ɛ/   set, sell, chef
/ʊ/   put, look, good
/ɔ/   caught, awful, bawd
/æ/   bat, sad, fan
/a/   far, father, cot
/ʌ/   gut, gull, rung
/ə/   the schwa vowel
       (the sound in 'the' when said fast or at the end of
       'sofa' when said fast)

The last vowel listed, often called 'schwa', is a vowel that occurs only in unstressed syllables in English. In most cases, when a syllable carries no stress, that syllable has the schwa vowel in it. Thus, this vowel is very pervasive in English. For example, in the word 'photograph' we have the following vowels and syllables: /fo-tə-græf/, with a schwa in the middle. However, in the word 'photographer', which adds '-er' to the end of the word 'photograph' and changes its stress pattern, we have the following vowels and syllables: /fə-tag-grə-fər/, with a schwa in the first, third and last syllables (for many people the last syllable really has no vowel, but a syllabic /r/). In 'photographer' the middle syllable has the vowel /a/, not schwa as in 'photograph'.

The use of schwa in English contributes a good deal to its characteristic "sound." In many languages (for example the Romance languages like French, Spanish, and Italian), unstressed vowels are not "reduced" to schwa but retain the quality of a full vowel. When English speakers speak these languages, they tend to reduce unstressed vowels to schwa and sound "mushy." On the other hand, many speakers of Romance languages when they are speaking English tend not to reduce unstressed syllables in English to schwa and therefore sound as if they are "overarticulating." In fact, it is just such factors that make for a "foreign accent" in a language.

We can arrange the regular vowels of English into the impressionistic space we described above, a space in which a vowel is treated as front or back, high or low, in terms of the position of the tongue in the mouth when the vowel is produced. Table 4-6 shows a picture of the vowel space and arranges the vowels in terms of whether they are high or low, front or back. I use features for these concepts.

Table 4-6 is to be read as follows: The vowel /ɪ/ is said to be [−back] [+front] [+high] [−low]; the vowel /a/ is said to be [+back] [−front] [−high] [+low]; the vowel /ɛ/ is said to be [−back] [+front] [−high] [−low] (that is, in the middle front of the mouth, neither high nor low); the vowel /ɔ/ is said to be [+back] [−front] [−high] [−low] (that is, in the middle back of the mouth); and the vowel /ʌ/ is said to be [−back] [−front] [−high] [−low] (that is, in the middle center of the mouth, neither high nor low, neither front nor back).

You can feel the differences between these vowels if you say them one after another. For example, if you say 'bit', 'bet', and 'bat' one after the other repeatedly, you feel the tongue drop from high to low in the mouth. Or if you say 'bit' and 'put' repeatedly, you will feel the tongue move from front to back in the mouth, staying high in the mouth. If you say 'bat' and 'father', you will feel the tongue also go from front to back, but now along the bottom of the mouth

TABLE 4-6. The Regular Vowels of English Arranged in an Impressionistic Space in Terms of Whether They Are Made at the Front or Back of the Mouth, or High or Low in the Mouth

	[−back] [+front] ————	[−back] [−front] ————→	[+back] [−front]
[+high] [−low]	ɪ (bit)		ʊ (put)
[−high] [−low]	ɛ (bet)	ʌ (gut) ə (schwa)	ɔ (bought)
[−high] [+low]	æ (bat)		a (father)

The vowels /ʌ/ and schwa are made in the middle of the mouth and are distinguished by the fact that the schwa vowel is unstressed and /ʌ/, like all other vowels, carries some appreciable degree of stress (it is sometimes called the stressed schwa).

(however, there is a great deal of dialect variation with vowels at the bottom of the mouth; some have more than the vowels I have listed above).

Tense vowels are the second type of vowel sound in English. The regular vowels above are all called **lax** vowels to distinguish them from the tense vowels. Phoneticians have argued for years about exactly what is happening when a tense or a lax vowel is produced. Tense vowels appear to involve a tensing of the tongue muscle and are produced in a slightly higher position in the mouth than corresponding lax vowels. The tense vowels have the feature [+tense], and lax ones (all the regular vowels above) have the feature [−tense]. The tense vowels of English can be placed in the same vowel space as the regular vowels. This is shown in Table 4-7.

As you can see from Table 4-7, there are only four tense vowels in English, one in the same position as /ɪ/, one in the same position as /ʊ/, one in the same position as /ɛ/, and one in the same position as /ɔ/. In English, these tense vowels are made by starting with the corresponding regular (lax) vowel and moving the tongue quickly upward and to the front or back of the mouth (producing a glide: the glide /y/ involves a movement of the tongue up and to the front of the mouth; the glide /w/ involves a movement of the tongue up and to the back of the mouth). Thus, the tense vowel /i/ is actually /ɪy/ (a combination of /ɪ/ and /y/); the tense vowel /e/ is actually /ɛy/ (a combination of /ɛ/ and /y/); the tense vowel /u/ is actually /ʊw/ (a combination of /ʊ/ and /w/); the tense vowel /o/ is actually /ɔw/ (a combination of /ɔ/ and /w/). In many other languages, like the

TABLE 4-7. The Tense Vowels ([+tense]) of English Arranged in an Impressionistic Space in Terms of Whether They Are Made at the Front or Back of the Mouth, or High or Low in the Mouth

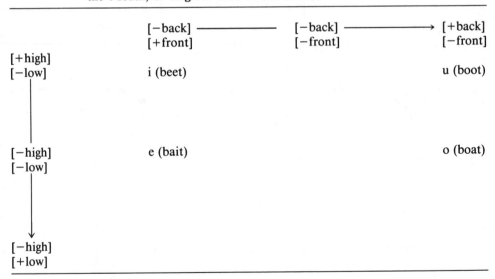

Romance languages, these tense vowels are not produced in this fashion, with these "off-glides," but start and stop at the same position in the mouth (slightly higher than the corresponding lax vowel). This is another factor that leads to a "foreign accent."

Diphthongs are the final type of vowel in English. Diphthongs are a combination of two vowels, said very quickly one after the other. They count as one sound, but they are longer than other vowels. The diphthongs in English are listed below:

/aɪ/   buy
/oɪ/   boy
/aʊ/   out

These diphthongs are sometimes described as having glides after the initial vowel, so /aɪ/ ('buy') is symbolized instead as /ay/; /oɪ/ ('boy') is symbolized instead as /ɔy/; and /aʊ/ ('out') is symbolized instead as /aw/. This way of doing things shows the diphthongs to be similar to the tense vowels, in English.

I mentioned in my discussion of consonants that in this chapter I have listed only features of sound that are distinctive in English. Vowels, like consonants, can take on a number of nondistinctive features as they adjust to the sounds around them in speech. However, there is also one salient nondistinctive feature that some English vowels always have: *roundness.* All English vowels that have the feature [+back] also have the feature [+round]. They are produced with a rounding of the lips. Thus, compare the back vowel [o] in 'low', where the lips are rounded, with the front vowel [i] in 'lee', where they are not. The feature [round] is always, in English, **redundant.** We can predict whether a vowel is [+round] or [−round] from knowing whether it is [+back] (in which case it is [+round] also) or [−back] (in which case it is [−round] also).

E X E R C I S E

Exercise K. Transcribe the following words in phonetic notation.

see	sofa	listen	jet
pill	photography	mushy	shout
look	sun	seat	toy
gull	moan	loot	gut
oat	lane	wait	organization
laugh	awful	caught	difference
far	boy	beat	elegant
sung	whine	hit	institution

4.13. THE SOUNDS OF ENGLISH

Table 4-8 lists all the sounds we have talked about in this chapter (except the vowels) and the features that characterize them. In this table, I add the feature [+ and −lateral] to distinguish /l/ (= [+lateral]) from /r/ (= [−lateral]). The sound /l/ is made with the tongue raised to the alveolar ridge, but the sides of the tongue are down, permitting air to escape laterally over the sides of the tongue. The sound /r/ is made variably by different speakers of English. Two people can make it differently in their mouths, and yet it comes out sounding the same. We will just say it is [−lateral] to distinguish it from [l]. The two sounds /r/ and /l/ are closely related in many languages (they count as variants of the same sound), though in English they are separate phonemes. Table 4-9 does the same for vowels.

TABLE 4-8. Phonetic Features of English Sounds (Except Vowels)

	p	b	m	t	d	n	k	g	ŋ	f	v	θ
Consonantal	+	+	+	+	+	+	+	+	+	+	+	+
Syllabic	−	−	+/−	−	−	+/−	−	−	+/−	−	−	−
Sonorant	−	−	+	−	−	+	−	−	+	−	−	−
Continuant	−	−	−	−	−	−	−	−	−	+	+	+
Nasal	−	−	+	−	−	+	−	−	+	−	−	−
Strident	−	−	−	−	−	−	−	−	−	+	+	−
Anterior	+	+	+	+	+	+	−	−	−	+	+	+
Coronal	−	−	−	+	+	+	−	−	−	−	−	−
Voiced	−	+	+	−	+	+	−	+	+	−	+	−
Lateral	−	−	−	−	−	−	−	−	−	−	−	−

	ð	s	z	š	ž	č	ǰ	r	l	y	w
Consonantal	+	+	+	+	+	+	+	+	+	−	−
Syllabic	−	−	−	−	−	−	−	+/−	+/−	−	−
Sonorant	−	−	−	−	−	−	−	+	+	+	+
Continuant	+	+	+	+	+	−	−	+	+	+	+
Nasal	−	−	−	−	−	−	−	−	−	−	−
Strident	−	+	+	+	+	+	+	−	−	−	−
Anterior	+	+	+	−	−	−	−	+	+	−	−
Coronal	−	+	+	+	+	+	+	+	+	+	−
Voiced	+	−	+	−	+	−	+	+	+	+	+
Lateral	−	−	−	−	−	−	−	−	+	−	−

TABLE 4-9. Phonetic Features of English Vowels

	i	ɪ	e	ɛ	æ	u	ʊ	o	ɔ	a	ʌ
High	+	+	−	−	−	+	+	−	−	−	−
Low	−	−	−	−	+	−	−	−	−	+	−
Back	−	−	−	−	−	+	+	+	+	+	−
Front	+	+	+	+	+	−	−	−	−	−	−
Tense	+	−	+	−	−	+	−	+	−	−	−

All vowels are [−consonantal] [+syllabic] [+sonorant] [+voiced]. The diphthongs would be represented by a two-column feature matrix of the one vowel followed by the other. I do not include the schwa vowel in the chart. It has the same features as the vowel /ʌ/, except that it is not stressed.

─────────────────────── E X E R C I S E ───────────────────────

Exercise L. What three consonants do the features listed below go with?

Consonantal	+	+	+
Syllabic	+/−	−	−
Sonorant	+	−	−
Continuant	−	−	−
Nasal	+	−	−
Strident	−	−	−
Anterior	+	+	−
Coronal	−	+	−
Voiced	+	−	−
Lateral	−	−	−

What three vowels do the features below go with?

High	−	−	+
Low	−	−	−
Back	−	−	+
Front	+	+	−
Tense	+	−	+

RECOMMENDED FURTHER READING

DENES, PETER & PINSON, E. N. (1973). *The Speech Chain.* Garden City, N.Y.: Anchor Books. (A lucid and short introduction to the physics of speech.)

LADEFOGED, PETER (1982). *A Course in Phonetics,* 2nd ed. New York: Harcourt Brace Jovanovich. (A readable classic book.)

CHAPTER 5

Morphology
The Shapes
of Words

5.1. INVENTING GRAMMAR

Fitting Language to the World

Language is used—among other things—to talk about the world. Thus, words must be fit to the world. Let's imagine (as we did in Chapter 3) that we are inventing a language. The simplest way to fit our new language to the world would be just to go around and name everything in the world: that person over there is named 'Sally', that cat over there is named 'Joan', that rock there is named 'Herman', the table over there is named 'Zandor', and so on. Obviously, this is foolish and isn't going to work.

It is foolish, first, because there are too many things to name. Second, it is foolish because we want to be able to talk about groups or *types* of objects (like people, cats, animals, rocks, chairs, furniture) and not just single isolated individual objects. Third, and finally, it is foolish because there are many things we want to talk about that we don't want names for: for instance, we want to talk about events and actions, but don't want a different name for each occasion on which one specific cat chases a mouse. So obviously we have to rise above and beyond names like 'Joan', 'Herman', and 'Sally'. We also need words for groups and types of objects (for example, 'cat' for all cats) and for types of actions (for example, 'chase' for all chasings).

So the real question becomes, what *types* of objects and actions, or anything else, for that matter, are worth having words for? It turns out that human beings are fundamentally interested in three major types of things. First, there are **happenings,** which we can separate into activities like eating and battling, where an actor controls the action, and **processes** like water flowing or people dying, where something happens but no actor controls the process. Second, there are

TABLE 5-1. Types of Things or States of Affairs that Exist for Humans

Happenings		Objects	States
Activities	Processes		
Eating	Flowing	Cats	Love
Fighting	Dying	Rocks	Sickness
(Actor controls action)	(No actor controls process)		(Conditions that objects are in)

objects (like cats and mice). Third, there are **states** or conditions things are in (like love, death, and sickness).

Table 5-1 summarizes the main sorts of things humans are interested in, and thus the main sorts of things their languages have words for.

─────────────────────── **E X E R C I S E** ───────────────────────

Exercise A. Starting in this section we will gradually invent a language that can talk about objects, states, and happenings (actions and processes). Of course, English can already do this. For each English sentence below, identify each underlined word as an action, process, object, or state term.

1. John became <u>sick</u> from <u>eating</u> <u>fish</u> and <u>died</u>.
2. John is <u>tall</u>.
3. <u>My</u> <u>small</u> <u>cat</u> is <u>black</u>.
4. John <u>made</u> the <u>water</u> <u>flow</u> down the hill.
5. Mary is <u>in love</u> with John.

From Words to Sentences: The Growth of Grammar. In inventing our language, we will need words for happenings (actions and processes), objects, and states, as well as proper names for individual objects we want to keep track of.

Happenings, in the typical case, are visible events involving *movement* or *change*. In a process, movement or change just happens to a participant ('Sally died', 'The water flows'); in an action there is also a participant (which we will call the *actor*) that instigates the change or movement ('Joan killed Sally', 'Mary pushed the cart', 'Sally ran away').

Let's say this is our *prototype* of a happening, the standard against we judge anything as a process or an action (the two types of happenings). Let's assume we go out and give words to these prototypical cases first, and call these words **process terms** ('die', 'flow') and **action terms** ('kill', 'push', 'run').

Objects are, in the prototypical case, visible, concrete things, which are, in fact, the participants in happenings. Let's call our words for prototypical types of objects **object terms** (like 'cat', 'person', and 'rock').

States are harder to define, since they are often inferred on the basis of indirect evidence (I may know you are sick or in love by how you look, though sickness and loving have more to them than just looking a certain way). We can say that prototypical states are the properties or conditions objects are in that change relatively slowly (like being sick, or tall, or in love), slowly enough that they can be taken to be characteristics of or identifying marks of the things that have them, at least for a time. I will call words for states **state terms.**

Imagine we have, among many others, the following words in our invented language:

Process Terms: DIE, FLOW, MELT, SINK
Action Terms: EAT, RUN, HIT, GIVE
Object Terms: CAT, DOG, PEOPLE, ROCK, CHAIR
State Terms: SICK, SLOW, TALL, LOVE, HATE

We want to say something about the world in our new language. We can't say anything yet, actually, because we have no agreed-on way to say it. Everyone who intends to use our language has to agree on how to say a message and distinguish it from other messages. For instance, if we want to use our words 'CAT', 'MOUSE,' and 'EAT' to say that a cat ate mice, we need some way to know who is the ACTOR (the eater) and who is the PATIENT (the one "done to," the eatee).

Now we can do this in three different ways, each of which will give us a different type of language. First, we could add some new words to the language, words meaning 'ACTOR' and 'PATIENT'. We could then allow people to put their words in any order they want, so long as the word ACTOR is next to the actor term (say right after it) and the word PATIENT is next to the patient term (again, right after it). I show this solution in sentence 1a.

1a. First solution (words for ACTOR and PATIENT):
CAT ACTOR MOUSE PATIENT EAT
CAT ACTOR EAT MOUSE PATIENT
or any other order as long as ACTOR is next to CAT and PATIENT is next to MOUSE

Second, we could, instead of adding new words, introduce little markers (sounds) that could be added to the existing words, little tags that would be attached to the ACTOR term to symbolize that it was the ACTOR and to the PATIENT term to symbolize that it was the PATIENT. Say we use the little tag 'er' for ACTORS and put it on the ends of words for ACTORS (for example, 'CATer'), and the tag 'em' for PATIENTS (for example, 'MOUSEem') and put it on the ends of words for PATIENTS.

Such little sounds that are parts of other words are called **morphemes.** In an English word like 'kissed', 'kiss' and 'ed' are morphemes, as are 'un' and 'help' and 'ful' in 'unhelpful'. Morphemes are the meaningful parts out of which words are made. Morphemes (like 'er' and 'em' in our invented language) that signal that a term is an ACTOR or a PATIENT are called **morphological cases (cases** for short). For clarity of display, I will write these case morphemes in lowercase letters and the object term to which they are attached in small capital letters (thus: 'CATer').

In 1b, I show the solution that involves adding CASE morphemes to object terms to signal whether they are playing the role of an ACTOR or a PATIENT in the action designated by the ACTION term in the sentence. Notice, once again, that word order is free to vary:

1b. Second solution (adding case morphemes):
CATer MOUSEem EAT
CATer EAT MOUSEem
('er' = ACTOR term; 'em' = PATIENT term)

Any other order is also possible.

As a third solution, we could just stipulate that the ACTOR term must always be placed (that is, said) first, the ACTION term second, and the PATIENT term last (or any other order—it doesn't matter which we use as long as we settle on one such order). I show this solution in 1c:

1c. Third solution (stipulate a word order):
CAT EAT MOUSE
(WORD ORDER stipulated: ACTOR ACTION OBJECT)

Something interesting has happened. Each solution is different, but, in fact, each has one thing in common with the others. Before we started trying to say 'a cat ate some mice' in our invented language, we had only words for *things in the world* (objects, happenings, and states). But now we also have devices that talk *not* directly about *things in the world,* but rather about *other words* in the sentence. The words 'ACTOR' and 'PATIENT' in the first solution, the cases 'er' and 'em' in the second solution, and the word order in the third solution do not signal anything directly about the world, rather they signal something about the word 'CAT' (that it names the ACTOR) and about the word 'MOUSE' (that it names the PATIENT).

Such devices—which may be separate words, morphemes that are parts of other words, or devices like word order—are called **grammatical** (or **functional)** words, morphemes, or devices. Words or morphemes that signal something directly about the world and not about other words in the sentence are called **lexical** (or **content**) words or morphemes. So the cost of moving beyond words to uttering them is in every case having to introduce grammatical machinery to help do the job.

Our three solutions are, in fact, not the only ones available. There is one more. Instead of placing little tags (morphemes) on the ACTOR term and the PATIENT term, we could have placed little tags on the action term, tags that AGREE with the ACTOR and the PATIENT. We do this by first placing all of our object terms into classes. The classes can be based on anything, but let's say we call all object terms that name masculine things *Class 1,* all object terms that name feminine things *Class 2,* and all object terms that name things that are neither masculine nor feminine *Class 3.* Then we can introduce morphemes that mean 'Class 1 (masculine) ACTOR' (say the morpheme 'he'), 'Class 1 PATIENT' (say the morpheme 'him'), 'Class 2 ACTOR' (say 'she'), 'Class 2 PATIENT' (say 'her'), 'Class 3 ACTOR' (say 'it') and 'Class 3 PATIENT' (say 'itm'). We then attach these morphemes, not to the object terms themselves but to the action term.

Then, for 'Mary kills John', we could say 'MARY JOHN sheKILLhim' (where 'sheKILLhim' is said as one single word). Any order of words is still possible: even in the order 'JOHN MARY sheKILLhim', we still know that the feminine term 'Mary' is the ACTOR because of the 'she' on the action term, and that the masculine term is the PATIENT because of the 'him' attached to the action term. Of course, this will not work well if both the ACTOR and PATIENT terms come from the same class (are both masculine, for instance), but languages don't seem to care about this—the solution works well enough in most cases. And in these cases, anyway, the language could fall back on a stipulated word order (say ACTOR ACTION PATIENT if the ACTOR and PATIENT are both in the same class).

When a language puts a tag (morpheme) on one term (like the action term here) to tell us something about another term in the sentence (the ACTOR and PATIENT terms in our example), these tags are said to *agree* with the terms they are telling us about. So the 'she' and 'him' in the word 'sheKILLhim' are said to agree with the ACTOR and PATIENT terms, respectively. While I have used English pronouns for the agreement morphemes, and, indeed, it is not uncommon for languages to use pronouns for this purpose in just this way, languages need not use pronouns. They can use any marks or tags they want.

Languages need not adopt just one of our solutions; they can mix and match them. So it is common to have both case morphemes on the ACTOR and PATIENT terms and agreement morphemes on the ACTION term.

Singular/Plural and Tense (Past/Present). We have managed to make clear *who ate whom* in our new language. But what about making clear that the cat ate more than one mouse? And what about making clear that the eating was in the past, not the present?

The sorts of solutions we discussed above are once again viable. We can add a word for PLURAL next to the object term we want to say is plural; we can add a morpheme that means plural to the object term (say 'pl'); or we can stipulate a word-order solution, like 'repeat the word that you want to pluralize'. We could also use agreement on the action term to signal which participant is plural (for example, 'Mary boys she-kisses-them'). English usually adds the morpheme '-s' to a word to signal that it is plural ('cats') and uses the absence of any ending to signal that the word is singular ('cat').

The same options are open for notating past versus present. We can add a word for PAST and for PRESENT and place them near the action term, or we can add a morpheme meaning PAST or one meaning PRESENT to the action term. A word-order solution here is less likely (it is hard to think of a reasonable one). The distinction between PAST (which really means past of the act of uttering the sentence) and PRESENT (which really means concurrent with the utterance of the sentence) are called **tense** distinctions, and PAST and PRESENT are said to be **tenses.**

Some languages have tense marking for PAST, PRESENT, and FUTURE. Many languages actually make a distinction between past and nonpast or present and nonpresent. In English we use the past tense for past actions ('John left') and the present tense for a variety of nonpast situations (for example, 'Tomorrow, John leaves' = future; 'John leaves each Tuesday' = habitual; 'He fades back and throws to the forty-yard line' = present in a sports cast). Thus, we are actually making a distinction between past and nonpast (but for convenience, I will continue to use the term 'present tense' when talking about English). English also uses a separate word for FUTURE and PREDICTION (that is, 'will').

Mixing and matching solutions means we can get some real complexity. For example, English uses word order for ACTOR and PATIENT, and yet uses morphemes for plural ('s' as in 'cats') and PAST ('ed' as in 'kissed'), except in words like 'mice' and 'knew', where it uses one word for singular mouse ('mouse') and a separate word for plural mouse ('mice'), one word for present knowing ('know') and a different word for past knowing ('knew'). On the other hand, for future it uses a separate word ('will'). Thus, we get 'A cat will eat some birds' (word order for ACTOR, 'cat', and PATIENT, 'birds'; separate word for FUTURE, 'will'; morpheme for PLURAL, 's'). Of course, since you speak English, this looks uncomplicated to you—but if you think about it, you'll see it is quite complex and strange.

——————————————— **E X E R C I S E** ———————————————

Exercise B. Divide each word in the sentences below into their constituent morphemes. Label each morpheme as a grammatical or lexical morpheme. Indicate which morpheme is an agreement morpheme.

   1. Boys like unhappy kittens.
   2. The princess loves her sisters.
   3. The parents punished the unhelpful kids.
   4. The drivers will drive until noon.

Aspect and Definiteness. Languages make another very important distinction that relates to time beyond tense (past/present). This distinction is called **aspect** and concerns the *internal temporal constituency* of an action or situation. A language will almost always offer the speaker the opportunity to treat an action or situation either as a *bounded entity* in time or as *not bounded* in time, but rather ongoing in time (either by extending for a long time, being repeated over and over, or being habitual). The former of these is called **perfective aspect** (treating an action or situation as a bounded entity, as if it were a point in time); the latter is called **imperfective aspect** (treating an action or situation as if it were not bounded, but rather ongoing through time).

Thus, if I say of my cat 'Wicked,' 'Wicked is eating a mouse' or 'Wicked was eating a mouse', I am, in the first case, treating the action of eating as ongoing in the present, and in the second case as ongoing in the past. Thus, these are in the imperfective aspect (usually signaled in English by a form of 'be' and a following verb with the morpheme 'ing' on it). On the other hand, if I say '(Now) Wicked eats a mouse' (imagine a sports cast) or 'Wicked ate a mouse', I am treating the action as bounded, like a point in time, in the present (the former) or in the past (the latter). Thus, these are in the perfective aspect.

Notice that the perfective/imperfective distinction is *not* a matter of how reality works—to eat always takes time. It is just that the language allows us to treat it (eating) either as a point bounded in time (now he eats/then he ate) or as stretching through time (he is eating/he was eating). One should note, however, that action verbs in the simple present tense ('He eats', 'Joan eats a mouse'), except in sports casts, normally do not have a perfective meaning ('he eats everyday' means he eats all the time, habitually, and, thus, is imperfective).

As an aside, let me point out that the term 'perfective aspect' should not be confused (though it often is in books on grammar) with the term 'present perfect' or 'past perfect'. The present perfect in English is seen in a sentence like 'John *has arrived* from Viet Nam'. This form is used for a past event that still has relevance to the present (if the event was felt to be of no current relevance, we would have said 'John arrived from Viet Nam' in the simple past). For the present perfect, English uses the helping verb 'have' plus a main verb ('arrived' in the example above). Not all, or many for that matter, languages do this. The past perfect is 'John *had arrived* from Viet Nam' and is used to name a happening that is in the past (here John's arriving) of some other happening that is itself in the past (this other happening is left implicit in our example sentence, but consider 'John had already arrived from Viet Nam when his child was born'—here John's arrival is past of his child being born and this is, in turn, past of the act of speaking).

A final grammatical distinction we will look at here is that between definite and indefinite object terms. This is the difference between 'A cat ate some mice' (where 'cat' and 'mice' are indefinite) and 'The cat ate the mice' (where 'cat' and 'mice' are definite). An object term is definite if its referent (what it refers to in the world) is already known either from being mentioned in the previous discourse or from the mutual and shared knowledge of the speaker or hearer. It is indefinite if its referent is not already known but is being mentioned for the first time and is not part of the shared knowledge of speaker and hearer.

Thus, if I say 'The cat ate some mice', I assume as speaker that you as hearer can identify what cat I am talking about, either because we have already talked about this cat or because we both know about her (and I know you know). I make no such assumption in the case of the mice. Rather, by using 'some mice', I am saying that you don't already know, cannot already identify, who these mice are.

We can comment now on another trick we have pulled off, almost without trying. We started by saying that we could not just have proper names for things (like 'Joan' and 'Sally') because there were too many things in the world. We needed words for *types* of things (like cats and mice). But now, in sentences uttered in given contexts where we say things like 'The cat ate some mice', we are actually referring to or talking about specific things (that cat, those mice), not just types of things (cats and mice in general). And we are getting to talk about specific things (that cat, those mice) without having to have proper names (like 'Sally' and 'Wicked') for them all.

Many languages do and many do not overtly mark the distinction between definite and indefinite (though all languages assume that such a distinction is being intended and inferred as people speak).

In our invented language, we could add words or morphemes for tense, aspect, and definiteness, creating quite a complex system if we liked.

——————————————— E X E R C I S E ———————————————

Exercise C. It is extremely difficult to say in detail where English uses the definite article ('the') and where the indefinite (the indefinite article is either 'a' or 'an' for singular nouns, and 'some' for plural nouns). Second-language speakers of English whose native languages do not have articles have a difficult time mastering the English system. For each article (underlined) in the sentence below, say why you think English uses this particular article in this position, what it means, and what it would mean to substitute any of the other articles (*the, some,* or no article) for it.

They say that <u>the</u> Russians are a threat to the U.S., but I know <u>some</u> Russians who like Americans; in fact, <u>the</u> Russians in the living room are rather nice, so <u>Russians</u> really aren't all that hostile, are they? (NOTE: in the last case, 'Russians' has no article; treat this as a type of article, namely 'zero' or nothing.)

Historical Change: From Words to Morphemes and Back Again

The different solutions we have seen above look quite diverse. But they are more closely related than you might think. We can only see this relationship if we consider how languages change through time.

Imagine that we have a language that favors adding separate words for the various grammatical notions we have discussed above. It has a word for ACTOR (let's say it is 'TOR'), a word for PATIENT (let's say it is 'PAT'), a word for PLURAL (let's say it is 'AL'), a word for PAST (let's say it is 'AST'), a word for DEFINITE (let's say it is 'THAT'), and a word for INDEFINITE (let's say it is 'SOME'). I pick these words because usually such words in a language are relatively short. So we can have a sentence like 2a in our language:

2a. THAT CAT TOR SOME MOUSE AL PAT EAT AST
  (Gloss: the cat actor some mouse plural eat past;
  Translation: the cat ate some mice)

We can assume that this language is free word order, except that the word for ACTOR (namely, 'TOR') must follow the actor term, and the word for PATIENT (namely, 'PAT') must follow the patient term. 'THAT' and 'SOME' precede the OBJECT terms they go with, and the word for PLURAL (namely, 'AL') follows the OBJECT term it goes with. Thus, we can see that the words in this sentence bunch together as '(THAT CAT TOR) (SOME MOUSE AL PAT) (EAT PAST)', where I have enclosed in parentheses words that go together and function as a unit (what we call a **phrase**).

In all languages, grammatical words tend to be given less stress or emphasis than content words, because in general they carry less salient information. Imagine that children begin to change the language by destressing or otherwise deemphasizing the grammatical words in sentences. Then, for 2a, we would eventually get 2b, by a process of language change. I have put words with stress or emphasis in small capitals and words with little or no stress in lowercase letters. For clarity, I place words that bunch together (which constitute phrases) in parentheses:

2b. (that CAT tor) (some MOUSE al pat) (EAT ast)
  (Gloss: the cat actor one mouse plural eat past;
  Translation: the cat ate some mice)

Words with little or no stress tend to be said faster and faster, and eventually children, over time, will say them as if they were part of another word (usually the word carrying stress that they go with, which are bunched in the same parentheses). When this happens, a new generation of children may not know that a sound sequence like 'TOR' was ever a separate word and may be unwilling to use it as a separate word, only using it as glued onto other words. It has become a morpheme, in fact, a **bound** morpheme, in that it can never be used as a free-standing form by itself or separately from other words.

When children make a destressed word (like 'TOR') part of another word, they tend to reduce its sounds, so 'TOR' might become 'OR', and 'PAT' might become 'AT.' 'THAT' might reduce to 'THA' and 'SOME' to 'OM'. We would then get the following (in the gloss I connect the translations of morphemes that are part of a single word together with hyphens):

2c. (thaCATor) (omMOUSEalat) (EATast)
   (Gloss: the-cat-actor some-mouse-plural-patient eat-past;
   Translation: the cat ate some mice)

Children are, in fact, always trying to speed up languages as they acquire them, since they want their language to be efficient and fast. They also want it to be clear and informative. And their attempts at speeding it up can eventually come into conflict with this need for the language to be clear and informative (if the increased speed causes meaning to become obscured). When they have invented morphemes, as they have just done, they will continue to reduce these morphemes, to integrate them yet more fully into the words they have collapsed them into. This will gain them yet more speed and efficiency.

At the stage represented by 2c, each morpheme has a clear shape and one clear meaning ('tha' = THAT; 'or' = ACTOR; 'om' = SOME; 'al' = PLURAL; 'at' = PATIENT; 'ast' = PAST). So the language is also clear and informative. But imagine that a generation of children begins to reduce 'alat' ('al' + 'at' = PLURAL + PATIENT) in the word 'omMOUSEalat' to just to 'a:t' (with a long 'ah' sound) and then yet further to just 'a'. And imagine they also reduce 'ast' (PAST) in 'EATast' to just 'st'. Then we would get

2d. (thaCATor) (omMOUSEa) (EATst)
   (Gloss: the-cat-actor some-mouse-plural/patient eat-past;
   Translation: the cat ate some mice)

Something important has happened here. We have lost a clear one-to-one mapping between pieces of words (morphemes) and meanings, which we had in 2c. In the word 'omMOUSEa', the morpheme 'a' now has two meanings: PLURAL and PATIENT. And, of course, we cannot tell what part of 'a' means PLURAL and what part means PATIENT (as we could with the previous 'alat'), since it has no parts. It just means PLURAL PATIENT. The two meanings are fused together, and thus meaning is not as clearly displayed as it was before. At this point, the words and the sentence they are in (2d) is fast and efficient, but we are beginning to sacrifice a bit of clarity and informativeness. Languages, however, are willing to go quite far in this direction (but, of course, not indefinitely far).

Languages that keep a clear one-to-one correspondence between their morphemes and meanings (as in 2c) are called **agglutinative** languages. Languages that often fuse meanings together (as in 2d) are called **fusional** or **inflectional** languages. Languages that tend to have separate words (as in 2a and 2b), rather than morphologically complex words, are called **analytic** or **isolating** languages.

Imagine that these changes continue—new generations of children continue to reduce further the sounds in grammatical morphemes (perhaps because the stress is carried by the content morpheme, and so the grammatical morphemes are not salient to the ear). Perhaps 'or' (= ACTOR) becomes just 'o' and perhaps 'st' (= PAST) becomes just 's'. Then we would get

> *2e.* (thaCATO) (omMOUSEa) (EATS)
>   (Gloss: the-cat-actor some-mouse-plural/patient eat-past;
>   Translation: the cat ate some mice)

Often in the history of languages, unstressed vowel sounds at the ends of words begin to disappear. More generally, sounds, vowels, or consonants at the ends of words tend to deteriorate and disappear. Imagine, then, that this happens not only to 'o' (ACTOR) and 'a' (PLURAL PATIENT) but even to 's' (PAST). All these, over time, quit getting said, and disappear from the language. Then we would get

> *2f.* (thaCAT) (omMOUSE) (EAT)
>   (Gloss: the-cat some-mouse eat;
>   Translation: the cat eats/ate some mouse/mice some mouse/mice eats/ate the cat)

We would now have lost the morphemes for ACTOR, PATIENT, PLURAL, and PAST. Furthermore, the language can no longer allow the ACTOR and PATIENT terms ('thaCAT' and 'omMOUSE' in our sentence) to occur in just any order in relation to each other and the ACTION word (as we have assumed up to now they could). This is because, having lost the ACTOR and PATIENT morphemes, there is no way to know whether the cat ate a mouse/mice or a mouse/mice ate the cat (since PLURAL is missing, we also do not know whether it is 'a mouse' or 'mice'; in fact, we probably don't know any longer whether it is 'the cat' or 'the cats').

To get over this problem, let's assume that children introduce a rule that stipulates ACTOR PATIENT ACTION word order; that is, one must say sentences in this language now with the words in this order. So the sentence in 2f will be taken to just mean 'the cat or the cats eat or ate a mouse or mice' (we still have no PLURAL or PAST).

New generations of children may now go on to add a new word for PAST, or may just leave the language without any tense markers (the language could always just specify a time in the past, if it had to, by saying YESTERDAY, YEARS AGO, and so forth). They may add a word for PLURAL, or perhaps leave the language with no such marking. Let's imagine they add a word for PAST (say FINISH), and a word for PLURAL (say ALL). Then we would get

2g. (thaCAT) (omMOUSE ALL) (EAT FINISH)
(Gloss: the-cat one-mouse plural eat past;
Translation: the cat ate some mice)

We are beginning to arrive back where we began. We have moved from a free word-order language, with lots of separate words, through a language with morphemes but a clear one-to-one relationship between morphemes and meanings, to a language without such a clear one-to-one relationship, and finally to a language with less morphemes and rigid word order. I show our progression below, a progression that would, of course, have taken hundreds or thousands of years:

2a. (THAT CAT TOR) (SOME MOUSE AL PAT) (EAT AST)
(free word order)

2b. (that CAT tor) (some MOUSE al pat) (EAT ast)
(free word order)

2c. (thaCATor) (omMOUSEalat) (EATast)
(free word order)

2d. (thaCATor) (omMOUSEa) (EATst)
(free word order)

2e. (thaCATo) (omMOUSEa) (EATs)
(free word order)

2f. (thaCAT) (omMOUSE) (EAT)
(rigid word order: ACTOR PATIENT ACTION)

2g. (thaCAT) (omMOUSE ALL) (EAT FINISH)
(rigid word order: ACTOR PATIENT ACTION)

Of course, children could introduce new words for ACTOR and PATIENT, thus freeing once again the word order of the language from having to do this job. Imagine they introduce 'BY' for ACTOR and 'TAKE' for PATIENT. We would get, at last

2h. (thaCAT BY) (omMOUSE ALL TAKE) (EAT FINISH)
(free word order)
(Gloss: the-cat actor some-mouse plural patient eat past;
Translation: the cat ate some mice)

This is virtually where we began (different words, but same overall pattern or form, that is, the same syntax as the language we started with). Languages undergo just these sorts of changes all the time. However, you cannot assume that the changes start where we started. They can start at any point in the progression we have described. It is actually a circle, and you can get back to any point from which you started by following such changes as reducing the stress or saliency of words, reducing unstressed or unsalient words to morphemes, reducing the sounds that carry morphemes within words, losing morphemes, stipulating a word order, adding words again, freeing word order, and so on, over and over again.

─────────────── E X E R C I S E S ───────────────

Exercise D. Sentence 2 below is a fast-speech version of sentence 1. Sentence 3 is a version of sentences 1 and 2 that is common in several non-standard dialects of English:

1. He will get her for that.
2. He'll-get-er for that. ('He'll-get-er' is said as one word.)
3. My brother, he'll-get-er for that.

Now imagine that in addition to 3, some dialect began to say something like sentence 4 quite regularly (meaning that my brother will get Susan for something she did):

4. My brother he'll-get-er Susan for that.

While no dialect in English that I know regularly says things like sentence 4, this does happen in many languages and is certainly a possible change in English, for some dialects. Imagine that such a change happened and that, in fact, 4 became the normal and usual way in that dialect to say that 'my brother is going to get Susan'. Once this dialect has moved to saying things like 4, how would you describe the morphemes 'he' and 'er' in this dialect? How do you think this dialect would say 'My sister is going to get Johnny for that'? How do you think it would say 'My brother is going to get Johnny for that'? What hypothesis does this example give you about the historical origins of (some) agreement morphemes in language?

Exercise E. The data below is from Hungarian. The morphemes in a word are connected by a hyphen (thus, for example, 'haz-ban' is one word with two morphemes in it). Answer the questions below the data:

a haz	the house	a haz-ak	the houses
a haz-ban	in the house	a haz-ak-ban	in the houses
a haz-uk-ban	in their house	a haz-ik-ban	in their houses

1. What is the morpheme for 'house'?
2. What is the morpheme for 'in'?

3. What is the morpheme for PLURAL?

4. What is the morpheme for 'their'?

5. What is the morpheme for DEFINITE? (in English both 'the house' and 'their house' are DEFINITE; that is, both 'the' and 'their' make the noun phrase they are attached to DEFINITE).

6. The form 'a haz-ik-ban', meaning *in their houses,* is odd given the rest of the data. What is odd about it? How do you think 'a haz-ik-ban' used to be said at some earlier stage of the language? Why do you think that it ended up being said the way it is?

States

So far we have said nothing about states. What if we want to introduce states into the language we have been building? Not surprisingly, we have several choices. However, the choices are somewhat different here.

Take a state like *being tall. Being tall* is a relatively permanent and stable state, one that does not change quickly (tall things tend to stay tall). So we could treat tallness as a special sort of object term and introduce the word 'TALL' as an object term, just like 'CAT' and 'ROCK'. We could, then, also introduce a word, let's say 'HAVE', meaning *to possess.* Just as someone (say Mary, a person) can possess a cat, and we could say 'Mary has a cat', so we might then say, for the meaning *Mary is tall,* MARY HAS TALL (much like English 'Mary has tallness'), where we are treating 'TALL' as an object term, and Mary is thought of as having tallness in something like the way she can have a cat, a bruise, or a haircut. English takes this solution sometimes (though not with *being tall*). We can say 'Mary has a cold', as if the cold were an object (it is really a condition or state Mary is in, however).

To see another sort of solution, consider a state like *being happy.* This is a state that can change relatively rapidly. It is rather mobile. So we could introduce 'HAPPY' as a special sort of happening term (a process term like 'dying'). We could then say, in our new language, of Mary when she is happy, 'MARY HAPPY' (just as we could say of Mary dying: 'MARY DIE'), and of Mary when she was happy in the past, 'MARY PAST HAPPY' (just as 'MARY PAST DIE'). These are to be interpreted as if English were to say 'Mary happies' (meaning *Mary is happy*) or 'Mary happied' (meaning *Mary was happy*). Of course, Mary's being happy is not really a happening, but a state Mary is in, but we are treating it, sort of by courtesy, as if it were a happening.

English does not do this for *being happy,* but it does it for mental states people are in, like 'Mary *loves* John', 'John *hates* Bill', 'Susan *knows* French'. These latter we treat just like they were actions, as if in loving John, Mary is doing something to him, but they are in reality no such thing. 'Mary loves John' does not really pick out an act that Mary is doing in the world, rather it picks out the fact that Mary is in the state of, or has the property of, *being in love* with John. Again, however, language is free to treat anything as if it were something else, free to take what perspectives it likes (within the limits set by our human biology and the human need to communicate effectively).

Finally, as a third sort of solution, we could introduce for some or all states another category of words, besides action terms and object terms, namely *state terms*. Words like 'HAPPY', 'SICK', 'TALL', and 'ANGRY' can just be state terms and will be considered to hook up to the conditions things are in or the properties things have. English often does this, connecting the state term to an object term in a sentence by use of the little word 'be', which also signals the tense (past or present): 'Mary *is* happy' or 'Mary *was* happy', where 'happy' is a special term for a state Mary is in.

Most languages, if they have special state terms (like English does), also treat some states as if they were objects and give them object terms and treat some states as if they were happenings (processes or actions) and give them happening (action or process) terms, as we did in our first two solutions above.

Two Major Types of Morphemes

We have seen above how the *grammatical* words or morphemes in a sentence organize the way in which the other words or morphemes in the sentence, the *content* words and morphemes, tie to the world, the speaker and hearer, or to the previous discourse. Grammatical words and morphemes relate not directly to the world (as content words do) but say something about other words in the sentence (for example, that some object term is naming the ACTOR or PATIENT), or about the relationship of the sentence they are in to the previous discourse (for example, 'the' says that the referent of an object term has already been mentioned in the previous discourse), or about the way the sentence relates to the speaker and hearer (for example, that the happening happened in the past or present of the speaker's utterance). They therefore organize how the sentence is internally structured (how the words in it relate to each other) and how the sentence relates to other sentences in the discourse and to the speaker and hearer. That is why we call them *grammatical* words or morphemes.

Let's leave aside for a moment free-standing grammatical words like 'the' and concentrate on grammatical morphemes that are bound to other words (like the plural marker 's' on 'boys' or the past-tense marker 'ed' on 'kissed'). All the bound grammatical morphemes we have looked at so far (for tense, aspect, singular/plural, or definite/indefinite, which is free-standing in English in the guise of 'the' and 'a', but a bound morpheme in lots of other languages) represent only one type of grammatical morpheme. There is also another major type of bound grammatical morpheme.

All of the bound grammatical morphemes we have looked at so far are called inflectional morphemes. This name distinguishes them from another type of bound grammatical morpheme we have not yet discussed: **derivational morphemes.**

Inflectional morphemes (all the ones we have seen so far) do not really change the meaning of a word they attach to. They just tell us something about how that word relates to the other words in the sentence, or to the previous discourse, or to the knowledge of the speaker and hearer. But some grammatical morphemes in a language do change the meaning of the word they attach to, and these are called derivational morphemes.

Inflectional morphemes, like the plural '-s', the present (also '-s' in the third-person singular, no '-s' added elsewhere), and past '-ed' in English, just give us *different forms* of the *same word* when they attach to a word. Thus, 'kisses' (present) in 'Mary *kisses* John' and 'kissed' (past) in 'Mary *kissed* John' are different forms of one word 'kiss' (note 'I kiss', 'you kiss', 'he/she/it kisses', 'we kiss', 'you kiss', 'they kiss' in the present and 'I kissed', 'you kissed', 'he/she/it kissed', 'we kissed', 'you kissed', and 'they kissed' in the past).

Derivational morphemes, on the other hand, when they attach to a word, change that word into a different (but related) word. For example, suppose that I want to say, in English, that someone did something over again (for example, that they painted a room over again). I could just say 'They painted the room over again', using separate words. But English also allows me to add a morpheme to an action term to mean *do over again.* This morpheme is 're-', which is attached to the beginnings of action words, as in 'repaint'. So I can say 'They repainted the room'. 'Paint' and 'repaint' are not different forms of the same word, rather they are different (but related) words. 'Paint' and 'repaint' have different meanings (the first means *to cover something with paint,* the second *to cover something with paint that has already been covered with paint).* 'Re-' is a derivational morpheme (it derives one word from another word, as in 'repaint' from 'paint').

A morpheme like 're-' changes the meaning of the word it is attached to. To *repaint* is a different thing than to *paint* (to "repaint a wall" there must have been paint on the wall already; this is not so in the case of painting a wall). On the other hand, an inflectional morpheme like the plural '-s' on 'cats' does not change the meaning of the word 'cat' at all. Many cats and one cat are all just members of the feline species. The plural '-s' just tells us that the sentence is about more than one cat. An inflectional morpheme like the past '-ed' on 'kicked' does not change in any way the sort of action kicking is; it just situates this action in relation to the act of utterance differently than 'kicks' does.

Derivational morphemes, then, can change the meaning of a word. They can also do something else. They can change the *category* of a word, the type of word it is. For example, English allows me to take any action term (say 'bake' as in 'bake a cake') and add the morpheme '-er' to the end of it. When I do this, I change the action term 'bake' into an object term, 'baker'. This new object term means *a person or thing that engages in the action designated by the action term to which '-er' was attached* (thus 'baker' means *one who engages in the act of baking).*

So the morpheme '-er' attaches to a word of one category (an action term, a term designating an action) and makes it into a word of another category (an object term, a word designating an object). This new word, 'baker', thanks to the derivational morpheme '-er', can be used wherever object terms can be used: for example, 'A baker hit John'. The morpheme '-er' has effectively turned an action word into an object word.

So derivational morphemes either change the meaning of a word or change the type of word it is. On the other hand, inflectional morphemes simply relate the word to the other words in the sentence, to the discourse, or to the speaker and hearer's knowledge. The distinction is subtle at points, and linguists argue all the time over exactly how to draw it.

EXERCISES

Exercise F. Divide each of the underlined words in the sentences below into their constituent morphemes and say for each morpheme whether it is an inflectional morpheme or a derivational morpheme.

1. John is mistrusting of bankers.
2. You have repainted the room beautifully.
3. He has computerized all the information we use.
4. John's unhelpfulness is discouraging his students.

Exercise G. Is the morpheme 'ful' in 'beautiful' and 'truthful' a derivational morpheme or an inflectional morpheme? How does this morpheme work; that is, what sorts of words is it added to, what sorts of words does it create from them, and what effect does it have on meaning (if any)?

Grammatical Categories

So far, we have constructed our imaginary language so that it has object terms, happening terms (action and process terms), and state terms. We have distinguished between grammatical words and morphemes on the one hand, and content words and morphemes on the other.

But English (and many other languages) does something very odd in this regard. The word 'pretty' is quite similar in meaning to 'beauty'. English treats 'beauty' as if it were an object term, saying things like 'Mary has beauty' (compare to 'Mary has a book'—'have' is used to connect objects to people who own them). But English does not do this for 'pretty'. Rather, English treats 'pretty' as a state term, not an object term. So we do not say 'Mary has pretty', but rather we say

'Mary is pretty' (but not 'Mary is beauty'). Furthermore, we can say 'Mary is a pretty person', but *not* 'Mary is a beauty person'. So we treat 'pretty' as a state term and 'beauty' as an object term. Why?

To get at the root of this problem, we need to see that, in fact, there are *two separate ways* we can talk about object terms, action terms, and state terms. First, we can define them in terms of how they hook up to the world (in terms of their meanings). Object terms designate types of objects, action terms designate types of actions, and state terms designate types of states or conditions things are in. This is how we have been talking about these terms so far.

A second way we can define these categories of words (object, action, state words), however, is by looking at what formal properties they have, not what meanings they have in relation to the world. By 'formal' properties I mean the ways in which these different sorts of terms are treated in sentences, the relationships they enter into with other words and morphemes in the sentence. For example, object terms can be accompanied by morphemes or words that signal whether the object term designates one thing (singular) or more than one thing (plural). On the other hand, action terms can be accompanied by morphemes or words that signal whether the action is in the past of the act of speaking or concurrent with it (present). Action terms do not take marking for singular and plural, and object terms do not take marking for past and present.

These sorts of relationships (object terms with singular or plural marking; action terms with past and present marking) are what I will call **formal** properties. They are formal because they involve structural or patterned relationships into which forms enter ('form' is a word used to designate words or morphemes). Formal properties involve not just talking about the meaning or function of the form, but rather about relationships into which the form enters with other forms (like the fact that action terms can take present and past morphemes and object terms cannot).

To see this second way of discussing object, action, and state terms, consider the different formal properties these terms have—the different ways they are treated in sentences, the different relationships they enter into. Table 5-2 lists the various patterned, structural, or formal relationships (they all mean the same thing) into which object terms, action terms, and state terms enter. We have discussed all of these above. Any given language may display all of these or only some of them, and there are others we could have mentioned. Furthermore, as we have seen, a language can use morphemes, separate words, or sometimes word order to signal these relationships.

Given a list of formal properties as in Table 5-2, we can define object terms not by what they designate in the world, but by their having the formal properties listed (that is, taking singular and plural marking; taking definite and indefinite marking; taking marking as ACTOR or PATIENT). The same is true for action terms and state terms. A word can be *treated* as an object term, an action term, or a state term just by being allowed to have the formal properties associated with these

TABLE 5-2.   Formal Relationships (Patterns) into which Object Terms, Action Terms, and State Terms Enter

OBJECT TERMS	ACTION TERMS	STATE TERMS
Marked for singular or plural (e.g., cat/cats)	Marked for tense: present or past (e.g., kiss/kissed)	Occurs after BE (e.g., 'is happy')
Marked for definite or indefinite (e.g., the boy/a boy)	Marked for aspect: perfective or imperfective (e.g., kissed/kissing)	Can be placed in front of an object term (e.g., 'a happy boy')
Marked for being an ACTOR or PATIENT (e.g., SVO order in 'Mary hit John'; or case in 'She hit him')	Marked for agreement with ACTOR and/or PATIENT (e.g., 'John likes Mary', or 'JOHN heLIKEher MARY')	Cannot be directly marked for past or present tense (e.g., 'Mary is/was happy', but not 'Mary happies' or 'Mary happied')

categories (by the company we let it keep, regardless of whether it has the right meaning or function).

Imagine I have a word 'glub'. You have no idea what it means, but I tell you the following sentence is grammatical: 'Mary felt the glubs'. Since 'glub' here is marked for definiteness (the presence of 'the'), plurality (the following '-s') and occurs where PATIENTS normally do (after the ACTION term), then 'glub' counts as an object term. This is a perfect example of how *formal* definitions work: You have no idea what 'glub' means, but you know by the way it patterns or works in the sentence that it counts as an object term.

You might say, "Well, at least I can conclude it names an object or thing, can't I?" No, not really. It doesn't matter. If I told you 'grub' meant *the presence of a dead ancestor,* so that our sentence meant that Mary felt the presences of dead ancestors, 'grub' would still count as an object term, whether or not it makes any real sense to consider a presence of a dead ancestor as an object (which it probably doesn't).

It is as if we defined, in a given society, males and females by how they dressed, and for a time biological males always dressed as males and biological females always dressed as females. Then, all of a sudden, some biological males dressed like females and some biological females dressed like males. So we decided to *count* as a female anyone who dressed as a female (regardless of their biological gender) and anyone who dressed as a male as a male (regardless of their biological gender). Perhaps we did this because it was too much trouble, or too unimportant, to actually determine biological gender.

Likewise, any word gets to count as an object term if it wears the right clothes—shows the right formal properties. Thus, take a concept like 'honor'. English will allow it to wear the clothes appropriate to an object term: 'Mary received the *honor* due her' (note that 'honor' is marked as definite with 'the' and is placed after the action term the way PATIENTS normally are). English will also allow it to wear the clothes appropriate to an action term: 'Mary *honored* her mother' (note that 'honor' is marked for past tense with the ending '-ed' and occurs after the ACTOR and before the PATIENT, where action terms normally do). If we add the derivational morpheme '-able' to 'honor', English will allow it to wear the clothes appropriate to a state term: 'Mary is *honorable*', '*Honorable* people don't lie' (note that 'honorable' occurs after BE and can be placed in front of an object term; further it cannot have tense placed on it: *'Mary honorabled'; here and elsewhere I use an asterisk to mark sentences, words, or phrases that are unacceptable—see Chapter 6). It does not matter much exactly what sort of thing, action, state, or whatever you really think 'honor' is in the world. The language dresses it different ways for different purposes. And the word gets to be what it dresses like.

Since our terms are now defined formally, and not in terms of what they designate in the world, the names we have used for them (object, action, and state terms) are not very appropriate (since they refer to what these terms designate in the world). So we can substitute new and more neutral names. We will call object terms **nouns;** we will call action terms **verbs;** and we will call state terms **adjectives.**

A noun is *not* to be defined as the name of a person, place, or thing (in terms of meaning). This would be to define it in terms of what it designates in the world (what it means). We have seen that this is not how English actually works (or most other languages). Rather, a noun is defined as a word wearing noun clothes, that is, as a word behaving in sentences like a noun (that is, behaving the way terms that prototypically do designate objects behave). A word is a noun just so long as it has the formal properties of nouns.

One and the same word can be both a noun and a verb if it is allowed to wear both sets of clothes. Thus, consider the sentence 'The great *honors* greatly *honored* Mary'. Here the first 'honor' is a noun because it is wearing noun clothes, and the second 'honor' is a verb because it is wearing verb clothes. By the way, the first 'great' is an adjective because it is wearing adjective clothes and the second 'great' ('greatly') is what is called an **adverb,** since it is wearing adverb clothes (in the case of an adverb like 'greatly', these clothes amount to the following: can occur before a verb, can take the ending '-ly'. Other sorts of adverbs can wear somewhat different clothes). In fact, one way to think about adverbs is that they are just state terms that are connected to verbs rather than to nouns; state terms connected to nouns are what we have called adjectives.

This little scenario in which we have first defined categories of words by how they relate to the world (object, action, and state terms), attributed to them formal properties that they obtain by getting into sentences, and then turned around and redefined our terms in terms of these formal properties themselves (noun, verb, and adjective), may be more meaningful than may at first sight appear. This may be just the way children proceed in acquiring a language and the way languages have developed throughout history.

Perhaps children first learn that words like 'cat', 'dog', and 'rock' are nouns because they name prototypical objects in the world, and then later accept the fact that words like 'beauty', 'honor', and 'truth' are nouns because they act grammatically like (enter into the same sorts of relationships as, wear the same clothes as) nouns that actually do designate prototypical objects (like 'cat', 'dog', and 'rock'). Children don't actually need to ask philosophical questions about what sort of object, if any, 'truth' is (though they can grow up to be philosophers and ask the question). The same is true for action, process, and state terms.

Subject and Object: Grammatical Relations

The trick that language uses to set up the category of nouns, verbs, and adjectives (that anything that wears the right clothes gets to be what it dresses like) is also used to define another set of important grammatical notions. We have seen that any language needs to signal clearly in a sentence which participant is the ACTOR and which participant is the PATIENT. In English, we do this by placing the ACTOR first, the action word second, and the PATIENT third (for example, 'Mary kicked John').

Once a language treats ACTORS and PATIENTS in certain ways (gives them certain clothes), then other things can "mimic" them by putting on their clothes. Thus, we can say things like 'Mary loves John', where 'Mary' is in first position, like an ACTOR, and 'John' is in the position after the verb, like a PATIENT. Further, the verb ('loves') agrees with 'Mary' (by the presence of the '-s' attached to the end of the verb), just as it does in 'Mary kicks John', where we have a clear ACTOR ACTION PATIENT sentence.

But 'Mary loves John' is not an action and 'Mary' is not really designating an ACTOR (Mary is not really doing anything, rather she is feeling something) and 'John' is not really designating a PATIENT (John is not having anything done to him, in fact he may not even be aware that Mary has any attitude toward him). What is happening here is that 'loves' is wearing the clothes of an action term, though 'love' is not really an action. That is why we count it as a verb. 'Mary' is wearing the clothes of an ACTOR and 'John' is wearing the clothes of a PATIENT, even though Mary and John are not really ACTORS and PATIENTS here.

Just as we wanted labels for object, action, and state words that designated them without appealing to their meanings (and so invented the terms 'noun', 'verb', and 'adjective'), so here too we need more meaning-neutral labels for ACTOR and PATIENT. We will call anything that is wearing the ACTOR clothes in a sentence the **subject** of the verb of the sentence and anything that is wearing the PATIENT clothes the **direct object** of the verb of the sentence (for short, just **subject** and **object**). It is unfortunate that the word 'object' here is the same as the word for "thing, entity" (like cats, dogs, rocks, and chairs) that we used earlier (when we used the phrase 'object term', now replaced by the label NOUN). But the word 'object' in 'direct object' has nothing (in current practice) to do with the word 'object' in the phrase 'physical object'.

Subject and direct object are said to be **grammatical relations**—they are *relationships* that nouns or noun phrases have to the verb of the sentence they are in.

—————————————— E X E R C I S E S ——————————————

Exercise H.   English uses the morpheme '-ing' a great deal. This morpheme shows up on nouns, verbs, and adjectives. Label each underlined word in the sentences below as a noun, verb, or adjective and state what formal property or properties told you this.

1. The <u>shining</u> light hurt my eyes.
2. John is <u>shining</u> a light.
3. The <u>shining</u> of the light meant that the redcoats are coming.
4. The light was <u>shining</u> brightly.

Exercise I.   Consider the sentence 'John received a blow to the head from Sam'. Do you think children would learn this sort of sentence late or early? Why? English has ACTIVE ('Mary kissed John') and PASSIVE ('John was kissed by Mary') versions of most of its sentences. This sentence ('John received a blow to the head from Sam') is not a passive sentence, but how is it like a passive sentence? Do you think that passives are learned early or late by children? Why?

5.2.   WORDS

It turns out to be very difficult to define the notion of a word, despite the fact that we have been freely using this term throughout our discussion. In writing, English words are usually printed with spaces between them, but this is not true of the writing systems of all languages. And this characteristic is not at all helpful in dealing with speech or languages that have never been written down.

I will use the following, rather awkward, definition of a word: A word in English is any string of sounds that can be separated from what precedes and what follows it in a sentence by other words. A similar definition will work for most languages. This is fairly clumsy, and it uses the term 'word' in the definition itself. However, it will do for our purposes.

Thus, if you want to know whether the string of sounds 'the' in the English sentence 'Mary likes *the* boys' is a word, you can prove that it is a word by showing that other words can separate it from what precedes and what follows (for example, 'Mary likes *all* the boys' and 'Mary likes the *happy* boys'). On the other hand, consider 'ful' in 'unhelpful'. This string of sounds cannot be separated from what precedes it: 'unhelpful', but never *'unhelp<u>o</u>ful' (compare 'not *full* of hope', where 'full' is a word).

Another, related, test of a word is this: Hesitaters like 'you know' or 'hum' (which involve pausing as well) can precede or follow anything that is a word, but not anything that is not a word. Thus, consider 'the' again in 'Mary likes *the* boys'. The word 'the' here can be separated from what precedes and follows it by hesitaters: 'Mary likes, hum, the boys' and 'Mary likes the, hum, boys', but never, *'unhelp, hum, ful'.

These tests may seem trivial, but, in fact, they give some interesting results. Some things that might look like words turn out not to be words. In the sentence 'Mary likes'em' (the fast-speech version of 'Mary likes them'), you cannot separate 'em' from 'likes': *'Mary likes, hum, 'em' or *'Mary likes, you know, 'em'. Thus, ''em' is part of the word 'likes 'em' (it is a morpheme in that word) and not a separate word.

On the other hand, some things that seem not to be single words turn out to be single words. Take 'air condition' in the sentence 'Mary wants to *air condition* her room'. Here 'air' cannot be separated from 'condition': *'Mary wants to air, you know, condition her room'. So 'air condition' is in fact one word. Cases like 'air condition', where two forms that in other situations are separate words (namely 'air' as in 'I don't like the *air* in here' and 'condition' as in 'I *condition* my body') function together as a single word ('air condition') are called **compound words.**

Compound words in English often look just like *phrases*. A phrase is a combination of two or more separate words that pattern structurally and meaningfully together, as in 'the happy boy', but that do not function as a single word. A compound word, on the other hand, is made up of two things that in other contexts are separate words, but that function together as a single word ('air condition', 'blackboard', 'bluebird', 'pay phone', 'troublemaker', 'cover-up', 'breakup', 'waterbed', and many more—as you can see, they are written in a variety of inconsistent ways).

To see the similarities and differences between phrases and compounds in English, consider the compound 'blackboard' (a board made of a material like slate that is suitable for writing on with chalk, which is often black but may be other colors, like green) versus the phrase 'a black board' (a board, for example a piece of wood, that is black in color). Note that, using the compound word, the sentence 'My blackboard at school is actually green' is not a contradiction, while, using the phrase, the sentence 'The carpenter's black board is actually green' is a contradiction. This is so because the compound 'blackboard' does not mean *a board that is black* but *a board you can write on with chalk.*

In American English, the compound 'blackboard' and the phrase 'black board' are stressed differently. In the compound, the greater degree of stress (saliency, emphasis) is on 'black': BLACKboard. In the phrase, the greater degree of stress is on the word 'board': a black BOARD. This is generally true: Compounds take more stress on their first term and phrases take more stress on their last term (as long as it is a content word), though there are plenty of exceptions to this generalization in actual speech.

Alongside phrases and compounds, we can consider the case of **idioms**. Idioms are phrases that contain forms that pass as separate words, but the idiom has a meaning that does not follow from the meanings of these separate words. That is, in the case of idioms, we have separate words that have lost their individual meanings and have taken on a unitary meaning as a group. Thus, consider 'kick the bucket' meaning *to die* in 'Fred kicked the bucket'. Here 'kick' and 'the' and 'bucket' are separate words but do not have their normal meanings in this phrase. Rather, they take on a single unitary meaning as a group: *to die.* Other idioms are 'to let the cat out of the bag', 'to keep tabs on', 'to cry wolf', 'to have a cow', 'to do a slow burn', 'to go out of one's mind', 'to come back to one's senses', and so on through thousands of cases.

5.3.   A FORM-BASED DEFINITION OF MORPHEMES

Linguists often define the term 'morpheme' as *the smallest meaningful parts of a word (or the word by itself if it has no smaller meaningful parts)*. Thus, in 'unhelpful', 'un', 'help', and 'ful' are morphemes; and the word 'boy' is only a single morpheme long, while 'boys' is made up of two morphemes, 'boy' and 's' (for plural).

This definition defines 'morpheme' in terms of meaning (*smallest meaningful part*). But we have already seen that definitions couched in terms of *meaning,* rather than *form* or pattern, are liable to be somewhat problematic in dealing with human language. And, indeed, this definition runs into trouble.

Consider the word 'cranberry'. 'Berry' is clearly a morpheme here, with an obvious meaning (a little round fruit of a certain type). But what is 'cran'? It has no meaning ('cran' in 'cranberry' used to mean *crane*—a stork-like bird; people thought that the flowers on cranberry plants looked like little cranes). Yet 'cran' clearly seems to be a discrete part of the word 'cranberry'. Why do we say that it seems to be a discrete part of the word? Because 'berry' clearly is meaningful, and when we take it off 'cranberry' we are left with just 'cran'. Further, there are a series of words like 'strawberry', 'gooseberry', 'cranberry', 'raspberry', and 'blackberry', from which we can extract 'berry', which they all have in common. Of course, this leaves us with 'straw', 'goose', 'cran', 'rasp', and 'black', only the last of which is clearly meaningful (for example, what have 'strawberries' got to do with straw?).

Or consider the word 'conceive'. This word was borrowed into English from

Latin, where it had two clear meaningful morphemes in it: 'con' and 'ceive' ('con' meant *with* and 'ceive' meant to *take, grasp,* so the word meant *to grasp with the mind*). However, most English speakers have no idea what 'con' and 'ceive' mean, they only know that 'conceive' as a whole has a meaning in English. However, they sense that 'conceive' has two parts, because they know words like 'deceive', 'receive', and 'perceive', all of which share 'ceive' with 'conceive', though they have no idea what 'ceive' means. However, by the operation of comparing 'conceive', 'receive', 'deceive', and 'perceive', they can segment these words into parts: con-ceive; re-ceive; de-ceive; per-ceive (since they all share the part 'ceive'). This segmentation is purely formal (= form based: based on perceptions of patterns—the common presence of 'ceive'), not based directly on meaning, just as the segmenting of 'cran' out of 'cranberry' was a formal (form-based) operation.

While for most purposes the definition of morphemes as the smallest meaningful parts of words will work, we can see from these latter cases ('cranberry' and 'conceive') that we actually need a form-based, not a meaning-based, definition of morpheme. This form-based definition would be something like *the parts into which words can be segmented based on either meaning or patterns in the language* (like 'conceive', 'receive', 'deceive', 'perceive'). Once again, we see that language is a formal (patterned, structured) space for humans, not just a domain of meaning that ties to the world.

There is yet a further problem. All along, I have talked as if morphemes, like plural 's' or the derivational morpheme '-er', are attached to meaningful words. So, consider the word 'baker' (one who engages in the act of baking). Here, clearly, the suffix '-er' is attached to the word (verb) 'bake' to yield the word 'baker' (noun). And this is true of many such words ('runner' from 'run'; 'walker' from 'walk'; 'lover' from 'love'; 'player' from 'play', etc.). But now consider the word 'butcher' (a person who cuts meat), which clearly seems to end in the same '-er' morpheme. But once we take this '-er' off the word 'butcher', we get 'butch', which is, unfortunately, meaningless and not a word. Here, then, '-er' is attached to something that is not a word. We can call 'butch' a **root,** using the term 'root' for things that inflectional and derivational morphemes attach to. Roots are usually words, but not always (as 'butcher' shows). In many languages, unlike English, roots are often not words.

I will close this section by defining a few technical terms having to do with morphemes:

Bound morpheme: A morpheme that can never occur as a separate word ('-ness' in 'happiness', the '-s' morpheme for plural in 'cats', or the '-ing' morpheme for imperfective aspect in 'kissing')

Free morpheme: A morpheme that can occur as a separate word, though it may also occur as part of a larger word ('help' in 'help' or in 'unhelpful', 'rest' in 'rest' and 'resting', or 'boy' in 'boy' and 'boys')

Suffix: A morpheme that is added to the end of a word (the '-s' morpheme for plural in 'cats', the '-ed' morpheme for past in 'kissed', or the '-ness' in 'happiness')

Prefix: A morpheme that is added to the front of a word ('re-' in 'repaint' or 'un-' in 'unhappy')

Affix: A suffix or prefix (There are also "infixes," affixes that are added to the middle of a word, but English does not use these.)

——————————— **E X E R C I S E** ———————————

Exercise J. Divide the following words into their component morphemes. You need to consider both meaning and formal patterns.

deception	nation	morphemic
phoneme	nationalist	phonemic
butcher	reception	national
singer	morpheme	nationalistic

HINTS: The morpheme 'morph' means *form* or *shape* and the morpheme 'phon' means *sound*.

5.4.   FROM MORPHEMES TO SENTENCES

Through historical change, a form can, through time, move from being a word to being a morpheme. For example, the English morpheme 'hood' (as in 'statehood', 'parenthood', 'nationhood', 'neighborhood', 'childhood', 'knighthood', 'priest-hood') used to be a separate word, meaning *condition* or *state* or *body of people sharing the same condition.* Thus, we can imagine a stage in the language in which 'priest hood' was a phrase meaning *body of people sharing the condition of being priests* (= 'priestly condition'). This phrase may eventually have occurred commonly enough that the two words began to be treated as a compound word (= 'priest-hood'). Then, at the next stage of development, 'hood' may have been felt as a morpheme in a single noncompound word (= 'priesthood'), like '-ful' in 'helpful', still recognizably related to the word 'hood' (which we assume could still occur as a separate word in other cases, as 'full' does), but beginning to lose a bit of the robustness of its meaning and form. Then, let us imagine, 'hood' ceases to occur in any situations as a separate word and people no long really recognize its meaning. They see it just as a morpheme that occurs in words like 'knighthood' and 'childhood' and 'priesthood', changing the meaning of a noun like 'child' into the meaning *state of being a child*. Now 'hood' is a bound derivational morpheme.

For another example, consider what has been happening in Tok Pisin, an English-based pidgin language spoken in Papua New Guinea. Over the last decade or so, it has been becoming a creole. (For the terms 'pidgin' and 'creole', see Chapter 9—a pidgin is a simplified language used for trade or as common medium of communication among members of a society who do not share a single language; it is always a second language. Under certain conditions, children may have to learn this pidgin as their first, or native, language. When they do this, they add complexity to the pidgin, and the language they actually acquire is called a creole, not a pidgin, since it is more complex than the pidgin, in fact, as complex as any other language used as a native language.)

In earlier Tok Pisin, the phrase 'by and by' was used to signal the meaning *future,* as in 'By and by, he go', much like the English adverb 'Tomorrow, he goes' (since Tok Pisin is a pidgin based on English, it uses mostly English words for its vocabulary). Eventually, 'by and by' was said faster and faster: 'Bymby, he go', 'Baim, he go'. Then it was moved to in front of the verb: 'He bai go', where it was further reduced in form and used with reduced stress. At this stage it is functioning like a function/grammatical word (like English 'will' in 'He will go', for instance). Currently, children who speak the newer creole version of Tok Pisin reduce 'baim' (old 'by and by') further and treat it as just part of the verb, and presumably consider it a bound morpheme for *future tense,* the way that '-ed' in English 'kissed' is a morpheme for *past tense:* 'He baGO'. Thus, through time, Tok Pisin has moved from a phrase 'by and by' to a function word 'baim' to a bound prefix 'ba'.

Thus, we see that words in sentences, though separate forms, have a tendency over time to get more and more closely caught up with each other and eventually to fall together. They can, in fact, collapse, and eventually disappear altogether. Thus, in English, 'John has gone' can become 'John's gone', which is ambiguous between 'John has gone' and 'John is gone'. There is a process in English in many dialects by which a final /s/ sound in a consonant cluster (like the /ns/ at the end of 'John's') is deleted. This gives us 'John gone'. If this happened regularly (which in most dialects it does not), then the function word 'has' would have become a morpheme ('John's gone') and then disappeared altogether ('John gone'). Such things happen quite often in the history of all languages.

The discussion above teaches us that there is not as much difference between a sentence and a word as you might think. A sentence is made up of words that have, over time, a tendency to collapse into each other; a word is often made up of morphemes that used to be words. The sentence 'He is not happy' is made up of four words. But 'He's unhappy' is made up of only two. The sentence 'She will not own up to them' is made up of seven words; 'she'll disown'em' is made up of two, but means something quite similar and is at least as complex in meaning as the preceding sentence.

5.5. WORD FORMATION RULES

Morphologically complex words, like 'unhelpful' or 'repaintings', are put together in a rule-governed fashion. That is, we must state for each language what possibilities exist for building complex words (if any). In this section, we look at what is involved in such a description for English.

We have seen that grammatical morphemes come in two varieties: inflectional (like plural '-s', past '-ed', imperfective '-ing', etc.) and derivational (like 're-' in 'repaint', 'un-' in 'unhappy', or '-ness' in 'happiness'). A large part of describing how complex words are built in English is a description of how these grammatical morphemes work, as they are the key device used to build up complex words.

Consider the following morphemes: 'un-', '-ness', and the plural '-s'. What can we say about each of these? There are, in fact, two different morphemes in English that are pronounced as 'un-'. One attaches to adjectives, like 'happy', 'pleasant', 'real', and 'popular', to create new adjectives that mean the negation of the original adjective. Thus, this 'un-' means *not*. For example, from the adjective 'happy', I can get the adjective 'unhappy', meaning *not happy,* by attaching the prefix 'un-' to 'happy'.

The description of the 'un-' that we have just given can be stated as a rule for forming complex words with 'un-'. This sort of rule is called a **word formation rule.** Below, I give one way of stating the rule for 'un-':

'un-' (derivational bound prefix):

ADJECTIVE→ [un-ADJECTIVE]_{ADJECTIVE}
Meaning: [NOT ADJECTIVE]
for example, happy→ [un-happy]_{ADJECTIVE}

This rule says that an adjective (for example, 'happy') can have 'un-' attached to the front of it, and what you get is another bigger adjective ('unhappy'). Further, this 'un-' negates the original adjective and thus means NOT ADJECTIVE (not happy). Writing brackets around 'un-ADJECTIVE' and labeling these brackets with the subscript _{ADJECTIVE} is just a way to say that the complex combination of 'un-' and 'happy' is itself an adjective (for example, 'an unhappy boy').

Thus, we can look at grammatical morphemes (like 'un-' or plural '-s') as *rules,* rather than just forms. Each one actually specifies an operation or process that must be carried out (for example, attaching 'un-' to the front of an adjective) as well as the meaning that results (for example, NOT ADJECTIVE) from that operation or process.

Now to the second 'un-' in English. This 'un-' attaches to verbs, like 'buckle', 'tie', 'do', or 'hook', to form a new verb which means *reverse the process* named by the original verb ('unbuckle', 'untie', 'undo', 'unhook'). Note that this 'un-' attaches to verbs (not adjectives, like the preceding 'un-') and that it does not mean NOT ('untie' does not mean *to* NOT *tie something,* rather it means to *tie it in reverse, make the tie come undone*). We can look at this prefix in terms of the following rule:

'un-' (derivational bound prefix)

> VERB→ [un-VERB] $_{VERB}$
> Meaning: REVERSE THE PROCESS NAMED BY VERB
> for example, tie→ [un-tie]$_{VERB}$, meaning *reverse the process of tying*

The only way that we can tell one 'un-' from the other is through the fact that they are involved in different rules, that is, they attach to different things (one to adjectives, the other to verbs) and create different meanings (one NOT, the other REVERSE A PROCESS).

So grammatical morphemes can be looked at as rules, namely *word formation rules.* These rules are part of the **morphological component** of the grammar, the component responsible for accounting for the speaker–hearer's unconscious knowledge of what counts as a word in the language and what principles are involved in building up complex words (words with more than one morpheme in them).

Let's now consider how '-ness' and plural '-s' work. The suffix '-ness' (a derivational morpheme) is added to the end of adjectives (like 'happy', 'red', 'tall', or 'sad') and forms nouns ('happiness', 'redness', 'tallness', 'sadness'). It changes the meaning from *condition or state of being* (for example, tall), to *abstract thing based on that state or condition* (such as tallness). There is, of course, no real, objective difference between these meanings (a state or condition like *being tall* on the one hand, and *tallness* viewed as an abstract object) in terms of the way the world is; the language just treats them differently, uses them as different perspectives on or ways of looking at the world.

The plural '-s' (an inflectional morpheme) is added to the ends of nouns, which remain nouns (an inflectional morpheme never changes the category of a word, while derivational morphemes do sometimes do this). It adds the meaning PLURAL to them. We can state the rules for '-ness' and '-s' as below:

'ness-' (derivational bound suffix)

> ADJECTIVE→ [ADJECTIVE-ness]$_{NOUN}$
> MEANING: STATE NAMED BY ADJECTIVE IS TREATED AS AN ABSTRACT THING OR OBJECT
> for example, happy→ [happi-ness]$_{NOUN}$, meaning *state named by 'happy' is treated as an abstract object*

'-s' (inflectional bound suffix)

NOUN→ [NOUN-S]_{NOUN}

MEANING: PLURAL OF NOUN (ONE OR MORE OF THING DESIGNATED BY NOUN)

for example, cat→ cats, meaning *more than one cat*

Some derivational morphemes affect not just the category and meaning of the form they attach to, they also affect their pronunciation. Take a morpheme like '-ity' (as in 'activity'). This morpheme attaches to adjectives (like 'active', 'scarce', 'national', or 'real') to create nouns ('activity', 'scarcity', 'nationality', and 'reality'). However, note that the original adjective is pronounced somewhat differently than the derived form with '-ity'. Thus, the adjective 'active' is stressed on its first syllable (ACtive) but the derived noun 'activity' is stressed on the second syllable (acTIvity). The adjective 'national' is stressed on its first syllable (NAtional) but the derived noun 'nationality' is stressed on its third syllable (nationALity). There are also changes in the vowel sounds due to these stress shifts. These changes in stress are being caused by the affixation of '-ity'. The information that '-ity' causes stress to shift would have to be added to the rule for '-ity', along with the category change it causes (from adjective to noun) and the meaning change it makes (however we want to characterize this).

There are other types of word formation rules beyond those involving grammatical morphemes (derivational and inflectional). The most interesting of these, perhaps, are the rules for the formation of compound words, like 'blackboard', 'air condition', and 'mind-boggling'. The rules for forming compounds are somewhat different than the word formation rules we have seen above. Essentially, they are of the form "A noun followed by a noun can count as a single noun" (for example, 'sunspot') or "a noun followed by an adjective can count as a single adjective" (for example, 'headstrong' or 'skin-deep'). By a general process, compounds are generally stressed (have the most stress) on the first word in the compound (thus: SUNspot, not *sunSPOT).

We can state the rules for forming compound words in English as follows:

RULE 1.   RULE FOR COMPOUND NOUNS:

A noun, adjective, verb, or preposition followed by a noun can count as a single noun:

EXAMPLES:

noun-noun:	adjective-noun:	verb-noun:	preposition-noun:
apron string	high school	swearword	overdose
sunspot	smallpox	scrubwoman	uptown
schoolteacher	well-wisher	rattlesnake	afterthought

RULE 2.   RULE FOR COMPOUND ADJECTIVES:

A noun, adjective, or preposition followed by an adjective can count as a single adjective:

EXAMPLES:

noun-adjective:	adjective-adjective:	preposition-adjective:
headstrong	white-hot	overwide
skin-deep	wordly-wise	underripe
heartbroken	icy cold	ingrown

RULE 3.   RULE FOR FORMING COMPOUND VERBS:

A preposition followed by a verb can count as a single verb:

EXAMPLES:
outlive, overdo, underfeed, offset, uproot, overstep

These rules have several interesting properties. First, note that the compound always counts as the category represented by the last word in it. So a verb-noun ('rattlesnake') combination is a noun, and a noun-adjective ('headstrong') combination is an adjective, and a preposition-verb ('uproot') combination is a verb, and so forth.

Second, note that these rules are *recursive;* that is, they can apply back again to themselves. For example, say I take the adjective 'high' and the noun 'school' and form the compound 'high school'. By Rule 1 (for noun compounds) this counts as a single noun: [high school]. But since it is a noun, it can enter into our rules again. Let's say we take this noun ('high school') and combine it with the noun 'teacher' to get 'high school + teacher' (this is noun + noun). By Rule 1 this also can count as a noun: [[high school] teacher].

Or, consider 'bath room'. This is a noun + noun combination, which by Rule 1 counts as a noun. 'Towel rack' is also a noun + noun combination, which by Rule 1 can count as a noun. Since these are both nouns, by Rule 1 they could be combined as noun + noun to form a bigger noun: [[bath room] [towel rack]]. There is no limit to the process, and we can form ever bigger compound words (for example, 'American history high school teacher' or 'bath room towel rack designer training').

——————————————— **E X E R C I S E** ———————————————

Exercise K.   Write word formation rules for the following affixes: '-ly' ('beautiful/beautifully', 'nice/nicely', 'quick/quickly'), '-er' ('bake/baker', 'run/runner', 'sing/singer'), '-ful' ('beauty/beautiful', 'truth/truthful', 'lust/lustful'), and 'in-'

('active/inactive', 'correct/incorrect', 'curable/incurable', but note also 'possible/impossible', 'probable/improbable', 'polite/impolite', and 'legal/illegal', 'logical/illogical', 'legible/illegible'). HINT: You will have to add a statement about 'in-' changing its shape in certain circumstances in its word formation rule.

5.6. WORD STRUCTURES

Sentences have *structure* in that different words in a sentence bunch into phrases. Phrases are groups of words that are closely associated with each other in the sense that the language treats them as a single unit. They also have a unitary meaning. Thus, consider the sentence 'The happy boy kissed the sad puppy'. In this sentence, the verb 'kiss' names an action. The group of words 'the happy boy' names a participant in that action, namely the ACTOR. The group of words 'the sad puppy' names another participant in this action, namely the PATIENT. Therefore, we can group the words of this sentence as follows: (The happy boy) kissed (the sad puppy). Since we have called object words (words that name the participants in actions) "nouns," we can call a group of words that name a participant in an action (which function like a noun) a **noun phrase.** Thus, 'the happy boy' (which names the ACTOR participant) and 'the sad puppy' (which names the PATIENT participant) are noun phrases.

In Chapter 6 we will see evidence that in a sentence like our example 'The happy boy kissed the sad puppy' the verb ('kiss') and the following noun phrase ('the sad puppy') together constitute a phrase (a unit), which we will call a **verb phrase.** We can represent the structure of this sentence in a tree diagram, as in Figure 5-1, in which each phrase is labeled with its name.

FIGURE 5-1

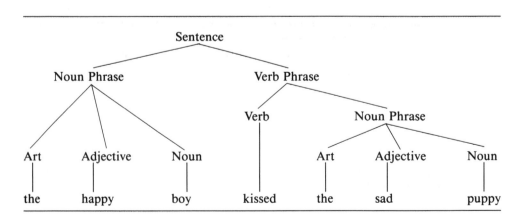

Figure 5-1 tells us that this sentence is composed of a verb, 'kiss', and a noun phrase, 'the sad puppy', which together make up a verb phrase: 'kissed the sad puppy'. This phrase, 'kissed the sad puppy', in turn, combines with the noun phrase 'the happy boy' to make a sentence (the whole thing). The diagram also tells us that each of our noun phrases is composed of an article (a name for words like 'the'), an adjective, and a noun.

Just as sentences have structure, so also do words, thanks to the operation of the word formation rules we studied in the last section. To see this, first consider compound words. We saw above that a compound word like 'high school teacher' is made by applying the compound rules several times. We first create the compound 'high school' and then, having done this, we create the bigger compound [high school] teacher. We can represent this in a tree diagram as well (Figure 5-2).

Figure 5-2 shows that the compound noun 'high school' (made of two simple nouns) is combined with the simple noun 'teacher' to form the complex compound noun 'high school teacher'. Below, in Figure 5-3, I give a diagram for the even more complex 'high school American history teacher'.

Tracing the groupings in this diagram (Figure 5-3), we can see that the large compound 'high school American history teacher' is made up of the compound 'American history' combined with the simple noun 'teacher' to yield the compound 'American history teacher' (note that this compound is ambiguous. Here it means *someone who teaches American history;* but it can also mean *a history teacher who is American.* In this latter case, it has the grouping [American] [history teacher], not [American history] [teacher], as in the above diagram). This, in turn, is combined with the compound 'high school' to yield the whole big compound.

It is not just compound words that have structure. All complex words do. Take a word like 'unhappinesses', which is made up of the following parts: un-happy-ness-es. We know that 'un-' (the one that means NOT) is added to adjectives and turns them into negative adjectives. We know that '-ness' is added

FIGURE 5-2

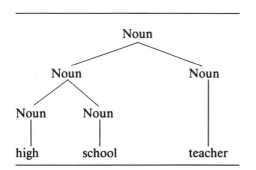

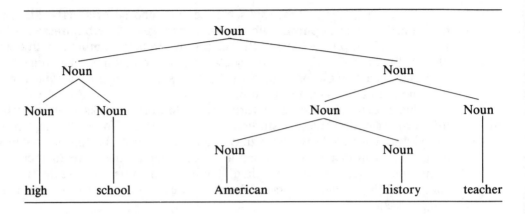

FIGURE 5-3

to adjectives also and makes them into nouns. Note that if we take the adjective 'happy' and first add '-ness' to it, we get the noun 'happiness'. We cannot add 'un-' to this now because it is a noun and 'un-' attaches to adjectives. However, if we take the adjective 'happy' and first attach 'un-', we get the adjective 'unhappy'. Since this is an adjective, '-ness' can attach to it to yield 'unhappiness'. Now we can add the plural '-s', which is added only to nouns, to this word. Thus, we see that the order in which the affixes must be attached is 'un-', '-ness', and '-s'. We can capture this constructional order by the tree diagram in Figure 5-4.

This tree (Figure 5-4) tells us that 'un-' and 'happy' are combined to create the adjective 'unhappy', and '-ness' is added to this to create the noun 'unhappiness'. Finally, plural '-s' is attached to this noun to yield the noun 'unhappinesses'.

FIGURE 5-4

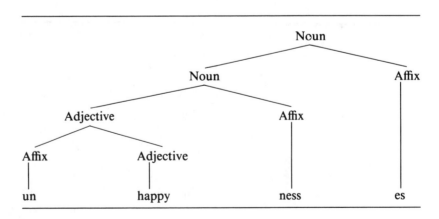

We see, then, that the structure of both words and sentences can be captured in hierarchical diagrams (the trees we have used here).

———————————————— E X E R C I S E S ————————————————

Exercise L.   Show how the following complex compound words (all compound nouns) are derived from the rules for compounds discussed in Section 5.5. Draw tree diagrams for each compound, as I have done in the examples in Section 5.6.

Example Answer.   Consider the second compound word, 'American high school teacher' in the meaning *a high school teacher who is an American.* It is put together as follows: The adjective 'high' and the noun 'school' have been formed into the compound noun 'high school'. Then this has been placed in front of 'teacher' to yield the compound noun: [high school] teacher. To this has been added the adjective 'American' modifying 'high school teacher', to yield American [[high school] teacher]. Note how I use brackets to indicate what has been combined with what (and, thus, what modifies the meaning of what). You can only figure out the structure of a compound by first ascertaining what it means (that is, what words modify what other words). The brackets we have used to make combinations clear can be directly translated into the tree diagram in Figure 5-5.

FIGURE 5-5

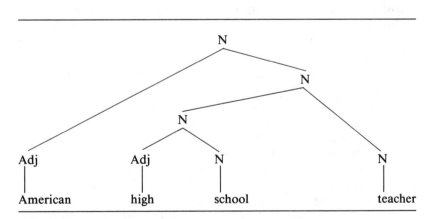

high school English teacher (one who teaches English in high school)
American high school teacher (done in example)
bath room towel rack designer
light house keeper (the house keeper is light in weight)
light house keeper (a person who keeps/takes care of a light house)

Exercise M. Draw trees for the following complex words, as in the examples in Section 5.6:

> bakers
> inactivity
> repaintable
> uncatchability (not able to be caught: un-catch-able-ity)
> uncooperativenesses

NOTES: 'able' is added to verbs to make them adjectives: catch/catchable. '-ity' is added to adjectives to make nouns: creative/creativity. 'in-' is added to adjectives to make negative adjectives: correct/incorrect. '-ive' is added to verbs to make adjectives: create/creative. 'un-' is added to adjectives to make negative adjectives: supportive/unsupportive. '-er' is added to verbs to make nouns: run/runner.

5.7. THE MENTAL LEXICON

Morphology is the study of the structure of words in a language. The **theory of grammar** is a theory of the unconscious knowledge each individual speaker–hearer has of his or her language, by virtue of which he or she knows what counts as a grammatical sentence in that language. This unconscious knowledge is, of course, stored in the speaker–hearer's head (mind/brain). Linguists view this linguistic knowledge as separated into different components or modules. There is a module devoted to the ways in which words can enter into phrases and phrases can enter into sentences. This component is the **syntactic component.** The component or module of unconscious, linguistic knowledge devoted to words and how complex words are built up constitutes the **morphological component.** Linguists assume that the words of a language are stored in a **mental lexicon** ('lexicon' is a fancy word for dictionary) in the speaker–hearer's head (mind/brain). These words are probably not listed in alphabetical order, like a written dictionary, and indeed are probably cross-listed in intricate and complex ways.

The word formation rules of the sort that we have studied here are listed in this mental lexicon. Thus, the rule for 'un-', or '-ness', or plural '-s', or any grammatical morpheme, is listed in the mental lexicon under the entry for that particular morpheme. We can assume that the rules for forming compound words are listed separately in a part of the mental lexicon devoted to more general morphological rules than those that constitute a single inflectional or derivational morpheme.

Since the compound word rules produce words no one has ever heard before, we cannot assume each compound word in the language is listed in the lexicon. Rather, we can assume that well-rehearsed and familiar compounds like 'blackboard' and 'air condition' are listed in the lexicon, with their meanings and pronunciations specified, but novel forms like 'kitty bag' (a doggy bag for cats) or 'house dog' (a dog that stays in the house) are created anew by the compound rule.

The compound rules still have a role to play for familiar forms like 'blackboard' and 'air condition', even though these words have their own entry in the lexicon that tells us they are words. The compound rules do not need to create these words anew each time they are uttered (we can simply look them up in the lexicon), but these compound rules do tell the speaker–hearer that such forms ('blackboard' and 'air condition') obey the general principles for acceptable (grammatical) compound words in the language.

That is, the compound rules have two functions: first, to *create* new combinations (like 'house dog') and second, to *represent* our unconscious knowledge of what counts as an acceptable compound word in the language, whether these happen to be new words like 'house dog' or familiar forms like 'blackboard'. We will see in the next section that even word formation rules tied to particular morphemes (like '-ness') also have this dual function of sometimes creating in actual speech new forms and sometimes just representing unconscious linguistic knowledge (what are and are not acceptable words in English).

5.8. PRODUCTIVITY

Consider the three word formation rules below, both of which we have considered above:

'er-' (derivational bound prefix)

> VERB→ [VERB-er]$_{NOUN}$
> MEANING: ONE WHO ENGAGES IN THE ACTION NAMED BY VERB
> for example, teach→ [teacher-er]$_{NOUN}$, meaning *one who teaches*

'-ness' (derivational bound suffix)

> ADJECTIVE→ [ADJECTIVE-ness]$_{NOUN}$
> MEANING: TREATS THE STATE NAMED BY THE ADJECTIVE AS AN ABSTRACT OBJECT
> for example, happy→ [happi-ness]$_{NOUN}$, meaning *the state of being happy treated as an abstract object*

'-ity' (derivational bound suffix)

> ADJECTIVE→ [ADJECTIVE-ity]$_{NOUN}$
> MEANING: TREATS THE STATE NAMED BY THE ADJECTIVE AS AN ABSTRACT OBJECT
> Phonology: The affixation of '-ity' affects the stress pattern of the word it is attached to in certain rule governed ways (which we will not deal with here).

for example, real→ [real-ity]_NOUN, meaning *the state of being real treated as an abstract object*

Further examples of '-ity':
  scarce/scar-ity
  curious/curios-ity
  sane/san-ity
  absurd/absurd-ity
  modern/modern-ity
  divine/divin-ity
  active/activ-ity

The affix '-er' will attach to any verb that names an action and produce a noun that names someone who does that action (bake/baker; golf/golfer; run/runner; love/lover; kiss/kisser, and so on). The only exception to this is that a form in '-er' is not very acceptable if another word already exists in the language with the meaning that the '-er' form would have. Thus, for example, if we take the verb 'steal' and add '-er', we should get 'stealer', but this is not very good, because a word already exists with this meaning, namely 'thief'. Likewise, 'cooker' can mean a pot that cooks food but not a person who cooks, since 'chef' already has that meaning.

This process by which a word that could exist from a word formation rule (such as 'stealer') is rendered less acceptable by the presence of another word in the language with the appropriate meaning (such as 'thief') is called **blocking.** Other examples of blocking are the fact that we cannot get 'ungood' (because of 'bad') or 'unbig' because of 'small' (despite the fact that the attachment of 'un-' to adjectives is quite general), or that we cannot get 'goodly' because of 'well' (despite the generality of '-ly' attaching to adjectives to make them adverbs—for example, bad/badly; sad/sadly; happy/happily, and so forth).

With the exception of blocked forms, the rule adding '-er' to verbs is completely general, applying to all the forms we would expect it to. When a word formation rule is general this way, it is said to be **productive.** With productive word formation rules, we can dream up novel forms that have never been said before. For example, I could call someone who xeroxes materials 'a xeroxer', or someone who looks into windows, 'a window looker iner'. That is, the affix ('-er') seems to attach quite freely to any action term.

The rule adding '-ness' to adjectives is also highly productive (for example, cold/coldness; nice/niceness; sad/sadness; red/redness; sore/soreness, and so on—for some rather novel forms, consider 'kittenness' or 'hard-to-get-along-withness'). In fact, '-ness' is yet more general than '-er', because blocking does not even apply to it. For example, despite the fact that 'glory' and 'fury' are nouns that designate the abstract object corresponding to the state of being glorious or furious, these words do not block 'gloriousness' (from the adjective 'glorious') or 'furiousness' (from the adjective 'furious'). So '-ness' is, if anything, even more productive than '-er'.

On the other hand, the suffix '-ity' functions very much like '-ness' (attaches to adjectives to create nouns with virtually the same meaning as '-ness' forms, namely, ABSTRACT OBJECT), but it is not nearly as general (productive). There are many words to which it seems it should apply but to which it does not. For example, while from 'nice' we can get 'nicety', from 'sad' there is no 'sadity' (but there is 'sadness'), from 'happy' no 'happity' (but there is 'happiness'), from 'red' no 'redity' (but there is 'redness'). There is 'certainty' (from 'certain'), but from 'sure' there is no 'surity' (but there is 'sureness') and from 'firm' no 'firmity' (but there is 'firmness'—note there is also 'infirmity'). While we have 'practicality' from 'practical', there is no 'radicality' from 'radical'. From 'stupid' we can get 'stupidity', but from 'smart' we cannot get 'smartity' ('smartness') and from 'dumb' we cannot get 'dumbity' ('dumbness'). From 'rare' we can get 'rarity', but from 'common' we cannot get 'commonity' ('commonness'). From 'rapid' we get 'rapidity', but from 'quick' we do not get 'quickity' (but we do get 'quickness'). Finally, from 'curious' we can get 'curiosity', but from 'spacious' we cannot get 'spaciosity' (but we do get 'spaciousness') and from 'gracious' we cannot get 'graciosity' (but we do get 'graciousness').

Thus, the affix '-ity' is much less productive (applies to fewer words than you would expect) than the affixes '-ness' and '-er'. Since we are viewing these affixes as *rules,* we can rephrase this by saying that the rule for attaching '-ity' is less general (has more exceptions), is less productive, than the rule for attaching '-ness' or '-er'. For any affix we must always ask just how productive it is. Some affixes are very productive (like '-ness' and '-er') and others are less so (like '-ity'); in fact, some are even less productive than '-ity'. Productivity is a matter of degree (for example, one can make up novel forms with '-ity', like 'uppity', but they are harder to make up than are new '-ness' forms—compare: 'taken for grantedness', which is fine, with *'taken for grantedity', which is terrible).

Often, when a rule attaching an affix is of low productivity, the words it produces do not have the meaning one would have predicted; that is, the meaning of such words is rather idiosyncratic. So, for example, 'niceness' just means the abstract object related to the state or property of being nice. But 'nicety', which we might expect would mean the same thing, actually means *a refined, subtle, or delicate point or distinction* (as in 'You've missed the niceties of my argument'). 'Specialty' from 'special' has a much more restricted and specialized meaning than 'specialness'. And 'frigidity' from 'frigid' means not just any coldness (as 'frigidness' would), but *sexual coldness.* This is typical of less productive word formation rules. Many of the forms they produce have rather idiosyncratic and specialized meanings.

Inflectional affixes tend to be quite productive, but they are not necessarily as productive as they might otherwise be. For example, the past-tense inflection '-ed' attaches to the vast majority of English verbs. But there are verbs that take different (and unproductive) past-tense formations (for example, sing/sang, know/knew, eat/ate), and these cannot take the "regular" past-tense ending (*singed, *knowed, *eated). We can see this as a kind of blocking. The presence of the irregular past-tense form 'sang' in the language blocks the operation of the regular word formation rule for past tense (the addition of '-ed'). And there are verbs like 'hit' and 'cut' that are the same in the past and present (note 'Everyday they hit me'/'Yesterday, they hit me' versus 'Everyday they kiss me'/'Yesterday they kissed me').

A consideration of productivity helps also to clarify the nature of word formation rules. We can ask the question, do speakers in uttering a complex word like 'happiness' or 'specialty' actually use the word formation rule and attach the affix "in their minds" as part of the process of producing speech? When they produce novel and creative forms like 'kittenness' or 'hard-to-get-along-withness', then it is quite plausible to believe that they have actually used the rule to produce the form in the act of speaking. Such novel forms are clearly not stored in the mental lexicon, but rather are made up "on the spot."

On the other hand, it is unlikely that when people produce well-rehearsed and often-used forms like 'happiness', 'sadness', or 'rapidity' or forms with rather specialized meanings like 'nicety', 'specialty', or 'frigidity' that they actually use the word formation rule each time. We will assume that these words are listed in the mental lexicon and simply "looked up" in the lexicon as people speak. They are not actually constructed on the spot from the word formation rule, as the novel forms are.

What is the function of the word formation rule in this latter case, the case where complex words are just listed as words in the lexicon, and not actively constructed by using the rule on the spot? The rule, in this case, is simply telling us something about the speaker–hearer's unconscious knowledge of (competence in) the language. Though speakers can simply access 'happiness', 'rapidity', and 'specialty' from their mental lexicons, they still unconsciously know that these words are made up of meaningful parts (happy-ness, rapid-ity, special-ty) and that these parts have certain properties. This knowledge is captured by the word formation rules.

So we see, once again, that word formation rules have two functions: First, they are "competence" rules, capturing the unconscious knowledge of the speaker–hearer of the language, and second, in some cases they can be actively used to construct novel or new forms (which may eventually enter the language and get listed in the mental lexicons of lots of speakers).

E X E R C I S E

Exercise N. Which of the following two affixes is more productive, '-ity' or 're-'? (Give evidence for your answer.) Which of the following affixes is more productive, 'un-' (as in 'unhappy') and 'in-' (as in 'inactive')? (Again, give evidence.) If you invented a new adjective, say 'glub', meaning *to feel hyper and excited,* and wanted to negate it, would you say 'Mary looks unglub today' or 'Mary looks inglub today'? Why?

5.9 MORPHO-PHONOLOGICAL RULES

We have seen that the attachment of some morphemes to words affects the pronunciation of the word that the morpheme attaches to. Thus, when '-ity' attaches to a word, it changes the stress pattern of the word and the pronunciation of its vowels. Sometimes there are yet other changes. For example, compare 'curious' and 'curiosity' or 'various' and 'variety'. This shows us that sometimes morphological processes (the operation of morphological rules, the attachment of grammatical morphemes) have implications for pronunciation.

While '-ity' affects the pronunciation of what it attaches to, it is also the case that some morphemes themselves vary in their pronunciation depending on what they are attached to. To see an example of this, consider the plural '-s' morpheme. So far I have represented morphemes, like plural '-s' or past '-ed', by how they are *spelled* in English. But obviously this need not be how they are represented in the minds' of speakers. A speaker could be illiterate and still know the plural morpheme in English. This speaker would have to represent the plural morpheme somehow in his or her mind, and this representation could not be determined by how it is spelled (since the person is, we are assuming, illiterate). More generally, writing is a rather late invention in language, and most of the world's languages are still not written. Nonetheless, morphemes are represented in people's minds, so that they can speak and understand, and this representation cannot in many cases have anything to do with writing (of course, once people know how to write, we cannot rule out that this influences how they represent things in their minds, even in regard to spoken language).

The plural morpheme in English is pronounced as an [s] sound in certain cases ('cats' = [kæts]); it is pronounced as a [z] in other cases ('cars' = [carz]); and it is pronounced as [əz] in yet other cases ('bosses' = [basəz]). The sound [z] is just like [s], except that in the case of [z] the vocal chords in the throat are vibrating, and in the case of [s] they are not. Thus, [z] is said to be a *voiced* sound and [s] is said to be a *voiceless* sound (*voiced* = vocal chords are vibrating). The sound combination [əz] is composed of two sounds, an unstressed vowel, called the "schwa" vowel (a vowel that shows up in many unstressed syllables in English) and the sound [z].

This variation in how the plural morpheme is pronounced is not random but is quite predictable, based on the sound that ends the word to which the plural '-s' morpheme is attached. If the sound that ends the word is a hissing sound (that is, [s, z, š, ž, č, ǰ]), the plural ending is pronounced [əz]. These "hissing" sounds are called **sibilants** or **sibilant sounds.** They are all similar to the sounds [s] and [z] (which are themselves sibilants), and the presence of the vowel [ə] helps to separate the hissing sound that ends the word from the [z] that signals the plural, allowing us to hear the plural marking more clearly.

For all other sounds (other than hissing sounds), if the sound that ends the word is *voiceless* (that is, involves no vibration of the vocal chords in the throat—[p, t, k, f, θ] are all voiceless), then the plural ending is [s]; if, on the other hand, the sound that ends the word is *voiced* (that is, involves vibration of the vowel chords in the throat—[b, d, g, v, ð], all vowels, the nasal consonants [n, m, ŋ], as well as [r, l, y, w]) are all voiced), then the plural is [z]. Clearly, this makes it easier to say the plural morpheme when it is attached to the end of a word. The plural agrees in voicing with the sound that ends the word, being voiced ([z]) if the sound that ends the word is voiced and being voiceless ([s]) if the sound that ends the word is voiceless.

The component of the grammar that is responsible for accounting for the knowledge that the speaker–hearer has about how to pronounce the language is the *phonological component,* which we surveyed in Chapter 3. Rules in this component must spell out the variation in pronunciation of the plural '-s' morpheme. To state the rule for pronouncing the plural morpheme, we must choose one of the three possible pronunciations ([s, z, əz]), as the *basic* pronunciation, or the basic version of the morpheme, and then state under what conditions this basic version changes to the other possibilities. That is, we must choose one of these variants as the way in which the plural morpheme is represented in the mind, allowing this representation to vary in actual pronunciation depending on the sound that ends the words to which it is attached.

In Chapter 3 we discussed how such choices are made, but let's just say for now that we choose /z/ as the basic version, and state a rule about when and how /z/ changes to either [s] or [əz] in certain cases (I am now going to start enclosing the "basic version," which I assume is the way in which the morpheme is mentally stored in the head, in slashes, thus, as '/z/', and the actual pronunciations, that is, the different versions that can occur in reality, in brackets, thus, '[əz], [s], [z]'). This rule can be stated as follows:

/z/, when it is attached to a word to signal the plural morpheme, becomes

> [əz] when the word to which it is attached ends in a sibilant (a hissing sound, voiceless or voiced)
> [s] when the word to which it is attached ends in a voiceless sound (other than a hissing sound)
> otherwise /z/ is just [z].

This rule says that the plural morpheme (represented in the head and in our rules as /z/) is, in its basic version, pronounced as [z]. However, when it is attached to a word ending in a sibilant, /z/ is changed to [əz] (which makes it easier to hear), and when it is attached to a word ending in a voiceless sound it is changed to [s] (which is itself voiceless and so is "assimilated" or made similar to the sound ending the word to which the plural morpheme is attached, which makes it easier to pronounce). If neither a hissing sound nor a voiceless sound ends the word (which only leaves voiced, nonhissing sounds), then the plural is said in its basic version as [z] (remember, I use slashes to enclose mental representations of the morpheme, thus '/z/', and brackets to enclose actual pronunciations of that morpheme, thus '[z], [s], [əz]').

We have not said why we chose /z/ rather than one of the other versions as basic (and, in fact, linguists still fight over the matter). But, you may ask, why pick any one pronunciation as basic and then change it to the other versions? Why not just say the plural morpheme (represented as PLURAL or what have you) has three pronunciations in three different situations? One reason is that the above rule changing /z/ to either [əz] or [s] in certain cases actually applies to other morphemes than the plural morpheme.

It also applies to the POSSESSIVE morpheme. Thus, in English, the possessive is pronounced as [əz] after hissing sounds (for example, 'the boss's pay' = [basəz]), it is pronounced [s] after other voiceless sounds (for example, 'the cat's paw' = [kæts]), and it is pronounced [z] after all other voiced sounds (for example, 'the car's hood' = [karz]). Thus, the rule above applies to the possessive as well. This will be accomplished if we just say that the basic version of the possessive in English is /z/, just like the plural, and let the rule above apply, adding that /z/ also undergoes the changes specified in the rule if it represents the possessive morpheme.

It is also the case that the English morpheme representing THIRD-PERSON SINGULAR SUBJECT AGREEMENT (that is, the morpheme in English that is placed on the verb to say that the subject is *third person*—not 'I', 'we', or 'you', but someone else—and singular) also obeys the rule above. This agreement morpheme is pronounced as [əz] if the verb ends in a hissing sound (for example, 'John *bosses* people around' = /bassəz/); it is pronounced as [s] after nonhissing voiceless sounds (for example, 'John *bats* last in the lineup' = [bæts]); and it is pronounced as [z] after nonhissing voiced sounds (for example, 'John *swims* every day' = [swɪmz]). Thus, the ENGLISH THIRD-PERSON SINGULAR SUBJECT AGREEMENT morpheme also obeys the rule above. This will be accomplished if we just say that the basic version of this agreement morpheme in English is /z/, just like the plural and possessive, and let the rule above apply, adding that /z/ also undergoes the changes specified in the rule if it represents the agreement morpheme.

In fact, we can now revise our rule as below, stating the conditions under which the mental representation /z/, whenever it represents any morpheme, is pronounced as [əz], [s], or [z]:

/z/, when it is attached to a word to signal some morpheme in English, becomes

> [əz] when the word to which it is attached ends in a sibilant (a hissing sound, voiceless or voiced)
> [s] when the word to which it is attached ends in a voiceless sound (other than a hissing sound)
> otherwise /z/ is just [z].

This rule is a **morpho-phonological** rule of English, that is, a rule that spells out how morphemes (thus the 'morpho') are pronounced (thus the 'phonological') in English. Such rules are part of the phonological component of the grammar, the component that captures the knowledge of the speaker–hearer in regard to the sound structure of the language (the ways things are pronounced and the rules that determine this).

The English past-tense morpheme '-ed' is also subject to a morpho-phonological rule. The rule is as follows, where I choose /d/ as the basic pronunciation of the past-tense morpheme:

/d/, when it is attached to a word to signal the past tense, becomes

[əd] when the word to which it is attached ends in an alveolar stop sound
[t] when the word to which it is attached ends in a voiceless sound (other than an alveolar stop)
otherwise /d/ is just [d].

An **alveolar** sound is a sound made by placing the tongue at the alveolar ridge of the mouth (the bony ridge behind the teeth), and a **stop** sound is any sound made by momentarily completely stopping the air from the lungs and then releasing it. The alveolar stops of English are /t/ and /d/. Thus, when /d/ is attached to a word ending in [t] or [d], the vowel [ə] is, once again, just as in the case of /z/, added to help differentiate the past /d/ from the [t] or [d] that ends the word. Otherwise, just as in the case of plural, possessive, and agreement (which are all represented by /z/), the /d/ is changed to /t/ to agree in voicing value (voiced or voiceless) with the sound that ends the word to which it is attached.

I will give one last example of a morpho-phonological rule. The morpheme 'in-', which is attached to the beginnings of adjectives to negate them (to mean NOT), and which thus functions just like 'un-', also has different versions. This time the versions depend on what follows the morpheme. We can assume that the basic form of 'in-' is /ɪn/. When /ɪn/ is attached to a word beginning in a *bilabial stop* consonant (a sound made by stopping the air with the lips: [p, b, m]), it is pronounced /ɪm/, as in 'impossible'. Here the /n/ of /ɪn/ has changed to an [m] to "agree with" the [p] that begins 'possible'. The sound [m] is itself a bilabial stop, like [p] and [b], but with nasal air coming out of the nose (it is *nasalized*).

When /ɪn/ is attached to a word beginning in a *velar stop* consonant, it is pronounced /ng/ as in 'inconsiderate' (a velar stop is a sound made by stopping the air with the back of the tongue placed on the velum, the soft part of the roof of the mouth back behind the central hard dome at the top of the mouth: [k, g, ng] are velar stops). Thus, the morpheme spelled 'in' is actually said in fast speech as /ɪng/ when it precedes a velar stop (that is, with the same /ng/ sound as ends 'sing' so it sounds like: 'ingconsiderate'). Here the /n/ of /ɪn/ is changing to [ng] to agree with the /k/ sound that begins 'considerate'. The sound /ng/ (which is a single sound, represented as [ŋ] in Chapter 3, despite the fact that I am writing it with two letters) is a velar stop just like [k] and [g], but with air coming out of the nose (it is *nasalized*).

I will not state this rule, although it is obvious that the /n/ of /ɪn/ is changing to be made in a position of the mouth similar to that of the sound that follows it. In this regard, consider the word 'illegal', which is represented in the mind as 'in-legal' (NOT LEGAL), but where the /n/ of the morpheme /ɪn/ has changed to [l] to agree with the [l] that begins the word 'legal'.

There are other morpho-phonological rules in English, but many other languages have many more than English and have morpho-phonological rules that are much more complicated.

We are proposing, then, that a morpheme will be listed in the lexicon in a "basic form," what we have called so far its "mental representation" or "basic form" and what is also sometimes called its "underlying" form. Thus, the underlying or basic form of the plural morpheme will be /z/, of the past-tense morpheme will be /d/, and of negative 'in-' will be /ɪn/. These basic forms are subject to the morpho-phonological rules of English and may have their pronunciations changed in certain cases.

Some of these morpho-phonological rules apply to several morphemes (as the rule for morphemes whose basic form is /z/ does). However, in some cases, a morphological rule applies to only one morpheme or fails to apply to a similar morpheme. Thus, the rule for /ɪn/ applies only to /ɪn/, and not to the similar morpheme 'un-'. For example, while we say 'impossible' with an [m], we say 'unpopular' with an [n], not *'impopular' with an [m]. Or, while we say 'illegal' with an [l], we say 'unlawful' with an [n] and not *'illawful' with an [l]. So the /n/ of the morpheme 'un-' does not change to [m], [ng], and [l] in the way in which the /n/ of the morpheme 'in-' (/ɪn/) does. So the rule does not apply to 'un-'.

Morpho-phonological rules obey the principles of the phonological component, which we studied in Chapter 3, but they are listed in the lexicon and associated with various morphemes. Thus, they have a foot in both the phonological component and the morphological component (as they should, since they spell out how morphemes are actually pronounced).

EXERCISES

Exercise O.   The data below is from Indonesian and Tagalog (one of the major languages of the Philippines). State how Indonesian forms the *plural* of nouns and how Tagalog forms the *future tense* of verbs.[1]

---

[1]The data in this problem is taken from the *Language Files*, 3rd ed., Department of Linguistics, Ohio State University (Reynoldsburg, Ohio: Advocate Publishing Co., 1985), p. 126.

Indonesian:

[rumah] house   [rumahrumah] houses
[ibu]   mother   [ibuibu]   mothers
[lalat] fly   [lalatlalat] flies

Tagalog:

[bili] buy   [bibili] will buy
[kain] eat   [kakain] will eat
[pasok] enter   [papasok] will enter

Exercise P. The data below is from a dialect of American English. I have written the data with the English spelling followed by a phonetic transcription of the word. (This system of transcription of sounds was introduced in Chapters 4 and 5.) The symbol [aɪ] stands for the vowel sound in 'write' and 'writer', the symbol [e] for the vowel sound in 'late' and 'later', the symbol [ɛ] for the vowel sound in 'red' and 'redder', and the symbol [æ] for the vowel sound in 'sad' and 'sadder'. The symbol [ᴅ] is explained after the data. The other symbols—all for consonants—are the same as English spelling. All that is relevant to the problem below is the distinction between vowel sounds and consonant sounds, not what symbols we use for these (vowels, which are the key sounds around which morphemes are built, are sounds made with an open mouth cavity; consonants are made with a relatively constricted mouth cavity).

write	[raɪt]	writer	[wraɪᴅr]	writing	[wraɪᴅɪŋ]
late	[let]	later	[leᴅr]	latest	[leᴅɛst]
red	[rɛd]	redder	[rɛᴅr]	reddest	[rɛᴅɛst]
sad	[sæd]	sadder	[sæᴅr]	saddest	[sæᴅɛst]

The sound written [ᴅ] is a *flap* sound made by quickly flapping the tongue against the alveolar ridge (the bony ridge behind the upper teeth). This data shows that certain words, like 'write' or 'sad', have two different morphological realizations (just the way the plural morpheme /s/ does). 'Write' is sometimes produced as [wraɪt] and sometimes as [wraɪᴅ], 'sad' is sometimes produced as [sæd] and sometimes as [sæᴅ]. State the morpho-phonological rule that produces this alternation. That is, when does [t]/[d] show up at the end of a morpheme/word and when does [ᴅ] show up? To state the rule here, you need to decide whether, taking 'sad' as an example, [sæd] or [sæᴅ] is the basic form of the morpheme/word, and which one is derived by rule.

Exercise Q. The data below is from a hypothetical language. The symbols [n] and [m] stand for *nasal* consonants (just like English [n] and [m]), consonants in which air comes out of the nose. The symbol [~] over a vowel means the vowel is *nasalized,* said with air coming out of the nose. Thus, these vowels and the nasal consonants [m] and [n] share the feature of being *nasal.* The symbols [n, t, k, p, m, l, f, d, r] stand for consonants, and the symbols [e, a, o, i, a] stand for vowels. You do not need to know more than this to answer the questions after the data.

[ẽ nato]	that fish	[e tek]	that cat
[et opot]	that girl	[ẽ mĩm]	that cow
[et ipi]	that table	[e lapit]	that rock
[et alat]	that child	[ẽ nalip]	that flower
[e fĩno]	that bottle	[e drapo]	that ground
[gõ mi et]	give me that	[no et]	not that

The morpheme that means 'that' obviously changes its pronunciation, as does the English plural /s/ morpheme and the English past-tense morpheme /d/. Which of the following would you take to be the basic form of the morpheme for 'that'?

/e/   /ẽ/   /et/

State a morpho-phonological rule or rules that will convert the basic form you have chosen into the other variants of the morpheme for 'that'.

Exercise R. Certain morphemes/words in English have two forms, as below:

wife [waɪf]	wives [waɪvəz]
leaf [lif]	leaves [livəz]
wolf [wʊlf]	wolves [wʊlvəz]
loaf [lof]	loves [lovəz]

The symbol [f] stands for the voiceless consonant that begins 'fish' (saying it is *voiceless* means the vocal chords in the throat are not vibrating); the symbol [v] stands for the voiced consonant that begins 'veal' (saying it is *voiced* means that the vocal chords are vibrating). Except for a difference in voicing, [f] and [v] are made in the same way. The data shows that a morpheme/word like 'wife' shows up in two forms: [waɪf] and [waɪv]. Choose one form as basic and state the rule that derives the other form (that is, state the condition in which the other form shows up). Why did you choose the basic form you did (that is, why did you choose either [waɪf] or [waɪv] as basic)?

RECOMMENDED FURTHER READING

ARONOFF, MARK (1976). *Word Formation in Generative Grammar (Linguistic Inquiry* Monograph). Cambridge, Mass.: M.I.T. Press. (Somewhat technical, a bit out of date, but a classic that is still well worth reading.)

BAUER, LAURIE (1983). *English Word Formation.* New York: Cambridge University Press. (A good description of how English forms words.)

COMRIE, BERNARD (1976). *Aspect.* New York: Cambridge University Press. (The best current introduction to aspect.)

COMRIE, BERNARD (1985). *Tense.* New York: Cambridge University Press. (The best current introduction to tense.)

COMRIE, BERNARD, (1989). *Language Universals and Linguistic Typology*, 2nd ed. University of Chicago Press. (Insightful view of how different languages work.)

HAWKINS, JOHN (1979). *Definiteness and Indefiniteness.* London: Croom Helm. (A thorough account of the use of the definite and indefinite articles.)

MATTHEWS, PETER (1974). *Morphology.* New York: Cambridge University Press. (A good descriptive and traditional approach to morphology.)

SPENCER, ANDREW (1991). *Morphological Theory: An Introduction to Word Structure in Generative Grammar.* Oxford: Basil Blackwell. (A technical, but thorough and up-to-date, introduction to morphology and its interrelations with phonology and syntax.)

CHAPTER 6

Syntax
The Structure
of Language

6.1. SENTENCES

A cat looks furry and sleek; water looks clear and wet. These are the *appearances* of these things. But a science like biology does not look at a cat as a furry and sleek object. Rather, biology looks at a cat as composed of various anatomical parts (its heart and lungs, blood and tissues, etc.) and ultimately of such small objects as cells and genes. A science like chemistry does not look at water as clear and wet, but rather as something that is composed of such small things as molecules and atoms. Further, biologists believe that cells and genes ultimately explain why cats look the way they do. And chemists believe that molecules and atoms explain how water looks, tastes, and feels to humans.

We can look at a cat as a *pattern* or *structure* of cells and genes, a pattern that helps explain aspects of the cat. And we can look at water as a pattern or structure of molecules and atoms, a pattern that helps explain aspects of water. These molecules and atoms, these cells and genes, are invisible to the naked eye. Nonetheless, they exist in the physical world.

Just like biologists studying cats or chemists studying water, linguists consider sentences to be composed of patterns or structures of things one cannot see with the naked eye or hear "with the naked ear." This pattern or structure helps explain properties of sentences, just like genes help explain properties of cats, or molecules help explain properties of water. However, while genes and molecules exist in the physical world, the patterns or structures of which sentences are composed exist in the mind.

We can view talk about cells and genes as a *theory* about cats and other living creatures. We can view talk about molecules and atoms as a *theory* about water and other material objects. Theories like these typically claim that the things they study, like cats or water, are really made up of smaller things, and that the ways in which these smaller things pattern together with each other ultimately explain the properties of the bigger things. This is also how linguists view sentences. I will call entities like cells and genes, or molecules and atoms, *theoretical entities.* I call them this *not* because they don't exist (they do exist), but because they are used to *explain* the properties of things that are more readily apparent and easier to observe than they are (things like cats and water, and the sentences one hears and understands).

However, something odd happens when we look at sentences this way. Consider the sentence 'I'll bet you.' This sentence can perfectly well be said and heard as one mushed-up single sound, something like 'abetcha'. This is a perfectly normal state of affairs. When we hear a sentence in an unknown foreign language, it always sounds like one mushed-up continuous sound with no discrete parts. However, English speakers know (even if they cannot read and write) that the sentence 'abetcha' is made up of four words, 'I', 'will', 'bet', 'you'. There is nothing in the sound waves produced when this sentence is spoken that tells hearers exactly where one word ends and another begins; no "hearing machine" could find these words. They simply are not out there in the physical world of sound. You hear a sentence, and as a fluent speaker and hearer of the language, you can "see with your mind's eye" the theoretical entities (like words) out of which the sentence is made. I am not saying that sentences are composed *only* of words—there are also other theoretical entities that go into sentences—but words are indeed theoretical entities.

While every fluent speaker of a language can unconsciously "see" (with their minds) the theoretical entities of which sentences are made (words), they cannot, however, bring these entities to consciousness very well. That is, they unconsciously know that sentences are made up of the theoretical entities we will study below, but they are not good at consciously thinking or talking about them. That is why linguists must, like all other scientists, work hard to discover the theoretical entities out of which sentences are made. The irony is that they are working hard to discover something that they already know unconsciously. Such ironies do not apply to biologists or chemists.

6.2. PHRASES

Noun Phrases

To start our consideration of the theoretical entities that compose sentences, consider the sentence below:

1a. Mary loves John

This sentence is composed of three *words.* Traditional grammarians called the word 'Mary' a NOUN and said it was the SUBJECT of the sentence. They called the word 'loves' a VERB. And they called the word 'John' a noun and said it was the OBJECT of the verb. We will gradually see what terms like NOUN, SUBJECT, and OBJECT really mean as we proceed. For now just call words like 'Mary' and 'John' *nouns,* and take this to mean no more than that such words can occur either immediately before or after the verb. And call the noun that occurs before the verb the *subject,* and the noun that occurs after the verb the *object.*

Notice now that the single word 'Mary' can be replaced by a string of words, for example, by the string of words 'the new professor of history', in such a way that we still get a grammatical sentence:

1b. *The new professor of history* loves John.

This string of words plays the same role—serves the same function—in 1b as 'Mary' does in 1a, namely it is the subject of the sentence. This string of words can also replace 'John', and now it plays the same role in the sentence as 'John' was playing (namely, the object of the verb):

1c. Mary loves *the new professor of history.*

'John' and 'Mary' in 1a are nouns. We see from 1b and 1c that the string of words 'the new professor of history' can play the same role as a single noun. Because this is the case, this string of words is called a **noun phrase** (**NP** for short). The string of words "hangs together," serves as a single unit, groups closely together, however we want to put it. A noun phrase is a group of words that occurs in the same place as and serves the same function as a single noun.

The string of words 'the new professor of history' has inside of it the noun 'professor'. We know this is a noun because it can occur right after or right before a verb by itself: 'Professors love John', 'Mary loves professors' (note that we have to put it in the plural because English does not allow nouns to occur alone unless they are proper names like 'Mary', plural nouns like 'professors', or nouns that name stuff or masses of things, like 'water' or 'rice'; otherwise the noun has to have a 'the' or an 'a' in front of it, as in 'the professor' or 'a professor').

The NP 'the new professor of history', in addition to containing the noun 'professor', has another little phrase ('of history') inside it. This is a PREPOSITIONAL PHRASE composed of the preposition 'of' and the object of the preposition 'history'. The preposition 'of' essentially allows the noun 'history' to link to or relate to the noun 'professor'.

The NP 'the new professor of history' also has an ADJECTIVE ('new') in it. Adjectives modify or further specify the meaning of nouns and can occur before the noun (as here) or linked to the noun by a "pseudo-verb" like 'be' (as in 'The professor is *new'*).

The only word left in the phrase 'the new professor of history' is the little word 'the', which is called an **article** or a **determiner** (we will use the latter term). It signals that the speaker assumes that the new history professor is KNOWN to the hearer, either on the basis of the previous talk or on the basis of mutual knowledge shared by the speaker and hearer. If the professor has not been assumed to be already known to the hearer, the little word 'the' would be replaced by the determiner 'a' (as in 'a new professor of history'). 'The' is called the **definite determiner,** and 'a' (which is 'an' in front of words beginning in a vowel) is called the **indefinite determiner.**

The noun 'professor' is said to be the HEAD of the NP 'the new professor of history' because it is the word around which all the other words cluster, the word whose meaning they all modify or otherwise relate to.

We can describe the structure of the string of words 'the new history professor' in terms of a tree diagram, as follows:

2.

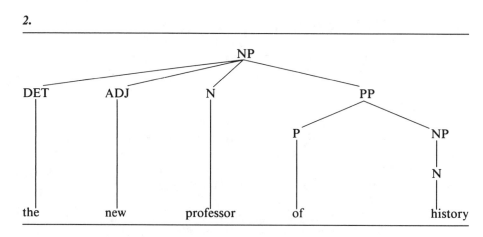

For convenience, I will use the term 'NP' for both single nouns (like 'history' or 'Mary' and 'John') and strings of words (like 'the new professor of history') occurring in the same place as nouns. NP, then, stands for a single noun or a string of words organized around a head noun. Phrases, as we see here and will see below, are single words (like 'Mary') or strings of words (like 'the professor of history') functioning like these single words and behaving as a *unit.*

——————————————— E X E R C I S E ———————————————

Exercise A. Considering the following sentences, say why defining a noun as "any word that names a person, place, or thing" and a verb as "any word that names an action or state (condition)" are poor definitions of nouns and verbs, at least in English.

1. The <u>honor</u> he received made his mother happy.   ('honor' = noun)
2. His colleagues <u>honored</u> him with a gold watch.   ('honored' = verb)
3. He <u>questioned</u> the man for an hour.   ('questioned' = verb)

4. His <u>question</u> got him in a lot of trouble. ('question' = noun)
5. The <u>punch</u> he took to the jaw knocked him out. ('punch' = noun)
6. Mary <u>punched</u> John in the jaw. ('punched' = verb)
7. <u>Love</u> is a wonderful thing. ('love' = noun)
8. John <u>loves</u> Mary. ('loves' = verb)

Verb Phrases

Consider again the sentence in 1a, repeated below:

1a. Mary loves John

We have seen that 'Mary' and 'John', though they just seem like simple words, are functioning like phrases, in the sense that they each could be replaced by a whole string of words (like 'the new professor of history'). Now we can ask, do any two of the three words in sentence 1a constitute a phrase (that is, is either 'Mary loves' or 'loves John' a phrase)? This is something about which English speakers have at best weak intuitions. But there are tests we can apply that show that the words 'loves John' make up a phrase in this sentence, and the words 'John loves' do not.

For example, notice that pronouns like 'he/him' or 'she/her' can "stand in" for NPs; that is, they allow us not to have to repeat a particular NP, as in:

3a. *Mary* thinks that *she* loves John

3b. *The new professor of history* thinks that *she* loves John

In 3a the pronoun 'she' stands in for 'Mary'. In 3b the pronoun 'she' stands in for 'the new professor of history'. The term 'pronoun' is, by the way, a bad term. Pronouns don't stand in for nouns, but rather for NPs (single nouns and phrases functioning like nouns). So they should really be called 'pro-NPs' instead of pronouns.

Now notice that English has a "stand-in" word (actually two word combinations) for the words 'loves John' in 1a:

4a. Mary loves John, and *so does* Bill ('so does' = 'loves John')

4b. Mary loves John, and Bill *does too* ('does too' = 'loves John')

'So does' and 'does too' stand in for a verb and what follows it. This string of words can be quite long:

4c. Mary gave presents to all the children in Children's Hospital and Bill *did too* ('did too' = 'gave presents to all the children in Children's Hospital')

English, on the other hand, has no "stand-in" words that will replace the subject and verb ('Mary loves' in 1a). Thus, the verb and what follows it constitute together a phrase. We will call it a **verb phrase** (**VP** for short).

Notice here how we used a test (the "stand-in word" test) to probe for the existence of the VP. NPs and VPs are, like words, theoretical entities. Of course, NPs and VPs are not too small to see; rather they are in the mind and thus not open to direct inspection, no matter how powerful the microscope.

Given the existence of VPs, we can diagram the structure of a sentence like 1a as below:

4.

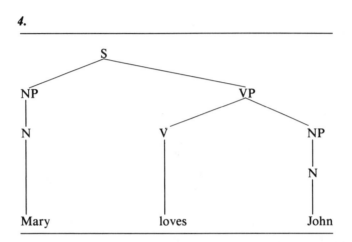

Phrase Structure Ambiguity

The sentence below has two different meanings:

5. John discussed violence on TV

5a. Meaning 1: John went on TV and discussed violence

5b. Meaning 2: John's topic was "violence on TV", though he may have been discussing this topic on the radio, or in a classroom, or anyplace else

Sentence 5 has two meanings because the words 'violence on TV' can be taken as two phrases (Meaning 1) or one phrase (Meaning 2). That is, in Meaning 2, the words 'violence on TV' constitute one phrase or unit (they name John's topic, which was "violence on TV"), while in Meaning 1 they do not constitute a single phrase (here 'violence' names John's topic and 'on TV' says where John talked about this topic). We can easily prove that in Meaning 2 the words are a single unit. If we try to interrupt these words with an adverb like 'yesterday', we lose Meaning 2 and have only Meaning 1:

6. John discussed violence *yesterday* on TV (only has Meaning 1, not Meaning 2)

   When we place 'yesterday' between 'violence' and 'on TV', we can no longer interpret these words as one phrase or unit. They can only be interpreted as two phrases: 'violence' (what John discussed) and 'on TV' (where he discussed it). This gives us Meaning 1. We also see here that phrases do not tolerate being interrupted by material that doesn't belong inside them.

   Sentence 5 can be assigned two different tree diagrams describing its structure, in one of which (7a) 'violence on TV' is two phrases, and in one (7b) these words constitute a single phrase (the symbol PP stands for "prepositional phrase"—these will be discussed later in this chapter):

7a. **Meaning 1:**

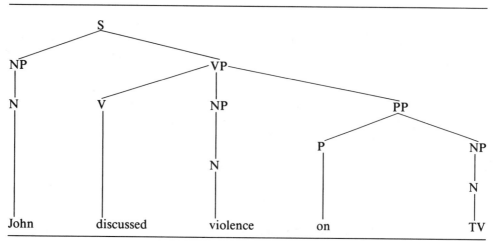

7b. **Meaning 2:**

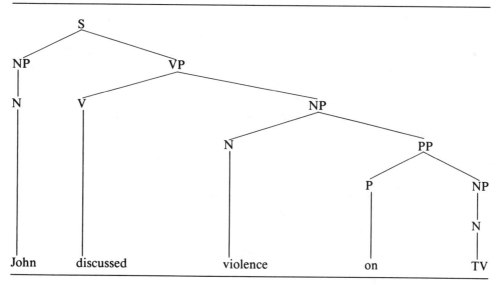

Note how in 7b the PP 'on TV' is inside (part of) the NP 'violence on TV' and that these words ('violence on TV') together make up a larger phrase, labeled "NP." In 7a, on the other hand, the PP 'on TV' is a separate unit from the phrase 'violence' (no single label is on top of the words 'violence on TV', rather, 'violence' and 'on TV' each have labels that separately connect to the VP).

─────────────────── E X E R C I S E ───────────────────

Exercise B. When a word, phrase, or sentence has two or more possible meanings, it is said to be *ambiguous*. A sentence like 'John looked at the bank' is ambiguous because it has an ambiguous word in it: 'bank' can mean bank of a river or bank as a financial institution. On the other hand, the sentence 'Old men and women like kittens' is ambiguous, not because it has any ambiguous words in it, but because the phrase 'old men and women' can be organized internally in two different ways; that is, the words in this phrase can be grouped together in different ways, either as '(old men) / (and women)' (where 'old' goes with 'men' and the women may not be old) or as '(old) / (men and women)' (where 'old' modifies 'men and women' and, thus, both the men and the women are old). The sentence 'John discussed violence on TV' is ambiguous because 'violence on TV' can be a single phrase or two separate phrases. Why are the following sentences ambiguous? (You do not have to worry about what trees for these sentences would look like in any detail.) Simply state your answer informally in English as best you can (however, feel free to make hypotheses about what trees would look like if this helps you think about the question, or to draw any sorts of structures or diagrams that help you spell out your answer).

Example Answer. Take sentence 5 below, 'John found Mary with a map'. No word is ambiguous in this sentence. One of its meanings is 'John used a map in order to find Mary' and the other is 'John discovered Mary holding a map'. In the first case, the phrase 'with a map' goes with or modifies 'found' (and, if we were to draw a tree, this phrase would be attached directly to the VP that dominates 'found'), and in the second case, the phrase 'with a map' goes with, forms a larger phrase with, 'Mary' (and, if we were to draw a tree, would be inside the larger NP 'Mary with a map', which would be the object of the verb 'found').

1. John dislikes visiting relatives.
2. John wrote a thesis on time.
3. The missionary is ready to eat.
4. Flying planes can be dangerous.
5. John found Mary with a map.   (done in example)

Tree Terminology

I now introduce some terminology for talking about tree diagrams. First, the tree itself is called a **phrase structure tree** (or a **phrase structure diagram**). The labels in the tree (S, NP, VP, N, etc.) are called the **nodes** of the tree. We make an important distinction between the two following technical terms: **immediately dominate** and (simply) **dominate**. A node (or label) is said to immediately dominate the nodes (or labels) right below it and connected to it by lines. So in 7b, the VP node immediately dominates the nodes V and NP, and this NP in turn immediately dominates the nodes N and PP. A node (or label) is said to dominate any nodes that are below it (right below or further down) and connected to it by lines, which may run through other nodes. Thus, VP in 7b dominates V and NP, N and PP, P and NP, and N—that is, everything you can get to by tracing down a line from VP to anything below it.

We talk about trees using female kinship terms. A node is said to be the **mother** of what it immediately dominates; thus in 7b, S is the mother of the NP and VP right below it, and VP is the mother of the V and NP right below it. Immediately dominated nodes are said to be **daughters** of the node that immediately dominates them, so NP and VP in 7b are the daughters of S, and V and NP are the daughters of VP. Daughters of the same mother are said to be **sisters.** Thus, NP and VP are sisters (they have the same mother, namely S), and V and NP are sisters (since they have the same mother, namely VP). Notice that S dominates everything in the tree, and VP dominates everything in the VP, though VP does not dominate S (since you cannot trace from VP to S by going downward), nor does VP dominate the subject NP (the subject is the NP right below S, and, again, you cannot trace from VP to that NP by going downward). It turns out that many properties of grammar depend on knowing where something is in a tree, what it dominates, and what dominates it.

————————————————— E X E R C I S E —————————————————

Exercise C.   Answer the following questions about the tree below:

1. Which nodes are immediately dominated by the underlined VP?
2. Which nodes does the underlined VP dominate?
3. Which node immediately dominates the underlined VP?
4. Which nodes dominate the underlined VP?
5. What nodes are the daughters of the underlined PP?
6. What node is the mother of this PP?

In your answers, you do not have to list the words at the bottom of the tree, but just the nodes above them. To answer these questions, you will probably want to redraw the tree and clearly label the nodes that answer each question.

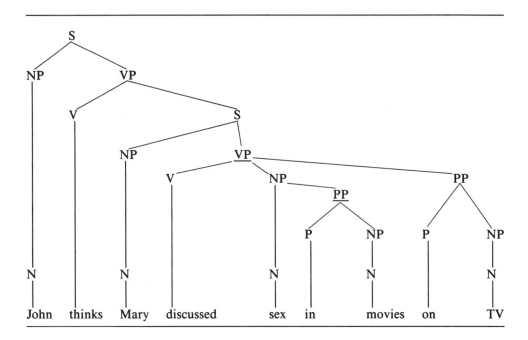

Phrase Structure Rules

We can formulate rules that state what phrase structure trees for English can and cannot look like. These are called **phrase structure rules.** For example, the following rule.

8a. S → NP VP

says that S (sentence) must immediately dominate NP and VP. And

8b. VP → V (NP) (PP)

says that VP must immediately dominate V and can *optionally* immediately dominate NP or PP or both (this optionality we state by placing node labels in parentheses). This allows for a tree like that in 7a, where the verb 'discuss' is followed by an NP ('violence') and a PP ('on TV'). It also allows for sentences where the verb is followed only by an NP ('John discussed *violence*') or only by a PP ('John spoke *on TV*') or where the verb is followed by nothing ('John spoke').

Of course, different verbs care about what does or does not follow them inside their VPs. A verb like 'eat' will allow an NP to follow it ('John *ate the meal*') or can occur with nothing following it ('John *ate*'). On the other hand, a verb like 'crush' must have an NP following it ('John *crushed the box*'). If no NP follows 'crush', then the sentence it is in is ungrammatical (*'John *crushed*'). By the way, linguists use an asterisk ('*') to mark phrases or sentences that their theories claim to be ungrammatical in a given language and that (they hope) native speakers of the language acknowledge to be unacceptable in the language. These preferences that verbs have about what can or cannot follow them are stated in a mental dictionary (called the *mental lexicon*) each of us has in our heads. Each verb in the language has its own entry in this dictionary, and this entry will state the preferences the verb has for what can or cannot follow it in its VP. We will study this dictionary below.

The rule below states what NPs can look like:

8c. NP→(DET) (Adj) Noun (PP)

This says that NPs must have a noun (for example, 'book') in them and can optionally have a determiner (*'the* book') or an adjective ('the *red* book', *'red* books') or a following PP ('the book *on the table'*). Any or all of DET, Adj, and PP can be present, but none need be. A single noun alone (like 'books', 'violence', or 'John') can also serve as an NP.

Finally, we need to state what a prepositional phrase can look like:

8d. PP→P (NP)

PPs are made up of a preposition followed by an NP ('on TV', 'in the red book', 'on the funny table in the kitchen'). Not all prepositions must have an NP following them, so the NP is optional: compare 'John went *in the house',* where the NP 'the house' follows the preposition 'in', and 'John went *in',* where nothing follows the preposition 'in'. In many cases, however, prepositions will not allow their following NPs to be absent (consider 'I looked *at the picture',* but **'I looked at'*). Once again, these preferences that different prepositions have will be stated in the mental dictionary, where each preposition will have its own entry.

Phrase structure rules "license" trees. If a tree fits the phrase structure rules, then it is an acceptable tree for English; if it does not fit them, it is not an acceptable tree. A string of words like 'Boy the loves the girl' has no acceptable tree because the phrase structure rule for NP stipulates that if a DET like 'the' is present it must precede the noun, not follow it. Strings of words for which there is no acceptable tree constitute ungrammatical sentences of English. We will always place an asterisk ('*') in front of ungrammatical sentences to indicate that they are ruled as ungrammatical by the grammar we are developing.

The trees 7a and 7b for the sentence in 6 ('John discussed violence on TV') are both acceptable by the phrase structure rules of English. In particular, note that the VP in the tree in 7a is licensed by the VP rule (8b): VP → V (NP) (PP), using both the NP and the PP options. The VP in the tree in 7b is also licensed by this VP rule, but chooses only the NP option, not the PP option. However, it then goes on to use the PP option in the NP rule (8c): NP → (DET) (Adj) Noun (PP), having a PP directly follow the head noun of the NP.

When a single sentence like 8 has two acceptable trees, it then has two meanings, since these trees, in addition to displaying the structure of the sentence, determine how the meanings of words are combined into the meanings of phrases and ultimately of the sentence as a whole.

Obviously, the phrase structure rules we have given here are too simple, and we will add to them and complicate them a little as we go on. But we will not give the full set of such rules for English. Discovering the phrase structure rules for English and all other languages, as well as discovering what the phrase structure rules of all languages do and do not have in common, is an important branch of research in linguistics.

We can use phrase structure rules to define terms like *noun, adjective, verb, subject* and *object,* terms we have so far just been borrowing from traditional grammar. A *noun* is any word that can occur where the phrase structure rules say N can occur. A *verb* is any word that can occur where the phrase structure rules say V can occur. A *subject* is any NP that fills the place of NP in Rule 8a (S → NP VP), that is, the NP right below (immediately dominated by) S. An *object* of a verb is any NP that fills the place of NP in Rule 8b (VP → V (NP) (PP)), that is, the NP right below (immediately dominated by) VP and to the right of the verb.

These are purely **formal definitions.** That is, terms like 'noun', 'verb', 'subject', and 'object' are defined by the places they fill in the pattern of theoretical entities (words and phrases) composing sentences, not by their meanings or communicative functions. Why would we want to do this? Because this allows us to define these terms independently from whatever their meanings or functions are (if they have any). This, in turn, allows us to see if any meaning or function does indeed attach to the entities (nouns, verbs, subjects, objects) we have so identified, without being prejudiced by what we have been previously taught to think these meanings or functions are.

For instance, traditional grammar often said that a subject was "what the sentence is about," that this was the meaning or function of the subject of a sentence. Now having a way to pick out subjects independently, we can go on to ask of all the things we have picked out as subjects, if they, in fact, have this meaning or function. Thus, we can test hypotheses about what subjects mean or how they function (and we may find out they have no meaning or function, or perhaps not the ones we thought they did). We will take up the matter of what subjects do and do not mean below and in Chapter 10.

———————————————— **E X E R C I S E S** ————————————————

Exercise D. What do the following sentences tell you about how good or poor the following definition for the term 'subject' is? "The subject of a sentence is the AGENT that carries out the action named by the verb."

1. John killed the boy.
2. The boy was killed by John.
3. John received a blow to the head.
4. John forgot the answer.

Exercise E. Draw trees for the following sentences, using only the most obvious meaning of each sentence. Be careful to consider what words modify the meaning of what other words, and thus what words belong in phrases together.

1. The old woman from the country loved the little boy from the city.
2. John hit the man with a wrench.
3. John hit the man with a scar.
4. John saw Mary in the park.
5. John saw Mary through binoculars.
6. John hit Mary on the head with a wrench.
7. John sat in the park on a bench at noon.

Do any of these sentences make you want to revise any of the phrase structure rules in any way?

6.3. CANONICAL PATTERNS AND RULES FOR CHANGING THEM

Canonical Patterns

The phrase structure rules above say that English is a SUBJECT VERB OBJECT (SVO) language. That is, its basic pattern is to have an NP (the subject) precede the verb and to have an NP (the object) follow the verb. Thus, in a sentence like 'The boy hit John', 'the boy' is usually ordered before the verb, and 'John' after the verb. The phrase structure rule for VP (Rule 8b above, which is: VP → V (NP) (PP)) says, in addition, that if a sentence has any prepositional phrases inside its VP, these will come after the verb and its object NP (if it has an object), as in the following sentences:

9a. The boy hit John *at the bank*

9b. *The boy hit *at the bank* John

10a. The boy hit John *at noon*

10b. *The boy hit *at noon* John

11a. The boy hit John *with an axe*

11b. *The boy hit *with an axe* John

However, PPs like those in sentences 9, 10, and 11 can also occur at the beginning of the sentence:

9c. *At the bank,* the boy hit John

10c. *At noon,* the boy hit John

11c. *With an axe,* the boy hit John

The sentences in 9c, 10c, and 11c represent special-purpose deviations from the normal pattern in 9a, 10a, and 11a, deviations that have a special communicative function. 9c, 10c, and 11c foreground or emphasize the PP by placing it at the beginning of the sentence, a particularly salient position. Notice that these sentences do not fit the phrase structure rules we have given, which say that S is composed of an NP followed by VP, and which allow for the PP to be at the end of the VP, not at the beginning of the sentence.

One way we can describe these facts is to say that 9a, 10a, and 11a represent a *canonical* (basic or "normal") pattern (which obeys the phrase structure rules of English) and that 9c, 10c, and 11c deviate from this pattern to do a special job. One common way linguists talk about this sort of deviation is to say that the PPs 'at the bank', 'at noon', or 'with an axe' have *moved* from their normal positions at the end of the VP to the front of the sentence. Thus, we can then state the following rule:

PP FRONTING RULE. PPs that are immediately dominated by (that is, that are daughters of) VP can move from their *normal* position at the end of the sentence (which is where the phrase structure rules say they normally occur) to the front of the sentence.

We are claiming, then, that a description of the special-purpose sentences in 9c, 10c, and 11c really involves also a consideration of the canonical sentence patterns in 9a, 10a, and 11a. The situation can be graphically depicted as below:

12.

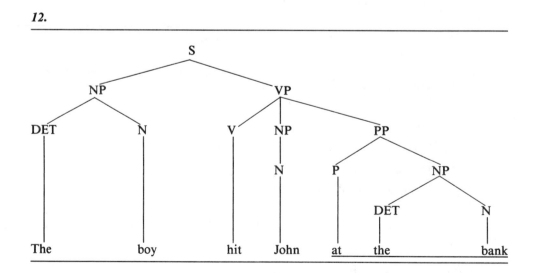

underlined PP moves to front of sentence by PP FRONTING RULE:

13.

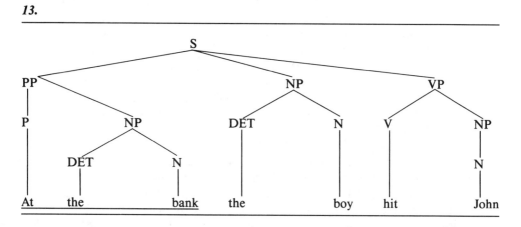

A rule like the PP fronting rule above is referred to as a **transformation** (or a **transformational rule**), because it transforms one tree into another one. Essentially, what PP fronting has done here is to start with a phrase structure tree that obeys the phrase structure rules and represents a canonical sentence pattern in the language and has transformed it into another phrase structure tree that does not obey the phrase structure rules and that represents a noncanonical pattern.

The phrase structure rules, thus, describe *only* the canonical or normal sentence patterns of the language, basically those for active, declarative sentences, as we will see. Deviations from this basic pattern are accounted for by transformations that rearrange or alter the basic sentence patterns to create more specialized patterns.

The tree in 12, which represents the canonical pattern, is called an **underlying structure,** and the tree in 13, which represents a deviation from the canonical pattern, is called a **derived structure.** The transformation is said to transform the underlying structure into the derived structure. The *whole* diagram made up of the two trees and the transformational rule that connects them is said to be a **transformational derivation.** The special-purpose sentence 'At the bank, the boy hit John' is said to have the *whole transformational derivation* as its **structural description.** We will see below that several transformations might apply to an underlying structure, one after another, producing a series of derived structures. The final derived structure (the one we are left with when we are done applying transformations) is also called a **surface structure.**

It is important to be clear on what we are saying here. Just as a cat, to a biologist, has a very complicated description in terms of its genetic structure, so to a linguist a sentence has a complicated structure in terms of (a) its underlying or canonical structure (which is a tree diagram organizing its words and phrases into a pattern that obeys the phrase structure rules; 12 is the underlying structure for sentence 11c, 'At the bank, the boy hit John'), (b) one or more transformational rules that may have applied to modify the underlying structure (in the example above, only the PP fronting transformation has applied), and (c) its various derived structures and its surface structure, which are also tree diagrams, and which may not obey the principles stated in the phrase structure rules (in the example above, only one transformation applied; its output is the derived structure in 13 and this derived structure is also the surface structure).

I am *not* claiming that to produce a sentence you first mentally produce an underlying structure, then apply a transformation, and then mentally produce a derived structure and utter its words. Rather, the theoretical structure above (12 and 13) is *all together* a single static representation or description of what you know about a sentence like 'At the bank, the boy hit John', and thus part of what you know about the language. It is meant to represent your linguistic *competence,* not your *performance* (see Section 2.2 in Chapter 2).

Linguists sometimes say that the phrase structure rules and the transformations "generate" structural descriptions for sentences (whole derivations like that in 12 and 13). This word 'generate' does *not* mean *produce,* it simply means *assign.* The rules "assign" structural descriptions (patterns of theoretical entities) to sentences. Because linguists use the word 'generate' this way, this sort of theory of grammar is sometimes called "Generative Grammar."

──────────────── **E X E R C I S E** ────────────────

Exercise F. For each of the pairs of sentences below, state which sentence represents the canonical pattern and which a special-purpose deviation from the canonical pattern. What purpose do you think that the special-purpose version in each case serves? Explicitly characterize the ways in which the pattern for the noncanonical sentence differs from the more canonical pattern (just describe this informally in English—there is no need to draw trees or formally state a transformation).

Example Answer. Take 6a and 6b. 6b represents the normal pattern, since it follows the regular SUBJECT ('John') VERB ('likes') OBJECT ('Mary') order of English. 6a represents a special-purpose deviation. 6b differs from the canonical pattern in 6a in that the object 'Mary' of 6a is in front of the sentence, not right after the verb, where objects usually are in English. Further, it is separated from the rest of the sentence by a pause (represented by a comma in writing). 6b is used when we want to call special attention to, or emphasize, the object (here 'Mary') for some reason.

1a. John loves Mary.

1b. Mary is loved by John.

2a. Into the house, ran John.

2b. John ran into the house.

3a. John will leave Mary.

3b. Will John leave Mary?

4a. John likes soup.

4b. John likes soup, doesn't he?

5a. I never liked John.

5b. Never did I like John.

6a. Mary, John really likes.   (done in example)

6b. John really likes Mary.

7a. John likes Mary, but he dislikes Sue.

7b. John likes Mary, but dislikes Sue.

The English System of Helping Verbs

English has a very interesting and intricate system of rules that determine other deviations from the canonical SUBJECT VERB OBJECT pattern. To understand these rules, we must first understand a bit about verbs and "helping verbs" in English.

English sentences always have at least one verb in them. This is the MAIN VERB of the sentence. However, the main verb may be preceded by up to three HELPING VERBS. There are three types of helping verbs. First, there are MODALS. The MODALS of English can simply be listed, as there are only a few of them: will/would; shall/should; may/might/must; and can/could ('John will eat the meal'). Second, there is the helping verb 'have' ('John *has* eaten the meal'). Third, there is the helping verb 'be' ('John *is* eating the meal'). Both *'have'* and *'be'* can also be used as main verbs as well; that is, they can be the only verb in the sentence or the last one preceded by helping verbs ('John *has* long hair', 'John may *have* long hair', 'John *is* happy', 'John may *be* happy').

As the examples in the last paragraph make clear, each helping verb affects the shape or form of the verb that follows it. Thus, note the changes in the examples below:

14a. John will *kiss* Mary   John will *eat* the meal

14b. John has *kissed* Mary   John has *eaten* the meal

14c. John is *kissing* Mary   John is *eating* the meal

English verbs can be classed as *regular* (like 'kiss') or *irregular* verbs (like 'eat'). Regular verbs take the normal past-tense ending '-ed' (as in 'John *kissed* Mary'). Irregular verbs take their own idiosyncratic past-tense endings (as in 'John *ate* the meal' or 'Mary *sang* the song'). I will use the term 'verb' for both helping verbs and main verbs. Modal verbs are followed by a verb in its "stem" form ('kiss', 'eat' in 14a). The stem form is the form in which the verb is listed in dictionaries. The helping verb 'have' is followed by a verb in its past participle form ('kissed', 'eaten' in 14b). Different verbs have different forms for their past participle, though for most verbs, like 'kiss', it is identical to the past tense (*'kissed'*), for irregular verbs, like 'eat', it varies from verb to verb ('eaten' for 'eat', 'sung' for 'sing', 'drunk' for 'drink'). If you want to know what the past participle of a verb is, and you are a fluent speaker of English, just put 'have' in front of the verb and what you produce is the past participle. If you are not a fluent speaker, you look it up in a book. The helping verb 'be' is followed by a verb in its present participle form ('kissing', 'eating'). The present participle is always the verb with the ending 'ing', so it is easy to recognize.

The English helping verbs always occur in the order MODAL, 'have', 'be', with a sentence being able to have one, two, or all three of them (or none). There are only two other things you need to know about English verbs: First, the *first* verb in a sentence, unless it is a modal, is inflected for tense; that is, it is placed in its present-tense or past-tense form to indicate whether the event described in the sentence occurred before the act of speaking (past) or at the time of speaking (present). You can always discover the present-tense and past-tense forms of verbs by putting the verb in a sentence where it has present or past meaning and where it is the only verb in the sentence (as in 'Now John *kisses* Mary/Now we *kiss* Mary' for the present, and 'John *kissed* Mary' for the past; or as in 'Now John *eats* the meal/Now we *eat* the meal' in the present, and 'John *ate* the meal' in the past). Note that verbs take the ending '-s' in the present tense when the subject of the sentence is singular and third person. 'Third person' means that a noun or pronoun (for example, 'he', 'him', 'she', 'her', 'they', 'them', 'it', 'John') does *not* name the speaker or hearer. When a pronoun names the speaker ('I', 'we'), it is called first person; when it names the hearer or hearers ('you'), it is called second person. In the present tense, verbs appear in the same form as their stem when the subject is anything but singular and third person (for example, 'We love Mary' versus 'John loves Mary'). If the first verb is a modal, then this modal indicates various other things beyond past or present time about the event the sentence describes, for instance whether it will happen in the future ('will'), whether it is only a possibility and not a reality ('may'), and many other subtle notions.

Second, the *last* verb in a string is always the main verb. If there is only one verb in the sentence, then this is the first and last, it is inflected for tense, and it is the main verb:

	MODAL	HAVE	BE		MAIN VERB	
15a. John	may	have (stem)	been (past participle)		kissing (present participle)	Mary

	HAVE	BE	MAIN VERB	
15b. John	has (present tense)	been (past participle)	eating (present participle)	sweets

	HAVE	BE	MAIN VERB	
15c. John	had (past tense)	been (past participle)	eating (present participle)	sweets

	MAIN VERB	
15d. John	eats (present tense)	sweets

	MAIN VERB	
15e. John	ate (past tense)	sweets

---------------------- **E X E R C I S E** ----------------------

Exercise G. Rewrite the following sentences and label each past participle form, past-tense form, present participle form, and main verb.

1. John sang for his supper.
2. John should have left on time.
3. John is living a fast life.
4. John has planned this trip.
5. John will have stayed for a week by now.
6. Mary will be going to Paris this spring.
7. John lives for his children.

Rules Concerned With Helping Verbs

English sentences that contain no helping verb (like 15d and 15e above) have a very interesting property. If one chooses to emphasize the assertion being made by such sentences, then a helping verb *does* show up—a stressed form of the verb 'do'. Thus, consider 16a and b, and 17a and b:

16a. John eats sweets. (Challenge: He does not).

16b. (Answer to challenge): John DOES eat sweets! (emphatic)

17a. John ate sweets. (Challenge: He did not).

17b. (Answer to challenge): John DID eat sweets! (emphatic)

The small capital letters above indicate that the word is stressed (said with higher pitch and more loudness). To account for this, I make the following assumption: *in underlying structure, all sentences* of English have at least one helping verb in them. If they do not have a MODAL, a 'have', or a 'be', then, at the very least, they will have the helping verb 'do'. If, however, this 'do' is not stressed to emphasize the assertion being made, then it disappears, leaving behind only the main verb by itself.

To see how this works in detail, consider the following revised phrase structure rules, which we will use to describe the *underlying structures* of English sentences:

18a. S→ NP AUX VP

18b. AUX→ $\begin{Bmatrix} \text{MODAL} & \text{(HAVE)} & \text{(BE)} \\ \text{DO-PRESENT/PAST} \end{Bmatrix}$

18c. MODAL→ (choose one of) can, could, may, might, must, shall, should, will, would

18a says that every sentence is made up of an NP subject, followed by an AUXILIARY node (AUX for short), followed by a VP. This AUX node is new, and it exists to hold onto (dominate) helping verbs. 18b tells us what the AUX node can contain. The curly brackets in 18b mean *or*. Thus, 18b means that the AUX node can contain *either* a MODAL optionally followed by the helping verb 'have' or the helping verb 'be' or both of them together, *or* it can contain instead just the helping verb 'do', in either its present-tense form ('does') or its past-tense form ('did'). 18c tells us what count as MODALS. We assume that the phrase structure rules otherwise are the same as given earlier. These rules produce underlying structures like that given in 19 and 20.

The following paragraph was inadvertently omitted from the first printing of this book, and will be restored in subsequent printings. It should be inserted at the bottom of page 205 before the paragraph beginning "Finally, we have to have..."

To deal with other possible auxiliaries in English, we need to add two more rules for what AUX can contain , in addition to Rule 18b above: AUX --> BE-PRESENT/PAST, allowing us to produce underlying structures for sentences with just the helping verb "be," such as "John is (or was) eat sweets," which the inflection rule will change to "John is (or was) eating sweets," and AUX --> HAVE-PRESENT/PAST (BE), allowing us to produce underlying structures for sentences with just the helping verb "have" or both "have" and "be," such as "John has (or had) eat sweets" and "John has (or had) be eat sweets," which the inflection rule will change respectively to: "John has (or had) eaten sweets" and "John has (or had) been eating sweets." For examples in the text I will use Rule 18b; you will get a chance to make use of one of these additional rules in doing exercise H below.

19.

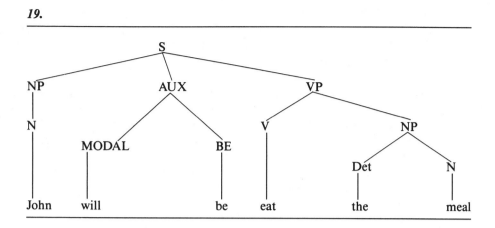

('eat' will become 'eating' by a rule to be discussed below)

20.

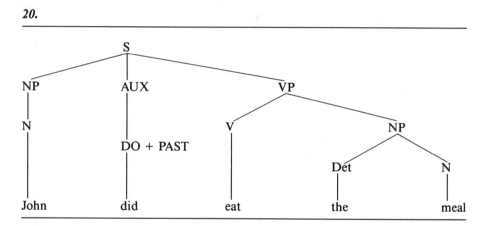

Obviously, 19 is not an English sentence as is. We have to have a rule to place each verb in its correct form. Let's call this rule the **inflection rule** (because the endings on verbs, like '-ed' for past tense or '-ing' for present participles, are called **inflections**). This rule places any verb following the helping verb 'have' into the past participle form, and any verb following the helping verb 'be' into the present participle form. Thus, the 'eat' following 'be' in 19 will be placed into its present participle form: 'eating'.

Finally, we have to have a rule either stressing 'do' if we want to emphasize the assertion being made by the sentence, or deleting the 'do' if we do not wish to emphasize the assertion being made. I give this rule—a transformational rule (since it changes one tree into another one)—below:

***DO* RULE.** To emphasize an assertion, stress the first helping verb in the sentence, or 'do' if there is no other helping verb. Otherwise, delete unstressed 'do'. Before deleting it, pass its tense (past or present) to the main verb directly following it.

For 20 above, if we retain 'do', we must stress it and get 'John DID eat the meal', which emphasizes the assertion being made. Otherwise, we delete 'do', giving its tense (in this case, it is past) to the main verb. We will then get 'John ate the meal'. Notice also that the *do* rule implies that we can stress any initial helping verb to emphasize the assertion being made: So we can get either 'John will eat sweets' (unstressed 'will', not emphasizing the assertion) or 'John WILL eat sweets' (stressed 'will', emphasizing the assertion).

Questions, Negatives, and Emphatics

We will now discuss how English forms **yes/no questions,** that is, questions that require yes or no for an answer. We will see that the simple *do* rule will help us a good bit in describing the syntax of English. Consider the examples of canonical sentences below (the "a" sentences) and their corresponding yes/no question forms (the "b" sentences):

21a. John is eating sweets

21b. Is John eating sweets?

22a. John will be eating sweets

22b. Will John be eating sweets?

23a. John ate sweets

23b. Did John eat sweets?

Sentence 21a fits the canonical SVO pattern of English, with helping verbs ('will' and 'be') preceding the main verb ('eat'), thus it has the form SUBJECT, HELPING VERBS, VERB, OBJECT. Sentence 21b does not fit the canonical pattern of English, since it starts not with the subject of the sentence but with a helping verb. It clearly is a special-purpose pattern, meant to signal that a question is being asked, a yes/no question.

It is also fairly clear what the rule for forming yes/no questions is:

YES/NO QUESTION RULE. Move the first helping verb in AUX to the front of the sentence.

This rule works to produce 21b from 21a by moving 'is' in 21a to the front of the sentence to produce 21b. The rule also works to produce 22b from 22a by moving 'will' in 22a to the front of the sentence to produce 22b. However, it must be remembered that it is really trees that are being changed here, not just sentences. The tree representing the underlying structure of 21a or 21b is modified by the yes/no question rule to produce the tree for the sentence in 21b or 22b, respectively.

In the case of 23a, something very interesting happens. The tree in example 20 above is the underlying structure for sentence 23a. The 'do' in the underlying structure has been deleted, leaving its past tense to 'eat' (producing 'ate' in 23a). However, assume that the yes/no question rule gets a chance to apply before the *do* rule has been applied. If the yes/no question rule applies, it will move the unstressed 'do' (in the tree in 20) to the front of the sentence to signal that a yes/no question is being asked. When this happens, the *do* rule can no longer apply, since the 'do' is no longer directly in front of the main verb and thus cannot any longer pass its tense to the main verb. Thus, we correctly produce a tree for the sentence in 23b, the yes/no question version of 23a. I give this tree below:

24.

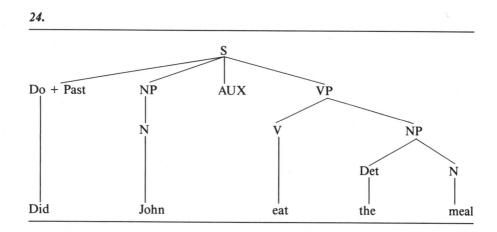

Note that 'did' is simply moved (from tree 20) to the front of the sentence, leaving an empty AUX node behind, to produce the tree in 24. In the case of the underlying structure in 19 above, once the yes/no question rule has moved the 'will' in AUX to the front of the sentence, it will leave 'be' behind in the AUX node.

We see here that the underlying structure in 20 can give rise to three different surface structures. We can stress 'do' and get 'John DID eat sweets' (17b); we can delete the 'do' and get 'John ate sweets' (23a); or we can apply the yes/no question rule and get 'Did John eat sweets' (23b).

We can get other results from the underlying structure in 20 as well. For instance, English has a rule producing negative sentences that can also apply to this underlying structure. Consider, for instance, the sentences in 25a and b, 26a and b, and 27a and b, where in each case the "b" sentences are the negations of the "a" sentences:

25a. John is eating sweets

25b. John is *not* eating sweets

26a. John will be eating sweets

26b. John will *not* be eating sweets

27a. John ate sweets

27b. John did *not* eat sweets

The rule for forming negative sentences in English is clear from this data:

NEGATIVE SENTENCE RULE.   Place 'not' after the first helping verb in AUX.

This rule places 'not' after 'is' in 25a to produce 25b; it places 'not' after 'will' in 26a to produce 26b (remember, this is really happening to full trees). In the case of 27a, once again we must consider the tree in 20, which is the underlying structure for 27a. Here the negative sentence rule places 'not' after the first (and only) helping verb ('did') and produces (a tree for) 27b 'John did not eat sweets'. The *do* rule cannot now apply, since 'do' cannot pass its tense to the main verb as it is now separated from the main verb by the word 'not'.

Finally, we can note that English allows other words to separate the 'do' in underlying structure from its following main verb, thus causing it to surface even when it is not stressed. For example, we can place a stressed 'so' or 'too' in a sentence to make it more emphatic. This produces sentences like the "b" sentences below from the canonical "a" sentences:

28a. John is eating sweets

28b. John is so eating sweets

29a. John will be eating sweets

29b. John will so be eating sweets

30a. John ate sweets

30b. John did so eat sweets

In 30b, the word 'so' has been placed after the 'did' in the tree in 20. Thus, 'did' cannot pass its tense to 'eat' and delete.

Applying the Rules Together

The rules we have given above can apply one after another to progressively deform a canonical or underlying structure, thereby producing derived structures that are more and more different in shape from the underlying structure. Consider, for example, the negative question 'Will John not be eating sweets?' Both the yes/no question rule and the negative sentence rule must apply to form this sentence. The underlying structure for this sentence is given by the tree in example 19 above. The negative sentence rule applies to place the word 'not' after the first helping verb, in this case 'will' ('not' is connected to the node AUX as its mother). This produces a new tree (one with 'not' in it), a derived tree. Then, the yes/no question rule applies to move the first helping verb ('will') to the front of the sentence ('will' is then connected to S as its mother). This produces yet another tree, another derived tree, and, since it is the last tree in this derivation, a surface structure. I show this derivation below, leaving out the trees (though you should imagine they are there, since these rules apply to whole trees, not just their bottom lines):

31a. UNDERLYING STRUCTURE: John will be eating sweets
31b. Negative rule produces: John will not be eating sweets
31c. Yes/no question rule produces: Will John not be eating sweets?

  Note how underlying structures (which are defined by the phrase structure rules) and transformational rules like the *do* rule, the yes/no question rule, and the negative sentence rule create a network of sentences that serve different communicative functions, but that are all related to the canonical pattern of English through being various transformations from the same underlying structure (which represents the canonical pattern of English). For instance, all the sentences in 32 are derived from the underlying structure in 19:

32a. John is eating sweets
   (declarative, makes a claim, canonical pattern)
32b. John IS eating sweets
   (emphasizes the assertion in 31a, derived by using the *do* deletion rule, which stresses the first helping verb or deletes 'do' when it is not stressed)
32c. Is John eating the meal
   (yes/no question, questions truth of 31a, derived by using the yes/no question rule)
32d. John is not eating the meal
   (negative sentence, denies 31a, derived by using the negative sentence rule)
32e. John is so eating the meal
   (emphatic sentence, emphasizes truth of 31a, derived by a rule that places 'so' after the first helping verb)
32f. Is John not eating the meal?
   (negative question, questions 31c, derived by using both the negative sentence rule and the yes/no question rule)

If we had formulated the transformational rule for negative contraction (for example, 'is' plus 'not' = 'isn't') and stipulated how it interacts with our other rules we could also have gotten

32g. Isn't John eating sweets?

E X E R C I S E

Exercise H. Give full derivations for the sentences below. That is, draw the underlying structure, apply each transformation you need to, and draw the surface structure. In the first case, draw a tree for each step (an underlying tree, a derived tree for each transformation that applies, and a surface structure tree). After that, you need not draw trees any longer, but just write out "terminal lines" of words (which you will assume have trees on top of them), as I did in 31 above.

1. Is John not eating the meal? (HINT: The terminal line of words of the underlying structure is 'John is eat the meal'.)

2. Is John eating the meal? (HINT: The terminal line of words of the underlying structure is 'John is eat the meal'.)

3. John left (HINT: The terminal line of words of the underlying structure is 'John did leave'.)

4. Did John leave? (HINT: The terminal line of words of the underlying structure is 'John did leave'.)

5. John is so eating the meal. (HINT: The terminal line of words of the underlying structure is 'John is eat the meal'.)

Content Questions (Wh-Questions)

So far, we have seen one type of question in English: yes/no questions. There is another type of question, one with many interesting properties, only a few of which we will be able to look at here. Consider the questions below:

33a. Whom has Mary kissed?
33b. Who has kissed John?

These sentences are called **content questions** (or **wh-questions**, because question words in English are all spelled with 'wh', except for 'how'—'who', 'where', 'what', 'why'—but they are all pronounced with 'hw' at the beginning).

Such questions require more than yes or no for an answer; one must answer them with some actual content (for example, either a name or a description).

The sentence in 33a clearly violates the canonical SUBJECT VERB OBJECT order of English. The object of the verb 'kiss' (the person who gets kissed) is named by the question word 'whom' and yet it is not after the verb, but in front of it. In fact, if the word 'whom' did occur after the verb we would still get a grammatical sentence, but one with a different function than 33a:

33c. Mary has kissed *whom?*
    (said with rising intonation and stress on 'whom')

33c is an "echo question." If someone says that Mary has kissed John, but I have failed to hear 'John', I can utter 33c in an attempt to get the speaker to repeat the name. But 33a can be used not just in this sort of context, when I have failed to hear what was said and need it repeated, but in any context in which I want to find out whom it was that Mary kissed.

Note too that in 33a the helping verb ('has' = have + PRESENT) has moved in front of the subject just as it does in yes/no questions. We can describe what is going on in 33a by saying that in underlying structure wh-words occur in the normal canonical places for NPs (as subjects and objects and objects of prepositions, for instance) but that they are moved to the front of the sentence by a rule (the **content question rule**). The yes/no question rule must also apply. Below I give the rule for forming wh-questions (the content question rule) and a derivation for 33a.

CONTENT QUESTION RULE. Move a wh-word from its canonical position to the front of the sentence

34. **Underlying Structure:**

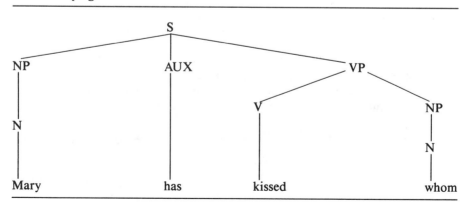

The yes/no question rule applies to produce

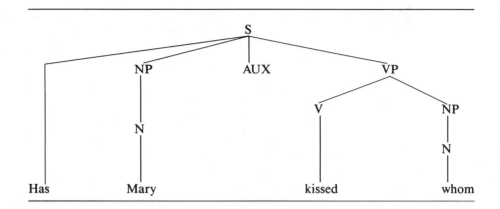

The content question rule applies to produce

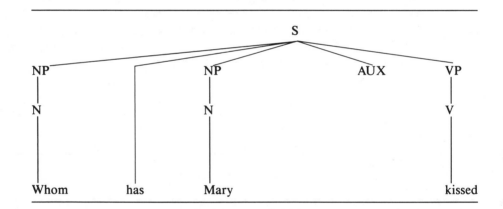

A derivation for 33b is given below. Note that the yes/no question rule has no real effect here, as the content question rule here undoes what the yes/no question rule accomplishes. This always happens if the wh-word is in subject position in underlying structure. For ease of reading, I leave out the trees:

35a. UNDERLYING STRUCTURE: Who has kissed John

35b. Yes/no question rule produces: Has who kissed John

35c. Content question rule produces: Who has kissed John?

—————————— E X E R C I S E S ——————————

Exercise I. Give a derivation, like the ones you did in Exercise H above, for the sentences below (draw a tree for the underlying structure and for the surface structure; you can use terminal lines of words for the intermediate steps, just assuming these have trees on top of them).

1. Whom will John have spoken to?
2. Whom did John kiss?

Exercise J. How would you change the content question rule to handle the following data?

1. Which girl will John speak to?
2. Whom will John speak to?
3. To whom will John speak?
4. To which girl will John speak?

Exercise K. English used to make a clear distinction between 'who' and 'whom', and some speakers still do. In particular, many people still make this distinction in writing. However, in everyday speech, most people do not use 'whom' anymore except in one situation, which is shown below:

1. Who will Mary kiss?   (used to be 'whom')
2. Who will kiss Bill?
3. Who will John speak to?   (used to be 'whom')
4. Who will speak to John?
5. To whom will John speak? (used to be and still is 'whom')

What was the old rule for using 'who' and 'whom' (the one still used often in writing)? What is the new rule? Why do you think that 'whom' is retained in a sentence like 5? Sentences 3 and 5 mean the same thing. Which do you think is more common? Why?

Form and Function in Syntax

We can learn something very important about the relationship between form and function in language from the content question rule. So far, we have labeled our transformational rules with names for their functions (yes/no question rule, content question rule), that is, in terms of what they can be used to communicate. But notice that these rules are also used in cases where they do *not* have the function in terms of which we have labeled them. We saw above that the yes/no question rule, which has the effect of moving a helping verb to the front of the sentence, also occurs in content questions, not just in yes/no questions. In fact, it does not occur just in questions (of whatever type). It also operates in other cases as well, cases which have nothing to do with asking a question:

36a. John will never give up.

36b. Never *will* John give up

37a. John has seldom said nice things

37b. Seldom *has* John said nice things

Thus, we cannot really say that the yes/no question rule, the movement of the helping verb to the front of the sentence, has the function of signaling that a yes/no question, or even a question of any sort, is being asked.

Furthermore, the content question rule, which has the effect of moving a wh-word to the front of the sentence, also operates in structures that have nothing to do with asking a question, namely in *relative clauses:*

38a. The man (Mary has just kissed whom) loves Susan →

38b. The man whom Mary has just kissed loves Susan

While we will not discuss relative clauses in detail, note that in 38b 'whom' is the object of 'kissed' (the person who gets kissed) and has moved from after 'kissed' in underlying structure (roughly as in 38a) to in front of the subject of 'kissed', namely 'Mary'.

We learn here that transformational rules really should not be labeled by names for functions (like asking a yes/no question or asking a content question). They are formal operations (deviations from canonical form) that actually operate in a number of different sentence types. The relationship between form and function in language is not simple and direct, but rather a very complex matter. We will see this throughout the rest of this chapter and in other parts of this book as well. It is for this reason that the yes/no question rule might better be called the **subject/helping verb inversion rule** and the content question rule might better be called **wh-movement.** Here we are labeling the rules by the sorts of forms (patterns) they create, not by the communicative functions (meanings) they signal.

The Unboundedness of Wh-Movement

Wh-movement (content question formation) has the interesting property that the wh-word can be moved indefinitely far across the sentence. Consider a very long sentence like that in 39a:

39a. John thinks that the President is going to appoint Sam to the job

Clearly 'Sam' is the object of the verb 'appoint'. Now substitute 'whom' for 'Sam':

39b. John thinks that the President is going to appoint *whom* to the job?

Now 'whom' is the object of 'appoint' and we have an echo question. The 'whom' here can move to the front of the sentence to form a content question:

39c. *Whom* does John think that the President is going to appoint to the job?

The speaker of English realizes that though 'whom' is in the front of the sentence here, it is still the object of 'appoint'. Objects usually occur after the verb, and we assume that they always, in fact, occur after the verb in underlying structure, though they may be moved from that position by various rules.

Obviously, we could put more and more material between the front of the sentence and 'whom', and the 'whom' would still be able to move to the front to form a grammatical question:

40a. John thinks that Sue said that the President is going to appoint *Sam* to the job
40b. John thinks that Sue said that the President is going to appoint *whom* to the job?
40c. *Whom* does John think that Sue said that the President is going to appoint to the job?

We could keep adding material to make the sentences longer and longer. The wh-word can move over any number of words to get to the front of the sentence. Because of this, the wh-movement rule is said to be "unbounded" or an "unbounded" rule.

Embedded Sentences

Many of the above examples have involved long sentences with complicated structures. We do not have the time and space to study these here. But I will point out some basic facts about the way in which English can embed one sentence inside another one. Consider the two sentences below:

41a. John thinks something
41b. Mary loves Bill

The sentence in 41b can be embedded inside the one in 41a by replacing the object of 'thinks' ('something') by the sentence in 41b. When this is done, we often introduce the embedded sentence by the word 'that', which is called a **complementizer,** though 'that' is usually optional. We get

41c. John thinks that Mary loves Bill

We say that the sentence 'Mary loves Bill' is embedded "beneath" the verb 'think'.

There is another type of embedding besides the one using 'that'. The embedded sentence can have, in its AUX, the word 'to':

42a. John wants something
42b. Mary loves Bill
42c. John wants *Mary to love Bill*   (42b is embedded in 42a)

When the little word 'to' shows up, the verb following it ('love') is said to be an **infinitive** (**nonfinite** is another word for the same thing; the verb appears in its stem form). When 'to' does show up, another thing can happen. The subject of the embedded sentence can be missing, in which case it is understood to be identical in meaning to the subject of the preceding verb under which the embedded sentence is embedded:

43a. John wants something
43b. John loves Bill
43c. John wants *to love Bill*   (43b, minus its subject, is embedded in 43a)

Here, in 43c, the embedded sentence is understood to be 'John to love Bill' but 'John' is missing. Some people dislike calling things like 'Mary to love Bill' in 42c or 'to love Bill' in 43c "sentences" (even if we call them "embedded sentences"), because they think of 'sentence' as meaning *something that could be said by itself* and they point out you could not utter 'Mary to love Bill' by itself. However, by 'sentence' we mean any verb with its associated subject and object (and the subject can sometimes be "missing" because it is understood as being identical to an NP that has already occurred).

Embedded sentences can have transformations apply to them just as if they were standing alone. For example, we can apply the negative sentence rule to the embedded sentence in 42c to get

42d. John thinks that Mary does *not* love Bill

And, finally, consider the verb 'wonder'. 'Wonder' can have a sentence embedded beneath it to which wh-movement (the content question rule) has applied:

44a. John wonders something

44b. Mary loves whom? → Whom does Mary love?

44c. John wonders *whom Mary loves?*   (44b is embedded in 44a)

The embedded sentence beneath 'wonder' here is called an **indirect question** or an **embedded question**. Notice one very curious thing about it. Though the wh-word 'whom' has moved from the object position behind 'loves' to in front of the embedded sentence, subject/helping verb inversion (the yes/no question rule) has not applied, though this rule does apply to regular wh-questions. This rule never applies in embedded sentences in standard English, though it does in many nonstandard dialects, which would say for 44c, 44d below instead:

44d. John wonders *who does Mary love?*

If a sentence is embedded beneath 'wonder' and it contains no wh-word, then the special wh-word 'whether' or the word 'if' shows up in front of the embedded sentence (these are said to be embedded yes/no questions):

45a. John wonders something

45b. Mary loves Bill

45c. John wonders *whether (or if) Mary loves Bill*   (45b is embedded in 45a)

Some nonstandard dialects could say instead of 45c:

45d. John wonders *does Mary love Bill?*

─────────────── **E X E R C I S E** ───────────────

Exercise L.   Underline the embedded sentences in the following sentences. Then state exactly how the embedded sentence in each case differs from a nonembedded sentence.

1. John thinks that Mary plays tennis.
2. Mary's playing tennis is a good idea.
3. I want Mary to play tennis.
4. Mary wants to play tennis.
5. For Mary to play tennis would be a good idea.
6. Mary loves playing tennis.
7. The girl who plays tennis is happy.

6.4. GRAMMATICAL RELATIONS

So far, the terms 'subject' and 'object' have referred to particular NP positions (subject = NP directly under S and before the verb; object = NP directly below VP and after the verb). Now we will look at what really lies behind these terms.

Prototypical ACTOR ACTION PATIENT Sentences

In all languages of the world, there is a basic, prototypical sentence pattern in which an ACTOR acts on a PATIENT and where the action is named by a VERB. The English sentence in 46 is of this type:

46. The girl (ACTOR) beat the boy (PATIENT)

Since there are two NPs ('the girl' and 'the boy') in this sort of sentence, a language must clearly indicate *who* beat *whom,* that is, it must indicate whether the girl beat the boy or the boy beat the girl. English uses *word order* to do this job. The NP naming the ACTOR is placed before the verb, and the NP naming the PATIENT is placed after the verb. If we change the order of 'the girl' and 'the boy' in sentence 46 (and thus produce 'The boy beat the girl'), we will change the meaning of the sentence, in terms of who is the ACTOR (now the boy) and who is the PATIENT (now the girl).

All languages must distinguish between the ACTOR and the PATIENT in sentences like 46. For example, Welsh, like English, uses word order to distinguish between an ACTOR and PATIENT, but places them in the order VERB ACTOR PATIENT:

47. Lladdodd   draig   ddyn
     killed   dragon   man
     VERB   ACTOR   PATIENT
     'A dragon killed a man'

The two most common word orders across languages are ACTOR VERB PATIENT and ACTOR PATIENT VERB, with the order VERB ACTOR PATIENT being fairly common. Other orders are rare. Latin, on the other hand, does not use word order for the job of distinguishing between the ACTOR and the PATIENT. Rather, it has special endings (**inflectional affixes**) on its nouns. The ACTOR gets one ending, and the PATIENT gets a different one (note that Latin does not have articles like the English words 'the' and 'a'. Only the discourse context makes clear whether the speaker is talking about 'the girl' or 'a girl'):

48. Puell-a   ferīvit   puer-um
     girl-ACTOR   beat   boy-PATIENT
     'The girl beat the boy'

The ending 'a' on girl ('puell') tells us that the girl is the ACTOR; the ending 'um' on boy ('puer') tells us that the boy is the PATIENT.

Languages like Latin that handle the problem of specifying the semantic role of each NP in sentences like 46 through endings on nouns need not stick to a rigid word order. Such languages are free to vary the word order of their sentences. Thus, a Latin sentence like 48 above can be said with any word order and will remain grammatical. And in each case it means 'The girl beat the boy'.

Since word order is free to vary in Latin, different word orders can be used to communicate different meanings beyond the bare facts of "who beat whom." For example, Latin speakers could indicate to their hearers what information in the sentence they took to be old or given information (assumed to be already known to the hearer) by placing it in the beginning of the sentence; and they could indicate information that they took to be new or not already known by placing it at the end of the sentence. But English does not have this freedom, since it uses its basic word order to indicate the semantic relation each noun has to the verb, that is, to signal who acted on whom. It is not that English cannot indicate what is given or assumed information versus what is new, but it must do so in a somewhat different way from Latin. We will see more of this matter in Chapter 10.

Sentences With One NP

The picture in the preceding section seems straightforward enough. But it turns out that things are not exactly what they seem. A very interesting problem arises when we consider sentences with only one NP in them, like those in 49a and 49b:

49a. The boy lied   [the boy = ACTOR]
49b. The boy died   [the boy = PATIENT]

Clearly, the boy plays a quite different role in 49a and 49b. In 49a he is an ACTOR. In 49b he is not an ACTOR, but a PATIENT. Now, if in a sentence like 'The girl beat the boy' (46 above), English places 'the girl' before the verb to indicate that it is the ACTOR and places 'the boy' after the verb to indicate that it is the PATIENT, we should wonder why English puts the NP naming the boy in 49b in the position before the verb, where it puts the ACTOR in a sentence like 'The girl beat the boy'. Why doesn't English put it after the verb, where it puts the PATIENT in 'The girl beat the boy', producing the sentence below:

49c. *Died the boy

However, almost all languages choose to treat 'the boy' in sentences like 49a and 49b the same, ignoring the difference in semantic role. Since there is only one NP in sentences 49a and 49b, there is really no need to use word order or a special ending to indicate the relation of this NP to the verb or to distinguish it from another NP in the sentence (there is no other NP). The meaning of the verb itself clearly indicates what semantic role the NP is playing.

But then another problem arises: Given that in these one-NP sentences there is no problem identifying the semantic role of the NP, then why doesn't English allow the single NP to occur in any order in relation to the verb; after all, no ambiguity could arise (as it could in 46 above, where if we allowed any order, then we wouldn't know who did what to whom). But, of course, English does no such thing. Sentences 49a and 49b are grammatical only when the NP precedes the verb. Variations like 'Lied the boy' or 'Died the boy' are ungrammatical.

This is what is going on: Faced with sentences like those in 49a and 49b in which there is only one NP, most languages actually use the ending or position they use for the ACTOR in ACTOR VERB PATIENT sentences (like 46 above) for this single NP as well. There are a small number of languages (called **ergative languages**) that make just the opposite choice and use the ending or position they use for the PATIENT in ACTOR ACTION PATIENT sentences for the single NP in single-NP sentences.

But the vast majority of languages choose to extend the ACTOR position (for example, before the verb in English) or ending (for example, the '-a' on 'puella' in Latin) to the single NP in single-NP sentences, whether it is an ACTOR or not. There is a cost, however, for doing this: The ending or the position can now no longer be taken to mean ACTOR, because in sentences like 49b the single NP ('the boy') is not an ACTOR. We might say that the ending or position takes on a life of its own. We discuss that life in the next section.

Subject and Object

The ending or position that English and Latin give to 'the girl' in sentences like 46 ('The girl beat the boy'), or 'the boy' in sentences like 49a ('The boy lied') and 49b ('The boy died') is not, in fact, indicating the ACTOR, at least not directly. It is indicating the *subject* of the sentence, a much used, abused, and misunderstood term.

Leaving aside the ergative languages mentioned above, the subject of English and Latin sentences (and most other languages) can be defined as follows:

> The *subject* of a sentence is that NP that has the ending or is in the position that an NP naming the ACTOR in a prototypical ACTOR ACTION PATIENT sentence has or is in.

In English, NPs naming ACTORS in prototypical ACTOR ACTION PATIENT sentences are placed before the verb. Thus, we call any NP in English that is placed before the verb a "subject," whether or not it refers to an ACTOR. In Latin, NPs naming ACTORS in prototypical ACTOR ACTION PATIENT sentences take a special ending ('a' for nouns in the same class as 'girl'). Thus, any noun with this special ending is said to be the "subject" of the sentence, regardless of whether it names an ACTOR or not. We can equally well go on to define the term 'object' of a sentence (often called the **direct object** of the verb), along the same lines:

> The *object* of a sentence is that NP that has the ending or is in the position that the NP naming the PATIENT in a prototypical ACTOR ACTION PATIENT sentence has or is in.

In English, the NP naming the PATIENT in a prototypical ACTOR ACTION PATIENT sentence is placed after the verb; thus, we will call any NP in English that is placed immediately after the verb the "object" of the sentence. Some of these NPs, in fact, do not name PATIENTS:

50a. The girl built *a house* (PRODUCT)

50b. The girl threw *the ball* (THEME) to the boy (GOAL)

50c. The girl saw *the boy* (GOAL)

50d. The girl reached *Africa* (GOAL)

50e. The girl stole $100 (THEME) from John (SOURCE)[1]

Subject and object, then, do not name any one semantic role, like ACTOR or PATIENT. Since they are not associated with any single meaning, certain questions naturally arise: What are they? Why do languages have them? What function do they serve in the sentence? Subject and object are called **grammatical relations.** They are important notions in language, but we can only get a full view of what they really amount to as we develop our view of language more fully in the rest of this chapter and in Chapter 10.

---

[1]In Chapter 2, I pointed out that THEME is the semantic role of the NP that names something that moves, changes location or state, or is located. GOAL names the end point of a motion or process; SOURCE names the beginning point of a motion or process. Thus, in 50e, John is the SOURCE because he is where the money was at the beginning of the robbery.

Finding Subjects and Objects in Languages

We have appealed to semantic concepts (concepts like ACTOR and PATIENT) in defining subject and object. But there is another way to approach the problem. There are tests that linguists apply to discover what constitutes a subject in a given language. These tests are purely *formal;* that is, they refer to structures and patterns ('form') in a language, not to meaning. They allow us to identify what counts as a subject or an object in a language without in fact having to make any reference to semantic notions like ACTOR and PATIENT. This is important because it allows us to come to terms with those languages (like the ergative ones) in which the subject is not the NP that names the ACTOR in prototypical ACTOR ACTION PATIENT sentences.

The first test is based on **reflexive** sentences. Reflexive sentences contain two NPs, one of which is a reflexive pronoun. Reflexive pronouns refer to the same person or thing as the other NP in the sentence, as in sentence 51a below (where the reflexive pronoun is underlined):

51a. The girl loves <u>herself</u>

The reflexive pronoun ('herself') signals that this NP ('herself') refers to the same person as does the preceding NP, 'the girl'. Thus, sentence 51a means something like *The girl loves the girl* where both phrases 'the girl' are understood to refer to the same girl. In no language can the subject (regardless of where in the sentence it is positioned) be represented as a reflexive pronoun. Thus, in English, 51b below is ungrammatical (such sentences can occur, in some dialects of English, as emphatic reflexives, but not as normal unemphatic sentences):

51b. *Herself loves the girl

If you were faced with a language and did not know which NP in its sentences designated the subject, you could try to get a translation of the meaning *The girl loves herself,* or of any reflexive sentence like this one. The NP that is *not* represented by a reflexive pronoun would be the subject. You could then check how this NP was inflected (for example, what ending it had) or positioned in the sentence (what its word order was in relation to the verb, for example). This would give you a guide to identify subjects in other sentences.

The second test is this: If we conjoin two sentences together using the conjunction 'and', and the second sentence contains an NP that refers to the same person or thing that an NP in the preceding sentence refers to, then this redundant NP can be left out (dropped from the sentence), provided it is the subject of its sentence. It cannot be left out if it is the object:

52a. The girl hit the boy and *she* (= the girl) killed him

52b. The girl hit the boy and __ killed him

53a. The girl hit the boy and the dog bit *him* (= the boy)

53b. *The girl hit the boy and the dog bit __

In 52a, 'she' refers to the girl in the previous sentence ('The girl hit the boy') and so is redundant. It is the subject of its sentence (*'she* killed him'). So it can be left out (52b). In 53a 'him' refers to the boy in the previous sentence ('The girl hit the boy') and so is redundant. But it is not the subject of its sentence ('The dog bit *him'*). Thus, it cannot be left out (53b is ungrammatical). There is, of course, no logical reason why a language, or even English for that matter, could not do something like 53b. It's just that no language does. Thus, if a language can leave out an NP in one sentence because it is redundant with one in a previous conjoined sentence (a sentence connected by 'and' or 'but' to a preceding one), then that NP that is left out is the subject.

Tests like these two (there are many more) are usually consistent for almost all languages. That is, they nearly always pick out the same NP as subject (for example, the reflexive test and the conjoined sentences test pick out the same NP, the one before the verb in English, or marked by endings like 'a' in Latin). In a few languages they don't, and problems arise for the linguist. For example, in Tagalog, a language spoken in the Philippines, some tests for subject pick out the NP in Tagalog sentences that is marked with the preposition 'ng' (a mark for ACTORS), and other tests pick out the NP marked by the preposition 'ang' (a mark for TOPICS). So here the tests are not consistent. Such problem cases are rare, but very interesting nonetheless. Linguists look for just such cases in the hope of discovering new facts about language or deepening their knowledge of old facts (like what subjects really are in English and other languages).

—————————————— **E X E R C I S E** ——————————————

Exercise M. For this exercise, you need either to go to the library or get a "language consultant." If you choose the former, go to the library and get a descriptive grammar of a language you know nothing about, and then answer the questions below (do the best you can, given the grammar you have learned so far). If you choose the latter, find a native (or, at least, very fluent) speaker of a language you know little or nothing about, a speaker who is willing to help you learn about his or her language. Ask the consultant questions about his or her language so that you can determine the answers to the questions below (never tell your consultant that you think he or she is wrong, and never push the consultant to answer if he or she appears to be unwilling; do the best you can under the conditions you find yourself in). Make clear to the consultant that you want to know how people *say* sentences in the language, not how one *writes* them. It is all right to let your consultant write the sentence down for you when he or she has thought about how to say it and after he or she has actually said it. Once you have the sentence in writing, write down an English "gloss" (literal translation) beneath each word or morpheme in the sentence.

1. Determine if the language you have chosen to work on has a fixed word order in simple declarative sentences (for example, in sentences like 'The girl kicked the boy', 'The girl killed the boy', and 'The girl loved the boy'). If it does, what is it? If it does not, which orders are grammatical? What determines when you use which order?

2. How does the language you are working with indicate what a *subject* is in a sentence that also has an object in it (like *'The girl* killed the boy')? How does it indicate what the subject is in a sentence with no object (like 'The boy cried' or 'The boy died')? How does it indicate what the object of the sentence is (in a sentence like 'The girl killed *the boy*')?

3. How does the language you are working on form a yes/no question? How does it form a content question? Describe how the way your language does this differs from English.

6.5. CASE AND GRAMMATICAL RELATIONS

Case

Consider again the Latin sentence 48 above, repeated here:

48. Puell-a   ferivit   puer-um
    girl-ACTOR   beat   boy-PATIENT
    'The girl beat the boy'

Latin grammarians call the endings on Latin nouns (like '-a' on 'puell/girl' and '-um' on 'puer/boy') **morphological cases** (often called just **cases**). The ending that marks the subject (for example, the '-a' on 'puell/girl') is called the **nominative case.** The ending that marks the object (for example, the '-um' on 'puer/boy') is called the **accusative case.** Latin has, in addition to the nominative case ending and the accusative case ending, a few other case endings. These additional cases signal meanings that in English would be signaled by prepositions. Below, I outline the case system of Latin:

SUMMARY OF LATIN CASE SYSTEM

Nominative Case = case of the SUBJECT = position before the verb in English
Accusative Case = case of the OBJECT = position after the verb in English
Genitive Case = case marked by 'of' or ''s' in English:

54a. pater   puell-æ
father   girl-of
'the father of the girl' / 'the girl's father'

Dative Case = case marked by the prepositions 'to' or 'for' in English (when they mark the BENEFICIARY, the one for whom the action is done):

54b. Puell-a   davit   don-um   puer-*o*
girl-NOM   gave   gift-ACC   boy-DATIVE (= to)
'The girl gave the gift *to the boy*'

Ablative Case = case often marked by the prepositions 'from', 'with', or 'in' in English:

54c. Puell-a   fundebat   aqu-am   pater-o
girl-NOM   poured   water-ACC   bowl-ABLATIVE (= from)
'The girl poured water from the bowl'

Linguists want to be able to talk about Latin and English and other languages without having constantly to make reference to how they mark subjects and objects, whether by special endings or by word order, or other devices for other languages. And, in fact, we can generalize the traditional use of the term 'case', to treat English as if it too had a case system. First, note that English pronouns overtly show case distinctions, that is, they change their shape to distinguish between nominative case (the case associated with the subject) and accusative (the case associated with the object; accusative case is also used when the pronoun follows a preposition, as in 55c):

55a. She (NOM) killed him (ACC)
55b. He (NOM) killed her (ACC)
55c. John took Mary with him (ACC)

It is a small extension to say that English marks NPs (when they are not pronouns) as nominative by placing them in front of the verb and as accusative by placing them after the verb or after a preposition:

56a. The girl (NOM) killed the boy (ACC)
56b. The boy (NOM) gave a gift (ACC) to the girl (ACC)

'The girl' is marked as nominative in 56a by being placed in front of the verb, 'the boy' as accusative by being placed after it. In 56b 'the boy' is marked as nominative by being placed before the verb, 'the gift' as accusative by being placed after the verb, and 'the girl' as accusative by being placed after a preposition.

—————————————— E X E R C I S E ——————————————

Exercise N. Does the language you studied in doing Exercise M have an overt case system (like Latin) for its nouns? What about its pronouns (for example, 'He likes her', 'She likes him')? Describe your language's system for marking case. You can use the chart "Summary of Latin Case System" above as a guide, though your language may have more or fewer cases than Latin does.

The Relation of Case Marking to Grammatical Relations (Subject/Object)

Being able to talk about case in this general way allows us to compare languages like English and Latin, and other languages, and to see if we can find any generalizations that hold true across many or all languages. For example, consider the English sentences below, which raise a very odd and interesting problem:

57a. As for John, Mary thinks that <u>he killed the boy</u>

57b. As for John, Mary wants <u>him to kill the boy</u>

57c. Mary tried *[Mary]* <u>to kill the boy</u> (= Mary tried to kill the boy)

The underlined words in 57a ('he killed the boy') constitute a little embedded sentence inside a bigger one ('he killed the boy' is inside 'As for John, Mary thinks that . . .'). The subject of 'kill' in this little sentence is clearly 'he' and it is marked as nominative (both by its position before the verb 'kill' and by its shape, since it is a pronoun). However, 57b is odd. Here 'kill' is preceded by the little word 'to', which English uses when it does not want to indicate any tense (past, present, or future) of the verb, as opposed to the '-ed' on the end of 'kill' in 57a, which tells us the verb is PAST TENSE (past time), or the 's' on 'thinks' in 57a, which tells us the verb is PRESENT TENSE (present time). The words 'him to kill the boy' in 57b are just like a sentence (ACTOR ACTION PATIENT), except that there is no indication of tense. And surely we would expect that in this sentence the word 'him' would name the subject, since this word refers to the ACTOR and it is playing the same semantic role here as 'he' is in 'he killed the boy' in 57a. So why is the word 'him' here in the accusative case, the case normally used for objects, not subjects? In 57c we see another situation: The embedded sentence is 'to kill the boy', where the subject is missing and is understood to be 'Mary'. No NP can occur in front of 'to' here (*'Mary tried Mary to kill the boy' is ungrammatical).

It turns out that English, and many other languages as well, obey the following rule for case assignment:

CASE ASSIGNMENT RULE

Subjects of sentences that contain either a modal (like 'may' or 'will') or a verb marked for tense (past or present) are assigned nominative case. We will say that they are "assigned" this nominative case by the modal or the tense of the verb.

Subjects of sentences that contain infinitives (verbs not marked for tense or modality) usually receive no case and must therefore be missing from the sentence (as in 57c above), since we will assume that all NPs must have a case in order to overtly show up in a sentence.

In some exceptional situations, the subjects of infinitives are allowed to be present (as in 57b above). In these exceptional situations, they receive accusative case.

Objects of all verbs and prepositions are assigned accusative case. We will say that the verb or preposition "assigns" the accusative case to its object.

I will not detail when infinitives have accusative subjects (as in 57b) and when their subjects are missing (as in 57c), though the normal case is for their subjects to be missing. Examples of case assignment follow:

58a. She (NOM) thinks that he (NOM) killed the boy (ACC)

58b. Mary (NOM) wants him (ACC) to kill the boy (ACC)

58c. Mary (NOM) tried—to kill the boy (ACC)
    (subject of 'to kill' is understood as 'Mary', but this NP cannot be present overtly because it cannot get case, since 'to kill' has no tense and thus cannot assign nominative case)

The case assignment rule is somewhat odd, but the same sort of thing happens in Latin and many other languages. Once again, human language doesn't behave the way we might have predicted. We see here that case marking takes on something of a life of its own, just as subjects and objects did earlier. Though nominative is the case associated with subjects, there are exceptions, as in the situation above. The subject of 'to kill the boy' in 57b and 58b is 'him', which is in the accusative case (and would be so also in Latin in similar sorts of sentences), the case normally associated with objects. Such "problems" teach us something very important about human language: Any set of notions that language uses, like semantic roles (ACTOR and PATIENT), grammatical relations (subject and object), or cases (nominative and accusative), though they may be closely related to each other (often ACTOR = subject = nominative), tend to take on a life of their own and obey their own principles, so that the relation between them is never total or direct. One may find this complex, or even perverse, but that's just the way human language is, thanks to the hundreds of thousands of years of human evolution that gave rise to it. And, as will be seen in Chapter 8, babies don't have any great difficulty learning these different systems.

—————————————————— **E X E R C I S E** ——————————————————

Exercise O.   How does the language you worked on for Exercises M and N above say the sentences below? Compare to English.

1. John tried to win.
2. John wants to win.
3. John wants Mary to win.
4. John thinks that Mary won.

6.6. ARGUMENTS

So far we have talked about semantic roles (ACTOR and PATIENT), grammatical relations (subject and object), and cases (nominative and accusative). In the next few sections, we will look in more detail at how these systems are related to each other.

Argument Structures

The heart of any sentence is the *verb*. In Chapter 2, we saw that a verb can be viewed as a PREDICATE, with a certain number of PLACES that can be filled by NPs to make up a sentence. A predicate is a word that attributes a property to an object (for example, 'John *laughed*' or 'John is *tall*') or that attributes a relationship to two or more objects (for example, 'Mary *loves* John', 'John *gave* a book to Mary'). Thus, the verb 'beat' can be viewed as a two-place predicate, that is, a predicate that combines with two NPs, one an ACTOR and one a PATIENT, to make up a sentence. We can write this as follows:

59. beat [ACTOR, PATIENT]   (cf. The girl beat the boy)

which we will take to mean that 'beat' is a predicate with two places to be filled by NPs, one of which must be an ACTOR ('the girl' in 'The girl beat the boy') and one of which must be a PATIENT ('the boy' in 'The girl beat the boy').

The NPs that fill a predicate's "places" are called the **arguments** of the predicate. So we say that in 'The girl beat the boy', 'the girl' and 'the boy' are "arguments" of the verb 'beat'. We will therefore refer to the formula in 59 above as the **argument structure** of the verb 'beat'. We assume that this formula is part of the **lexical entry** of 'beat'. The **lexicon** is the mental list of the words in a language, a list that each of us stores in our heads ('lexicon' is a fancy word for 'dictionary', though the mental dictionary is organized differently than a dictionary in a book). Each lexical entry lists all the linguistic information we know about a word—for example, what part of speech it is (noun, verb, adjective, adverb), how it is pronounced, and what it means, as well as its syntactic properties. It is these syntactic properties that we are concerned with now. The argument structure of a verb tells us something about its meaning and, as we will see, also tells us something about its syntax.

The ACTOR argument and the PATIENT argument are **obligatory arguments** in the argument structure of 'beat'. This means that a sentence with 'beat' is ungrammatical unless it contains both of these arguments. In the sentence 'The girl beat the boy', 'the girl' and 'the boy' fill the ACTOR and PATIENT argument positions of 'beat', respectively. If either one were not present, the sentence would be ungrammatical:

60a. *'The girl beat'

60b. *'Beat the boy'

'Beat' can also take **optional arguments,** that is, NPs that can be added to sentences with 'beat', but whose absence does not cause ungrammaticality. These optional arguments are all preceded by prepositions if they are added to the sentence. For example, we could add an INSTRUMENT ('with a stick') or a LOCATION where the blows fell, or both, as in:

61a. The girl beat the boy *with a stick*

61b. The girl beat the boy *on the head*

61c. The girl beat the boy *with a stick on the head*

61d. The girl beat the boy *on the head with a stick*

We can add these optional arguments to the argument structure of the verb by enclosing them in parentheses to notate that they are optional, not obligatory:

62. beat [ACTOR, PATIENT, (INSTRUMENT), (LOCATION)]

The *first* argument listed in an argument structure (ACTOR in 62) we will call just that: the first argument in the argument structure (it is sometimes called the highest argument in the argument structure). It is the argument that becomes the *subject* of the sentence (in underlying structure). The second argument listed in the argument structure is the one that becomes the *object* (in underlying structure). The other arguments are usually optional, are marked by prepositions, and are fairly free in terms of the order in which they appear in sentences.

Optional Arguments Distinguished From General Time and Place Specifications

English has many different types of verbs, each with their own characteristic argument structures. For example, 'yell' requires at least one NP to make up a grammatical sentence, where this NP must name an ACTOR. This single NP is placed before the verb:

63. The girl (ACTOR) yelled

'Yell' can also optionally be combined with various prepositional phrases (PPs for short) that name either other participants in the action of yelling (optional arguments) or the general TIME or PLACE (LOCATION) the yelling took place:

64a. The girl (ACTOR) yelled *at the boy* (GOAL)

64b. The girl (ACTOR) yelled *at noon* (TIME)

64c. The girl (ACTOR) yelled *in the bedroom* (LOCATION)

Note that the PP in 64a, naming the GOAL ('at the boy') relates to the verb 'yell' quite differently than the PPs naming the general time and location ('at noon', 'in the bedroom') do in 64b and 64c, despite the fact that they all simply follow the verb 'yell'. 'Yell' means *someone produces a loud noise with his or her voice.* The noise may, but need not, be directed at some thing or person. If the noise is directed at a person or thing, that person or thing is the GOAL (target, end point) of the yelling. Notice, then, how 'at the boy' in 64a fills out or specifies part of the meaning of 'yell' by naming the person that the loud noise is directed at, the GOAL of the yelling. Though it is optional in the sense that a sentence with 'yell' is not ungrammatical if the GOAL is left out, nonetheless the GOAL further specifies or spells out a piece of the meaning of 'yell'.

However, this is not true of 'at noon' or 'in the bedroom' in 64b and 64c, which respectively name a general time and a location. All verbs in the language can combine with PPs naming time and location. These time and location specifications don't further spell out the meaning of 'yell' in the way in which 'at the boy' does in 64a (or even in the way the location 'on the head' does in 'The girl beat the boy on the head', where 'on the head' specifies not the general location of the beating—for example, in the park—but what part of the boy got beaten). General time and location specifications, when they don't further spell out the meaning of the verb, are not arguments of the verbs they go with.

Verbs have decided preferences about what prepositions will accompany their arguments. Comparing 'yell' to 'lie', we see that 'yell' will allow the person to whom the yell is directed, the GOAL of the yelling, to be singled out by a PP with either 'at' or 'to' (with its meaning being slightly different when we use 'to'). 'Lie' allows the GOAL to be picked out only by a PP with 'to'.

65a. The girl lied

65b. The girl lied to the boy (GOAL)

65c. *The girl lied at the boy (GOAL)

66a. The girl yelled

66b. The girl yelled to the boy (GOAL)

66c. The girl yelled at the boy (GOAL)

Here we see that verbs (like 'yell' and 'lie') place constraints on which prepositions can mark their arguments.

————————————— **E X E R C I S E** —————————————

Exercise P. Rewrite the following sentences, and label each NP or PP as an obligatory argument, optional argument, or a nonargument (general time or location specification). HINT: Be careful about 'resides' in 5—does the location 'in Africa' further spell out the meaning of this verb? Is this location obligatory here? Is it an argument?

 1. On Monday, John robbed Mary of $100.
 2. John gave a book to Mary yesterday.
 3. The girl asked her mother for her dinner.
 4. John inherited a million dollars on Monday.
 5. John resides in Africa.
 6. John put the flowers in the vase on Tuesday.
 7. John bought a rose for Mary.
 8. In the office, Mr. Smith lied to Mary.
 9. John received a message from his sister.

6.7. WORDS IN THE MIND

The Mental Lexicon

Linguists assume that people have a dictionary in their heads, which linguists call **the mental lexicon.** In this dictionary, people store all the words they know. This dictionary in the head is probably not organized like any written dictionary. In fact, it probably has a much more complex organization than any dictionary.

The lexicon must have an entry for each word in the language. Each entry must list at least the following: (a) the way the word is pronounced, (b) the meaning of the word, and (c) the syntactic properties of the word. The syntactic properties of the word include the word's part of speech (whether it is a noun, verb, adjective, preposition, or adverb) and, for verbs, the argument structure of the verb. We will concentrate here on the lexical entries for verbs. Specifically, we will concentrate only on that part of the lexical entry that details the argument structure of the verb.

Let's imagine that the lexical entries for 'yell' and 'lie' in the mental lexicon look like the following (we will fill in only part of the syntactic sections of the entry, leaving the other parts unspecified, as we are not now concerned with them. The only difference in the way we will write argument structures now is that we will add information about which preposition goes with which argument).

67a. 'yell'
    PRONUNCIATION:
    MEANING:
    SYNTACTIC SPECIFICATION:
        PART OF SPEECH: verb
        ARGUMENT STRUCTURE: 'yell' [ACTOR, (GOAL = at/to)]

67b. 'lie'
    PRONUNCIATION:
    MEANING:
    SYNTACTIC SPECIFICATION:
        PART OF SPEECH: verb
        ARGUMENT STRUCTURE: 'lie' [ACTOR, (GOAL = at)]

The lexical entry for the verb 'steal' would look like

67c. 'steal'
    PRONUNCIATION:
    MEANING:
    SYNTACTIC SPECIFICATION:
        PART OF SPEECH: verb
        ARGUMENT STRUCTURE: 'steal' [ACTOR, (THEME) (SOURCE = from)]

This entry means that 'steal' is a verb and that to make a sentence it combines with an NP that names the ACTOR (stealer), and it can also be combined with either an NP naming the THEME (thing stolen) or an NP naming the SOURCE (person who loses the thing stolen) marked by the preposition 'from', or with both a THEME and a SOURCE, as shown in the examples below:

68a. Mary (ACTOR) steals

68b. Mary (ACTOR) stole a book (THEME)

68c. Mary (ACTOR) stole from a church (SOURCE)

68d. Mary (ACTOR) stole a book (THEME) from a church (SOURCE)

———————————————— E X E R C I S E ————————————————

Exercise Q.   Give the argument structures for the following verbs: 'throw', 'put', and 'read'. You can use the data below to guide you:

1a. The girl (ACTOR) threw the ball (THEME) at the boy (GOAL)

1b. The girl threw the ball

1c. *The girl threw at the boy

1d. *Threw at the boy

2a. The girl (ACTOR) put the money (THEME) on the table (GOAL)

2b. *The girl put the money

2c. *The girl put on the table

2d. *The girl put

2e. *Put the money on the table

3a. The girl (EXPERIENCER) read the book (THEME) to the boy (GOAL)

3b. The girl read

3c. The girl read the book

3d. The girl read to the boy

3e. *Read the book to the boy

Semantic Role Assignment

In earlier sections we appealed to the idea that sentences have both underlying (canonical) structures and surface structures derived from the underlying structures by transformational rules. We now need to see how the argument structures we have been describing hook up with this picture.

We will assume that the underlying structure of a sentence contains not just words, but the *whole lexical entry* of each of the words in the sentence. Below, I give a simplified underlying structure for the sentence 'The man killed the dragon' containing only a *part* of the lexical entry for one word, namely the argument structure of the verb, since this is the part of the underlying structure that I want to concentrate on here (remember that in an underlying structure like the one below, 'did' is present, but, if it is not stressed, will delete and pass its tense to 'kill', giving us 'killed').

69a.

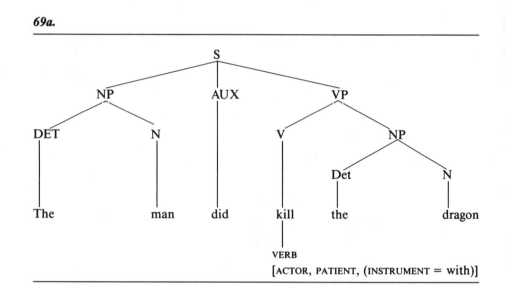

[ACTOR, PATIENT, (INSTRUMENT = with)]

The semantic roles in the argument structure of the verb must somehow be assigned to the NP arguments of the verb ('the man' and 'the dragon'), since these NPs actually bear the semantic roles. The rule that assigns the NPs in a sentence their semantic roles we will call **semantic role assignment.** This rule simply takes the first or highest semantic role in the verb's argument structure and assigns it to the subject (the NP before the verb and directly under S) and the next semantic role in the argument structure and assigns it to the object (the NP after the verb and directly under VP). Any semantic roles in an argument structure that are marked by a preposition will be assigned to the NP after that particular preposition. Thus, the argument structure for 'kill' says that 'kill' allows an optional INSTRUMENT role marked by the preposition 'with' (for example, 'The man killed the dragon with an axe'). This INSTRUMENT role would be assigned to the object of the preposition 'with' if it was present in the sentence (thus, to 'axe' in 'The man killed the dragon with an axe').

We assume that semantic role assignment operates before any transformations have applied. It will operate on 69a to produce 69b:

69b.

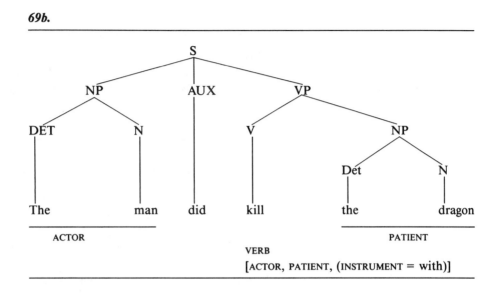

Notice that this very simple device of having the verb assign semantic roles to its NP arguments allows us to say why the following sentences are ungrammatical:

69c. *The man killed

69d. *The man killed the dragon the boy

'Kill' has two obligatory semantic roles to assign (ACTOR and PATIENT), but in 69c there is only one NP ('the man'). Thus, one semantic role has gone unassigned. Since both roles are obligatory in the argument structure for 'kill', this causes ungrammaticality. In 69d there are three NPs, but 'kill' has only two semantic roles (which do not require a preposition) to assign, so one of the NPs in 69d ('the boy') goes without a semantic role. This means it has no meaning in the sentence, thus the sentence is ungrammatical.

Once semantic roles are assigned, two things happen to an underlying structure like 69b (though in no particular temporal order—remember, we are actually talking about a static overall abstract description of a sentence that is true "all at once", though often it helps us to think about the description as if things happened one after another in time). First, the underlying structure is given a semantic interpretation or **semantic representation** by means of semantic rules. We have discussed some of the issues germane to semantic representation in Chapter 2. Second, transformations apply to the underlying structure to create derived structures and finally a surface structure.

Generalizations in the Lexicon About Argument Structures

Unlike 'kill' above, some verbs have three semantic roles that they can assign without a preposition. Consider a verb like 'give', which has two possible argument structures. In one, the subject is an ACTOR, the object is a THEME, and the GOAL/BENEFICIARY is marked by the preposition 'to':

70a. John (ACTOR) gave a book (THEME) to Mary (GOAL/BENEFICIARY)

However, 'give' also allows the GOAL/BENEFICIARY to be the object and the THEME to occur after the object with no preposition:

70b. John (ACTOR) gave Mary (GOAL/BENEFICIARY) a book (THEME)

In fact, what is true of 'give' here is true of many verbs that mean to *transfer something from someone to someone else* (for example, 'send', 'mail', 'tell', 'bring', 'throw', 'hand', and a number of other verbs). Such verbs are called **dative verbs** because the NP in English that has the option of occurring with 'to' or directly after the verb is marked by the dative case in a language like Latin.

Since these facts about 'give' are true of a number of other verbs, we can state a partial generalization, a generalization that holds true of many verbs that mean to transfer something from someone to someone else. We will assume that such generalizations are listed in the lexicon (these generalizations tell us what to expect when we look at the actual lexical entries of the words in the lexicon). This generalization we will call the **dative generalization:**

DATIVE GENERALIZATION.   Many verbs in English that mean for a THEME to be transferred by an ACTOR to a GOAL/BENEFICIARY have two argument structures of the following form:
verb [ACTOR, THEME, GOAL/BENEFICIARY = to]
verb [ACTOR, GOAL/BENEFICIARY, THEME]

There are a number of generalizations like this one that can be listed in the lexicon, generalizations that tell us about alternative argument structures for certain types of verbs. We will still have to say in the entry for each verb in English that might obey this generalization whether it actually obeys it or not, since there are some verbs that have the right meaning, but that do not obey the generalization. For instance 'tell' obeys the generalization, but 'report,' a verb with similar meaning, does not:

71a. I told the story to John

71b. I told John the story

72a. I reported the story to John

72b. *I reported John the story

Nonetheless, this generalization is part of the knowledge of English speakers. On the basis of it, they can make up new dative verbs:

73a. Bill telefaxed a letter to me in England

73b. Bill telefaxed me a letter in England

—————————————— **E X E R C I S E** ——————————————

Exercise R. The sentences below point to another lexical generalization in English, similar to the "*to*-dative" generalization:

1a. John bought a book for Mary.

1b. John bought Mary a book.

2a. Mary got a cab for John.

2b. Mary got John a cab.

List several other verbs that display these two possibilities. State the generalization here, along the lines we stated the dative generalization above. This generalization is sometimes called "the *for*-dative generalization." Find at least one verb that would seem like it should follow the generalization but does not.

6.8. BRINGING THE SYSTEM TOGETHER

I will now show how all the parts of our syntactic theory (case, semantic roles, argument structures, underlying structures, transformations, and surface structures) can be used together to explain an aspect of English grammar.

NP Movement

In this analysis I will explicitly make two assumptions that I have so far mentioned only rather indirectly:

Assumption A.   Every NP must get assigned a semantic role (unless the NP is just a meaningless "dummy" word—we will see what this means below).

Assumption B.   Every (nonempty) NP must be assigned a case, either nominative or accusative (we will see what 'nonempty' means below). Modals and verbs with tense assign nominative case to their subjects; verbs and prepositions assign accusative case to their objects.

Now consider the verb 'seems' in the following sentences:

74a. It seems that <u>Mary beats John</u>

74b. It seems that <u>John knows the answer</u>

'Seems' requires an embedded sentence (underlined in 74a and 74b) following it. Let's say that embedded sentences are assigned the semantic role FACT. Thus, 74a means that it seems as though the FACT 'that Mary beats John' is true.

Interestingly, it appears as though 'seems' does not assign any semantic role to its subject. The subject 'it' in 74a and 74b is meaningless (it does not refer to anything) but is just a dummy word to ensure that the subject position is not empty (something that English never allows if the verb has tense, that is, is not an infinitive).

The fact that 'seems' has no semantic role to assign to its subject is the reason a sentence like 'Bill seems that Mary beats John' is ungrammatical. 'Bill' is not a dummy NP and needs a semantic role, but 'seems' has none to give it. Only dummy meaningless words like 'it' in 74a and 74b or in 'It's raining' can go without a semantic role ('it' in a sentence like 'Mary liked it' is meaningful, it is the "neuter" third-person pronoun referring to an object).

Notice, however, that the verb 'seems' in 74a and 74b is tensed (present tense) and so can assign its subject, the dummy word 'it', nominative case. We can say that 'seems' has the following argument structure:

75. seems [0, FACT]

This means that 'seems' assigns no semantic role (0 = zero) to its subject and the role FACT to its object, which thus must be an embedded sentence since embedded sentences are what name FACTS in English. The underlying structure for 74a would be

76a.

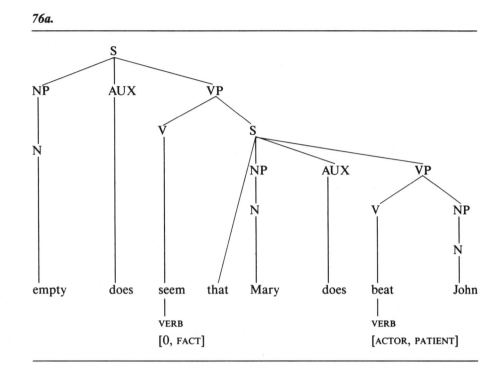

I assume that the underlying subject position of 'seem' is empty in underlying structure (since this position gets assigned no semantic role, it cannot be filled with NPs like 'Bill' or 'the boy', which need a semantic role to play). I further assume that a transformational rule fills this position with the dummy word 'it'. By semantic role assignment, 'seem' will assign its embedded sentence the role FACT. 'Beat' in the embedded sentence will assign its subject the role ACTOR and its object the role PATIENT. This will produce, after 'do' deletes and passes its tense to the following main verbs, 'It seems that Mary (ACTOR) beats John (PATIENT)'.

We have assumed that every NP must be assigned a case, and, indeed, in this structure every NP will get a case. Assuming that case is assigned after all transformations have applied, the subject of 'seems' (the dummy 'it') will get nominative case (since 'seems' has tense). The subject of 'beats' (which also shows tense), namely 'Mary', will also get nominative case. The object of 'beat'—'John'—will get accusative case. Thus, everything is fine.

Now notice what will happen if we make one very little change in the underlying structure in 76a. Imagine that we had made the verb of the embedded sentence an infinitive (untensed). Then 'to' would show up instead of any indication of tense and 'that' would disappear. Otherwise, the underlying structure would be unchanged:

76b.

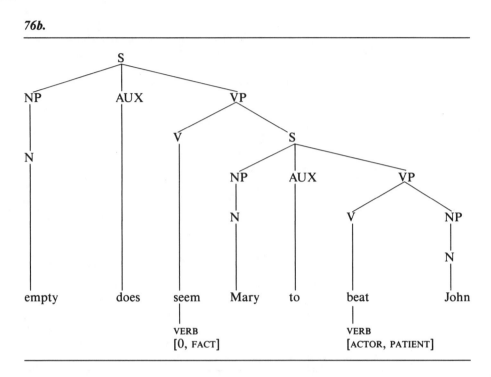

This underlying structure will not give rise to a grammatical sentence as it is. If we delete 'does', we will eventually get the surface structure for *'It seems Mary to beat John', which is clearly ungrammatical. The problem is that, as we saw above, in the normal situation, nontensed verbs (infinitives, like 'to beat') do not assign any case to their subjects, and thus their subjects are usually missing from the sentence (as in 'Mary tried to leave'). Thus, 'Mary', the subject of 'to beat', cannot get a case and should be left out of the sentence. But we cannot just leave it out, since it is playing the role of the ACTOR of the verb 'beat' and there is no other NP in the sentence identical to 'Mary' to tell us who this ACTOR is if we leave 'Mary' out of the sentence.

However, notice that the subject position of 'seems' is empty at the underlying structure, though anything that happened to fill this position could receive nominative case thanks to the fact that the following verb has tense ('does', which will pass its tense to 'seems' when it deletes).

Now, what if the NP subject 'Mary' *moved* from its position in front of 'to beat', where it cannot get any case, to the empty subject position of 'seem', where it can? This position has no semantic role (since 'seem' has no semantic role to give its subject), but that does not matter because 'Mary' has already received a semantic role (ACTOR) from 'to beat', a verb that gives its subject the role ACTOR and its object the role PATIENT. The NP 'Mary' can carry this semantic role along with it when it moves to the empty subject position of 'seem'.

If there is indeed a transformational rule that can move an NP into an 'empty' position (that is, a position that gets no semantic role), then 'Mary' could move from where it is to the subject position of 'seem', where it will get a case, which it needs (nominative, thanks to the tense of 'seem'). The transformation would carry out the operation I diagram below, moving the NP 'Mary' from its place in the tree in 76b to the empty subject position in front of 'seem' in that tree:

76c. empty does seem [Mary   to beat   John]
                      (ACTOR)   (PATIENT)

76d. Mary   seems [empty   to beat   John]
    (ACTOR)   (PATIENT)
       cf.: 'Mary seems to beat John'

I mark the position from which 'Mary' has moved as empty (to keep a record of where it came from). 76c is the terminal line of words from the tree in 76b, with semantic role assignment already carried out. In a complete description, 76c would have a tree on top of it. 76d is the terminal line of words you get when you move 'Mary' from where it is in 76b to the empty subject position of 'seem'. In a complete description, 76d would also have a whole tree on top of it.

In 76d, every NP has a semantic role. 'Mary' brings along the ACTOR role she got from 'beat', and 'John' has the PATIENT role from 'beat'. Further, now every NP can get a case. 'John' can receive accusative case as the object of 'beat' and 'Mary' can receive nominative case because, having moved, it is now the subject of 'seem', a tensed verb (and subjects of tensed verbs receive nominative case). Thus, after case assignment, we get the following terminal line of words (imagine that it has a tree on top of it):

76e. Mary   seems   [EMPTY   to beat   John]
    (ACTOR   (PATIENT
    NOM. CASE)   ACC. CASE)

Let's call this hypothesized rule **NP movement.** Notice that NP movement gives us an account of how in 76e 'Mary', while the surface subject of 'seems' actually has the semantic role that 'beat' requires it to have (ACTOR). Note that in a sentence like 'Mary seems to know the answer', 'Mary' is understood to be an EXPERIENCER (the one who might know), that is, to have the semantic role that 'know' requires its subject to have. In underlying structure (*'empty* seems Mary to know the answer'), 'know' assigns the role EXPERIENCER to its subject, 'Mary', and then 'Mary' moves to the subject position of 'seems' to pick up the nominative case that 'seems' has to offer and that 'to kill', being an infinitive, could not give it).

─────────────────── **E X E R C I S E** ───────────────────

Exercise S. Construct an argument for the existence of NP movement from the data below (that is, show how this data gives evidence for the claim that in a sentence like 1 below—'The soldiers seems to have dispersed'—'the soldiers' is the subject of 'dispersed' in underlying structure and has moved to the subject position of seems).

1. The soldiers seem to have dispersed.
2. *The soldier seems to have dispersed.
3. The soldiers dispersed.
4. *The soldier dispersed.
5. The soldier seems to have left.
6. The soldiers seem to have left.

───

Passive

In English, almost every canonical sentence of the form SUBJECT VERB OBJECT (as in 'Mary kissed John') has a **passive** version (as in 'John was kissed by Mary'). The passive means pretty much what the canonical version (called the **active**) means, though it has a different role in discourse (in the active sentence 'Mary kissed John', 'Mary' tends to be taken as the **topic,** what we are talking about, while in the passive version 'John was kissed by Mary', 'John' tends to be taken as the topic—see Chapter 10). Passive sentences always have the verb in its past participle form preceded by the helping verb 'be': thus, note 'Mary *knows* John' (active), with 'knows' in the present tense, and 'John *is known* by Mary' (passive), with 'known' in its past participle form, and preceded by the helping verb 'be' (in this case, 'be' is in its present-tense form, 'is'). In any passive sentence, the 'by-phrase' at the end is optional: Thus, both 'John was kissed by Mary' and 'John was kissed' are grammatical.

While most verbs that can occur in the pattern SUBJECT VERB OBJECT also have a passive version (as shown in 77 below), there are exceptions, some of which are shown in 78:

77a. John loves Mary→
Mary is loved by John

77b. The girl kicked the boy→
The boy was kicked by the girl

77c. Sue was watching the puppy→
The puppy was being watched by Sue

78a. John resembles Bill→
 *Bill is resembled by John

78b. This sock fits my foot→
 *My foot is fit by this sock

78c. This book costs $10→
 *$10 is cost by this book

There has been a great deal of controversy about how to handle passives within linguistic theory, which is why I bring it up only at the end of this chapter. At one time, passive was treated as a transformation (see Section 6.7) that from an underlying structure for a sentence like 'Mary kissed John' produced a tree for the sentence 'John was kissed by Mary' by switching the positions of the NPs 'John' and 'Mary', adding a helping verb 'be', placing the verb in its past participle form, and adding 'by' to the sentence.

A later account treated passive as a generalization in the lexicon, like the dative generalization discussed earlier. On this account, we list a generalization in the lexicon that says that many verbs in English have two possible argument structures: an active one of the form NP_1 verb NP_2; and a passive one in which the first of these NPs (the one labeled NP_1) occurs optionally in a prepositional phrase with 'by' and the second of these NPs (the one labeled NP_2) is the subject, as in NP_2 *be + past participle of verb* (by NP_2). Certain verbs (like 'resemble', 'fit', and 'cost' in 78 above) would be listed as exceptions to this lexical generalization.

A yet more current account treats passive verb forms (like 'was' 'kissed') just like the verb 'seem' above. In underlying structure, a passive form of a verb always occurs with an empty subject and cannot assign case to its object. Thus, the underlying structure for 'John was kissed by Mary' would be a tree for '—was kissed John by Mary', where the subject position is empty. The passive form of the verb 'kiss' ('was kissed'), just like the regular active form, can give the object NP 'John' the semantic role of PATIENT, but cannot give it any case. However, since the subject position is empty, 'John' can move to this position and get case (nominative) from the tense of 'was kissed' (which is past tense).

We see, then, that linguists have proposed various treatments of passive sentences. The question is still open, as is normal in any developing science. New evidence from other languages or new insights into English grammar may eventually lead us to newer, and deeper, insights in this area of grammar and many others as well.

RECOMMENDED FURTHER READING

BROWN, E. K. & MILLER, J. E. (1980). *Syntax: A Linguistic Introduction to Sentence Structure.* London: Hutchinson. (Illuminating description of the basic facts of syntax and their relation to morphology and discourse; not couched in terms of any one current theory.)

COOK, V. J. (1988). *Chomsky's Universal Grammar: An Introduction.* Oxford & New York: Blackwell. (A good short introduction to current Chomskian syntactic theory.)

GIVON, TALMY (1984). *Syntax: A Functional Typological Introduction,* vol. 1. Amsterdam & Philadelphia: John Benjamins. (A good introduction to the relationships between syntax and discourse, as well as to a variety of languages beyond English.)

HAEGEMAN, LILIANE (1991). *Introduction to Government and Binding Theory.* Oxford: Basil Blackwell. (A technical, but thorough, up-to-date, and clear introduction to current syntactic theory in Chomsky's "Government and Binding" framework.)

JESPERSEN, OTTO (1969). *Essentials of English Grammar.* University of Alabama Press. (A one-volume condensation of Jespersen's multi-volume *Modern English Grammar;* Jespersen is the greatest descriptive grammarian of English—true lovers of grammar love to spend an afternoon in the library browsing in the *Modern English Grammar.)*

MCCAWLEY, JAMES D. (1988). *The Syntactic Phenomena of English,* two volumes. University of Chicago Press. (An idiosyncratic but massively complete introduction to the details of English syntax.)

RADFORD, ANDREW (1988). *Transformational Grammar: A First Course.* New York: Cambridge University Press. (An excellent and accessible full-length textbook introduction to contemporary Chomskian syntactic theory. Be sure you have Radford's newer book; his 1981 *Transformational Syntax* is good but out of date.)

SELLS, PETER (1985). *Lectures on Contemporary Syntactic Theories.* Center for the Study of Language and Information, Stanford University. (A clear and lucid introduction to three current competing theories of syntax, including the theory dealt with in the Cook and Radford books above.)

CHAPTER 7

Psycholinguistics

Processing Language in the Mind

7.1. PSYCHOLINGUISTICS

Linguists study the structure of language and the relationships that exist between language, society, and culture. They study what people consciously and unconsciously know when they know a language. Linguists engage in their studies by collecting and analyzing data from real speech (or writing) or by asking people for their intuitions about the grammaticality of certain sentences or the meanings of a certain form, sentence, or text, or the acceptability of using language in a certain way in various social contexts.

The term 'psycholinguistics' is used for two different studies. Sometimes the term is used for work on language acquisition in children and adults. This is a study carried out by both linguists and psychologists. Though they bring somewhat different techniques and approaches to the study of language acquisition, work in this area is more and more a real combination of the two disciplines. (We will look at language acquisition in Chapter 9.)

The second study to which the term 'psycholinguistics' is applied is the study of how people put their unconscious linguistic knowledge (which linguists study) to *use* in speech and writing. The goal of psycholinguistics in this sense is a coherent theory of the ways in which language is produced and understood (comprehended). This chapter will use the term 'psycholinguistics' only for this type of work.

Psycholinguistics is largely a "laboratory" study. Psycholinguists run experiments in laboratories and often artificially manipulate the speech stream, collecting data that they subject to various statistical tests. They use their experimental manipulations of language to draw deductions about the mental mechanisms that underlie the production and understanding of speech (and writing).

Psycholinguistics is a separate discipline from linguistics, though linguists and psychologists often work closely together, especially in the emerging new discipline of **cognitive science.** Cognitive science combines work in psychology, mathematics, linguistics, philosophy, and computer science to study the nature of human cognition (human thought, belief and knowledge, and the ways in which it is put to use in the world). My purpose in this chapter will be to give the reader the "flavor" of work in psycholinguistics and a feel for how this work relates to the field of linguistics.

Before we look at some of the specific claims about the mind that psycholinguistics have put forward, we will overview the philosophy of mind that underlies much of the work in cognitive science and psycholinguistics.

7.2. THE NATURE OF THE MIND

Symbols, Computers, and the Mind

The cognitive scientist sees the mind as made up of *mental processes.*[1] These processes carry out manipulations of perceptions we receive from the world. They also carry out manipulations of the various ideas, thoughts, beliefs, and memories we can form or store in our minds. The cognitive scientist views all of these—perceptions, ideas, thoughts, beliefs, or memories—as various types of *representations* or *symbols.* These representations or symbols in the mind are *mental* representations or symbols. There are also symbols that exist outside the mind. We can understand mental symbols better if we first understand symbols outside the mind.

Symbols usually come in systems. Each symbol in the system stands for something, which counts as its interpretation. Thus, the system of colored lights in a traffic signal (red, green, yellow) is a system of symbols. Each color stands for a particular action to be carried out by drivers (stop, go, go carefully).

The richest symbol systems have an infinite number of possible symbols. An example of such a rich symbol system is architects' drawings, the sort of drawings one sees in blueprints of buildings. Such a drawing is made up of a set of elements, such as lines and vertices, each one of which stands for the various parts of a building. In such a complicated system, you need more than a mere list of what each symbol stands for. You need, rather, a set of *principles* or *rules* that tell you how to "translate" the symbols into the things they stand for (in this case,

---

[1]See Philip N. Johnson-Laird's two introductory books on cognitive science, *Mental Models,* 1983, and *The Computer and the Mind: An Introduction to Cognitive Science,* 1988, both from Harvard University Press; some of the discussion in this section is based on the latter book.

the rules of scale drawings and various other conventions that architects use to translate their scale drawings into buildings).

The set of symbols (called letters) by which we represent the sounds of words in spelling English is also a complex symbol system. All such complex symbol systems have three components: first, a set of primitive or simple symbols (like the letters of the alphabet: 'a', 'b', 'c', and so forth); second, principles or rules that specify how the simple symbols can be combined to form complex symbols (for example, that the simple symbols 'p', 'e', and 'n' can be combined, with spaces on either end, to represent the English word 'pen' in sentences like 'I lost my pen'); and third, a set of principles or rules that specify how to relate the simple and complex symbols to what they stand for (which are quite complicated in the case of English spelling; for example, these rules specify that the symbol 'a' stands for the sound /æ/ in 'fat', but for the sound /e/ in 'fate', because of the "silent" letter 'e' at the end of the word).

Any set of things (whether buildings, sounds, or numbers) can be represented by many different systems of symbols. For example, we call the symbols that represent numbers *numerals*. In English, we normally use numeral symbols that were originally devised by the Arabs (1, 2, 3, and so forth). But there are many other symbol systems that are used to represent numbers and many others we could invent. For example, one could use Roman numerals (I, II, III, IV, etc.).

Morse code is a symbol system for representing the letters of the alphabet. But Morse code is a special sort of symbol system: It is a *binary* notation, because it has only two primitive or simple symbols (a dot and dash). It combines various dots and dashes to represent any letter in the alphabet. There is also a binary notation for representing numbers. In fact, all a modern digital computer does is manipulate binary numbers (much like the dots and dashes in Morse code). We humans treat the binary numbers the computer is manipulating as symbols for things that interest us, like the names of people, or their Social Security numbers, or lists of addresses, words in an essay, or the pieces of a graphic image.

Many modern psychologists and philosophers think of the mind/brain in terms of a metaphorical comparison to a digital computer. They compare the mind to the *software* of a computer (the programs it runs), and the brain to the *hardware* of a computer (the electrical circuits it is made up of). In several respects, however, modern digital computers turn out not to be particularly good metaphors for the human mind/brain. Digital computers operate *serially,* computing one small step of a problem at a time. The human brain operates in a massively *parallel* fashion, carrying out many operations at one and the same time.

Furthermore, digital computers break down all their operations into *binary* decisions (simple yes/no, all-or-nothing decisions). However, the human brain is made up of nerve cells called *neurons* that produce impulses. These impulses are electro-chemical changes that propagate relatively slowly down nerve fibers and then leap the junction (or synapse) between one neuron and another via other electrical and chemical processes. The neurons in the brain can each be *activated* to *different degrees* depending on how greatly they are *stimulated* by other neurons that send them signals. They operate more in terms of a scale of *how much* (lots, little, somewhere in between) than in terms of simple binary yes/no decisions.

Computer scientists are currently designing computers that function more like the brain—in a highly parallel fashion and with units that can be activated to different degrees, rather than digitally (in terms of discrete yes/no, all-or-nothing decisions). Cognitive science is currently undergoing a great deal of ferment and controversy as scientists are becoming more and more convinced that the modern digital computer is a very limited, and often inaccurate, model of the mind. Much work is going on in neuroscience ("brain science"), and cognitive scientists are developing models of the mind that resemble more closely how neurons actually work and less how modern digital computers work.[2]

The Mind as a Symbol-Manipulating Device

A major tenet of cognitive science is that the mind is a device that constructs, stores, and manipulates *symbols.* The manipulations it carries out on its symbols are called *mental* or *cognitive processes.* We have no idea what sort of symbol system the brain uses. But whatever system it uses, it must relate these symbols to something to make the symbols symbols; that is, they must stand for something. In some instances they stand for things in the world (as in perception). But in other instances they stand for hypothetical states of affairs and imaginary entities, since we can think about what may exist or what doesn't exist just as well as we can think about what (we think) exists.

Consider visual perception. Continuous and ever-changing patterns of light fall on the eye. The mind must convert these patterns of light into symbols that stand for things like chairs, ocean waves, sky, and locations—for information about what is where, so we can move around the world and think about it. This information is not explicit in the patterns of light, but is recovered by several stages of processing by the eye and brain. This process assigns each symbol its interpretation, what it stands for (for example, lines, angles, shapes, and objects in the world). How we humans carry out this process is determined by our human biology. Another creature (a bee, for instance, or a frog) may carry out the process quite differently.

Mental phenomena depend on the brain, and cognitive scientists believe they can best be explained in terms of symbols. The number of different symbols

---

[2]William Allman's book *Apprentices of Wonder: Inside the Neural Network Revolution* and Israel Rosenfield's book *The Invention of Memory: A New View of the Brain* are both good introductions to the issues, as is Paul Churchland's article, "Cognitive Activity in Artificial Neural Networks," in Daniel Osherson and Edward Smith's *Thinking: An Invitation to Cognitive Science.* These sources are listed in "Recommended Further Reading" at the end of this chapter.

corresponding to images, beliefs, and memories is potentially infinite. But the brain cannot contain an infinite number of preexisting primitive or simple symbols—no more than a library can contain an infinite number of books. The vast diversity of mental symbols must be constructed out of finite means—out of a finite number of primitive or simple symbols. Nerve impulses and the other electro-chemical events in the brain can therefore be treated as the underlying simple symbols. That is, the firing of an individual brain cell (a neuron) could count as a simple symbol (like 'a', 'b', and 'c', and the other letters of the alphabet in the symbol system for representing spelled sounds). Patterns of firings of several or many of these neurons would represent complex symbols (like 'pen' in the English alphabet).

Cognitive scientists could talk directly about the firings of neurons, but the brain is far too complicated for this—we know too little about it, as of yet, to talk this specifically about what the brain does when it thinks. Thus, cognitive scientists usually talk about the mind manipulating symbols such as sound features (like [+voice] or [−consonantal]) or phonemes (like /p/ and /f/) or words (like 'pill' and 'bill'). But they assume that these ultimately are represented in some symbol system in the brain, encoded in the neurons in the brain.

─────────────────── **E X E R C I S E** ───────────────────

Exercise A. In traffic signals in the U.S., red is on top, yellow in the middle, and green at the bottom in a vertical row. Red means *stop,* green means *go,* yellow means (something like) *prepare to stop, and go with caution only if you have already entered the intersection; otherwise stop.* In their book *Telling Stories: A Theoretical Analysis of Narrative Fiction* (New York: Routledge, 1988), Steven Cohen and Linda Shires give the following example of symbol systems operating in the real world (they use the word 'sign' instead of 'symbol'):

> Syracuse, New York, offers an excellent example of the procedure by which the system of driving gives the colors red and green their distinct value as signs. An area of the city called Tipperary Hill with a large population of Irish descent has a traffic light which reverses the conventional locations of red and green colors (red is at the bottom and green at the top). Once this traffic light matched every other light in the city. But the neighborhood population kept shooting out the red light because it was over the green one. In this instance, the color symbolism of driving crossed that of political representation. Green traditionally signifies Ireland, while red signifies— on maps, say, or on army uniforms—Britain and the British Empire. Every time the city replaced the broken red light, someone smashed it out again, until finally the city yielded and placed the green light at the top, the red light at the bottom. To a stranger in this neighborhood, that traffic light could pose a problem of interpretation because it does not follow the

conventional alignment of color and location. In order to read the signal, one has to observe how other drivers read it, to see whether they follow the conventional meaning of the color alone or the color's unconventional location. In either case, interpretation is a public act; it involves knowing the system of conventions *and* negotiating the meaning of the sign with other drivers. (p. 4)

In the normal traffic light, the symbol system is redundant in the sense that both the color and the position of the light (for example, red and being on top) carry the same meaning. Why do most drivers pay attention to the colors and not to their positions (why would lights all of the same color, but in the three different positions, not work as well as lights of different colors)? Symbol systems are arbitrary in the sense that any color or position could have been assigned any meaning. But, how does your answer to the last question show certain limits on the arbitrary nature of symbols (that is, how does your answer show that we can't really use just any symbols for just any meanings?), and what do these limits stem from? What is the symbol system that the Irish of Tipperary Hill were using? Is it redundant in the way the normal traffic light symbol system is? (HINT: What does location symbolize in the symbol system they are using?) How does the fact that after years of driving I do not really know what yellow on the traffic light actually stands for demonstrate the point that Cohen and Shires make at the end of the excerpt above? What does this tell us about how symbol systems function in the social world? What would "yellow" mean if the law code said it meant *go, with caution, through the intersection only if you have already entered the intersection, otherwise stop,* but drivers always acted as if it meant *go cautiously through the intersection, stop only if you see red prior to getting near the intersection?* Why would it mean this?

7.3. RECOGNIZING WORDS IN THE STREAM OF SPEECH

To begin our discussion of the sorts of specific proposals psycholinguists make, we will look at the processes by which the mind recognizes words in the stream of speech. When a listener is exposed to speech, what comes in the ear are simply waves of sound in which there are, as a matter of physical fact, no nice discrete and separate sounds and words (unlike print, for instance). The human perceiver must discover the sounds and words of his or her language in these sound waves, turning continuous variations of air pressure (which is all sound waves are) into discrete sounds and words, that is, into the meaningful symbols of his or her language. By studying the details of how this is done, psycholinguists are led to interesting hypotheses about the structure of the human mind and the ways in which it operates.

For example, psycholinguists have found that if they artificially manipulate a word and excise one of its sounds (phonemes), replacing the excised sound with a buzz, listeners frequently fail to detect the distortion and "hear" the sound that is missing. Thus, if subjects are presented with /fotogr#f/ ('photograph' with the vowel of 'graph' replaced by a buzz, which I symbolize as '#'), they often say they have heard /fotogræf/ ('photograph'). They restore the missing sound, which is not actually in the speech stream.

From this sort of evidence, the psycholinguist can conclude that what people hear when they comprehend speech is not just due to what they actually hear (the "physical" evidence, so to speak, in the speech stream), but also what their minds expect to hear. Listeners are actively predicting what will be in the speech stream and actually placing it there, in a sense, in some cases. They are making these predictions based on their unconscious linguistic knowledge (in this case, their knowledge about the set of English words).

Given a result like the one we have just discussed, the psycholinguist wants to know how the mind carries out this restoration of the missing sound. What mental mechanisms in the mind account for this sort of performance and how do they relate to the sorts of linguistic knowledge the linguist studies?

One possible way to look at the matter is as follows: We will assume that a listener's mind contains various mental mechanisms, mental devices, or mental modules (I will use these all interchangeably), including both a module for recognizing sounds in the speech stream, which we will call a **phoneme recognition device,** and a mental lexicon, which is a list of all the words in the language the listener knows. These two modules are connected to each other and can "talk" to each other (communicate with each other).

As we have said above, when the speech stream comes into the ear, it is simply sound waves (different frequencies of air pressure translated into different degrees of pressure against the eardrum), not nice discrete phonemes. The phoneme recognition device discovers in these sound waves evidence for the occurrence of various phonemes. As it does so, it sends this information to the mental lexicon. As the phoneme detection device detects an /f/, for instance, in the speech stream (based on physical properties in the sounds waves), it sends this information to the mental lexicon (essentially says "I found an /f/, I think").

In the lexicon, each word gets "excited" when it recognizes any part of itself in the phonemes that the phoneme detection device is sending to the lexicon. When a word gets excited, it "shouts" back to the phoneme detection device that it might be the word that the speaker is saying. The phoneme detection device uses this information, together with the sound waves it is processing, to determine what phonemes, and ultimately what words, it is hearing. The more of its sounds the word recognizes, the more excited it gets and the louder it shouts to the phoneme detection device. As the listener hears a few phonemes, lots of words are shouting, but as he or she hears more and more phonemes, fewer words shout (as most of them fail to continue to recognize their own phonemes), and finally only one word is shouting and that is the word the listener assumes the speaker is uttering. This word, as we will see below, is then sent off to yet another device to be bundled into phrases and sentences.

To see how this works, assume that we have fed to the phoneme detection device the sound waves that encode /fotogr#f/, where the symbol '#' stands for a buzz we have placed in the word 'photograph' where the vowel /æ/ normally occurs. As the listener detects in the sound waves evidence for /f/ and then /o/, the phoneme detection device sends these phonemes to the mental lexicon. In the lexicon, all words beginning with /fo/ get excited and begin to shout out (for example, 'foe', 'phobia', 'photo', 'photograph', 'foal', 'phone', and many more shout out that the word coming into the phoneme detection device might be themselves). As the phoneme detection device detects /t/ following /fo/, words like 'foe', 'phone', 'phobia', and 'foal' stop shouting, but words like 'photo', 'photograph', and 'photon' are still shouting. Once the phoneme detection device detects the following sounds up to /g/, only 'photograph' is left shouting (words like 'photography' and 'photographer' have a different stress pattern than 'photograph', and the vowel in the first syllable of these two words is /ə/, the schwa vowel, and not /o/ as in 'photograph', so they have stopped shouting). At this point this word has "won" out over the other candidates. The phoneme detection device now has the information that this is the last word left in the mental lexicon that is a candidate for what it is hearing (trying to detect).

Thus, by the time the phoneme detection device is fed the buzz sound that has replaced the vowel /æ/ in 'photograph', it has already gotten the information that the word it is trying to detect is probably 'photograph'. Since this device is using information from the sound waves it is being fed and information that is being shouted to it from the lexicon to detect phonemes (make good guesses about what is in the speech stream), it detects /æ/ instead of a buzz. That is, it "hears" /æ/ instead of the buzz it was actually fed, thanks to the information it has received from the mental lexicon (the word 'photograph' shouting out to the phoneme detection device that it's probably the word being said).

This type of account postulates, then, several connected mental devices or mechanisms that actively manipulate the information in the speech stream and do not just passively take it in. Of course, terms like 'get excited' and 'shout out' are just metaphors and have to be spelled out in terms of operations going on in the brain (for example, in terms of sets of neurons firing and sending signals to other neurons). However, we can learn a lot about the mechanisms for producing and understanding speech by using psycholinguistic experiments to test hypotheses about the sorts of "devices" (modules) the mind might be using to process speech and the ways in which they might connect ("talk to") each other.

Figure 7-1 diagrams the sorts of mental mechanisms that the above account makes use of, and the ways in which they communicate with each other. This sort of 'picture' constitutes a **model** of a part of the system for understanding speech. We can test (and change, if necessary) such models by further experiments.

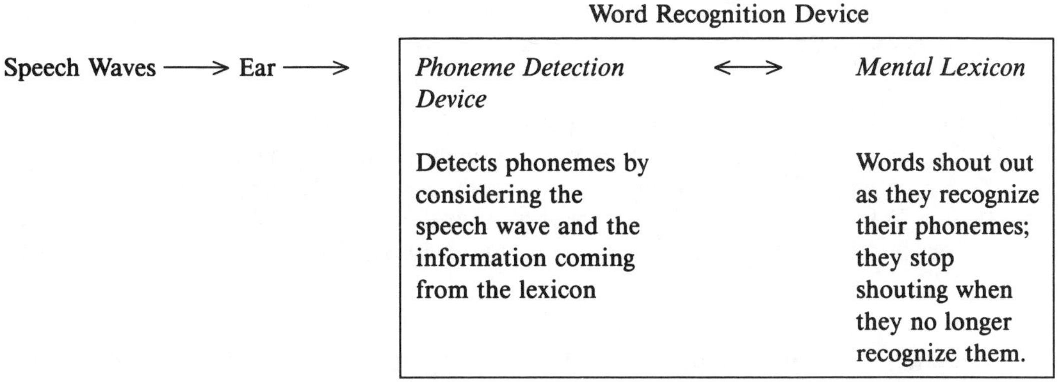

Word Recognition Device

Speech Waves ———> Ear ———>

Phoneme Detection Device	<———>	*Mental Lexicon*
Detects phonemes by considering the speech wave and the information coming from the lexicon		Words shout out as they recognize their phonemes; they stop shouting when they no longer recognize them.

FIGURE 7-1.   A model of the process by which humans recognize phonemes and words in the speech stream

In addition, there are two further ways in which we can deepen our understanding of such models. We can study the ways in which the brain works, with its billions of neurons and their intricate connections to each other. And we can seek to implement such models on computers and run artificial simulations of speech processing (feeding the computer system various words and sentences and seeing what it will do). Thus, studies in neuroscience (the study of the brain) and artificial intelligence (using computers to simulate various sorts of human intelligence) complement psycholinguistic studies.

Figure 7-1 shows the two mental mechanisms that we have been discussing (the phoneme detection device and the mental lexicon) as themselves component parts of a larger mental mechanism, which I have labeled the **word recognition device.** This larger device recognizes words (using the phoneme detection device and the mental lexicon as its component parts) in the speech stream.

———————————————— E X E R C I S E S ————————————————

Exercise B.   In Chapter 4, I pointed out that the sound features of any phoneme in a word are actually spread out throughout the word. Thus, in a word like 'arm', the nasal air that partly characterizes the sound /m/, which is a *nasal* sound, starts to occur on the sound /a/; that is, the speaker anticipates saying /m/ by starting to let air out of his or her nose as early as the sound /a/. This can clue a hearer to anticipate hearing a nasal sound soon (like /m/ or /n/ or /ng/). The /r/ sound influences the sound /a/ also, causing it to be said differently than it would in a word without a following /r/ (like 'on', which is pronounced /an/). How would these sorts of facts make you revise the model of recognizing words that is developed in Section 7.3?

Exercise C. If you tape record a sentence like 'I like boysenberries' and play it for people, they will sometimes momentarily think they have heard 'I like boys and berries'. Why? What about this sentence eventually makes clear to hearers that they have heard 'I like boysenberries' and not 'I like boys and berries'? What does all this suggest has to be added to our account of word recognition in Section 7.3?

Exercise D. If you tape record something like 'John and I love fruit. He especially likes blackberries. However, I like boysenberries' and play it for people, do you think they are less likely to momentarily think they have heard 'I like boys and berries' as the last part? Why? By the way, different psycholinguists answer this question differently, and there is controversy over the matter—so give your own answer. What does this tell us about how people recognize words in the speech stream?

7.4. RECOGNIZING SENTENCES

The Syntactic Processor

Obviously, speech is not just a stream of unconnected words. The listener must put the words together into phrases and sentences. Thus, we can assume that the word recognition device must pass the results of its work (the words it is finding) to another device that puts them into phrases and sentences. I will call this device the **syntactic processor.** In Figure 7-2, I add this device to Figure 7-1.

If you look at Figure 7-2, you will see that I have placed two question marks at the end of the arrow that leads back from the syntactic processor to the word recognition device. It is clear that the word recognition device "speaks to" the syntactic processor by giving it the words that it will place in phrases and sentences. But we can ask whether the syntactic processor "talks back" to the word recognition device. That is, can the syntactic processor let the word recognition device know what it is doing so that the word recognition device uses this information to help it find words in the speech stream?

To see how this would work, consider the following situation. A word like 'rose' is ambiguous. It can be a verb meaning *to stand up* (as in 'They all rose') or it can be a noun that names a flower (as in 'They bought a rose'). If the syntactic processor can talk back to the word recognition device and help it with its work, then it would be able to do the following sort of thing: In the case of a sentence like 'They bought a rose', when the syntactic processor has been handed the

Word Recognition Device

Speech Waves ——→ Ear ——→

Phoneme Detection Device	←——→	Mental Lexicon
Detects phonemes by considering the speech wave and the information coming from the lexicon		Words shout out as they recognize their phonemes; they stop shouting when they no longer recognize them.

? ?
↓

Syntactic Processor

Takes words from the word recognition device and puts them into phrases and sentences.

FIGURE 7-2. The word recognition device (made up of the phoneme detection device and the mental lexicon) passes words to the syntactic processor, which bundles them into phrases and sentences.

words 'they', 'bought', and 'a', it will have assembled these into the parts of a sentence. This sentence will have the structure shown below:

1.

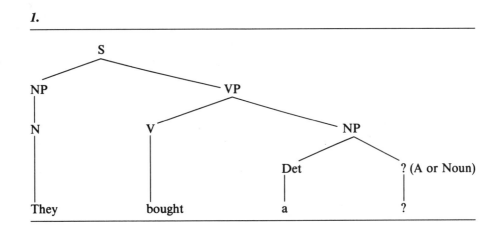

The syntactic processor, using the rules for English phrase structure, has assembled the words into a sentence where 'they' is the subject, the verb is 'bought', and this verb, which requires an object, has a noun phrase object beginning with the determiner 'a'. Given the rules of English phrase structure, the syntactic processor knows that what will follow 'a' must be either an adjective (as in 'They bought a pretty rose') or a noun (as in 'They bought a rose'). It certainly cannot be a verb (*'They bought a sit').

While the syntactic processor is doing this work, the phoneme detection device is receiving the sound waves for 'rose' (in the sentence 'They bought a rose'). As it hears /r/, all words beginning with /r/ get excited in the lexicon, as it hears /ro/, many "turn off," but many others get more excited (like 'row', 'road', 'roam', etc.). When it arrives at the end of the word, getting /roz/ ('rose'), there are, unfortunately, two words that are loudly excited: both 'rose' the verb (stand up) and 'rose' the noun (the flower), since the sound /roz/ is ambiguous.

The question is, can the syntactic processor tell the word recognition device, after getting the determiner 'a' (in 'They bought a rose') that what will follow 'a' cannot be a verb? This would turn off the verb 'rose' so that it never gets excited (even when the /r/ comes in). Thus, only the noun 'rose' will get excited at the end of the string of sounds /roz/ (since the verb 'rose' has never "turned on," thanks to the fact that it is a verb and the word recognition device has been told by the syntactic processor that what is coming up cannot be a verb).

This would seem to be a helpful process, but there is some evidence that it does not happen. That is, there is evidence that while the word recognition device talks to the syntactic processor (passes it words to work on), the syntactic processor does not talk back to the word recognition device and help it in its work.

We can see this if we consider for a moment a tricky task that psycholinguists use, a task called *cross-modal naming*. One version of this task works as follows: You present in speech a sentence to a subject, say 'They like cats'. At the end of the sentence, you flash a written word on a computer screen (say the word 'dog' or the word 'rice') and the subject is supposed to name (say) the word as fast as possible. The psycholinguist measures the "reaction time" of the subject (how long it takes him or her to name the word, which is always very fast, a matter of milliseconds, so it takes sophisticated equipment to measure this reaction).

It turns out that, in this task, subjects can name the visually presented word faster if the visually presented word's meaning has something in common with the meaning of the last word in the sentence they have just heard. Thus, subjects will react to the visually presented word 'dog' more quickly than the word 'rice' if they have just heard the sentence 'They like cats'. The word 'cats' in the sentence is said to "prime" the naming of the word 'dog' (and not 'rice'). This is happening presumably because when the word 'cats' in the sentence has become excited in the mental lexicon, it has caused words in the lexicon with partially related meanings to get somewhat excited themselves, and these are thus more ready to be recognized (and named in the task when visually presented). In fact, it is tasks like this that allow psycholinguists to probe how the mental lexicon is organized and how it works.

If the syntactic processor can help the word recognition device, we would expect that when presented with the spoken sentence 'They bought a rose' and the visual word 'flower', the naming of 'flower' will be speeded up by its semantic relation to 'rose' (the name of a flower) in the sentence. And it is. But if the syntactic processor has told the word recognition device *not* to consider the verb 'rose' (stand up) once having heard 'a' (in 'They bought a rose'), then if the visually presented word is 'stood' (not 'flower'), the naming of this word should *not* be speeded up (in relation to irrelevant words like 'car') since the verb 'rose' is not excited, having been turned off by the word recognition device thanks to what the syntactic processor has told it. However, it turns out that the naming of 'stood' after having heard 'rose' in 'They bought a rose' *is* speeded up, despite the fact that this sentence contains the noun 'rose' (a flower) and not the verb 'rose' (stand up). Thus, it appears that the word recognition device is considering both the noun and verb 'rose' when it hears 'I bought a rose', and therefore the verb can facilitate the naming of 'stood'.

So it seems that even when the word recognition device has heard the words 'They bought a' and passed these words to the syntactic processor, it still considers both the verb and noun 'rose' when it hears / roz /. Thus, it cannot know what the syntactic processor surely knows, that after the determiner 'a' a verb cannot occur and so the word being said in the speech stream cannot possibly be the verb 'rose'. Nonetheless, the verb 'rose' does get excited, along with the noun 'rose', and so can prime (speed up) the naming of 'stood', a word it is related to in meaning.

Evidence like this leads us to believe that the syntactic processor does not talk back to the word recognition device and help it out. What appears to happen is that the word recognition device, hearing the 'rose' of 'They bought a rose', comes up with both the noun 'rose' and the verb 'rose' and cannot decide between them (they are both shouting loudly as the phoneme detection device gets to the end of /roz/ ('rose')). The word recognition device passes both of these to the syntactic processor, and the syntactic processor, knowing it needs a noun and not a verb to finish its work in building the sentence ('They bought a'), throws out the verb 'rose' (because it doesn't "fit" in the sentence).

If we delay the presentation of the visual word a bit (say 200 milliseconds) after the spoken sentence has been heard, then the effect we have been discussing disappears. In this case, only the "right" meaning of 'rose' primes the visual word. Thus, given the sentence 'They bought a rose', the word 'rose' here will prime (speed up) the naming of 'flower' (which it is meaningfully related to), but not 'stood' (which it is not meaningfully related to). The time we have allowed to lapse between the spoken sentence and the visually presented word has allowed the word recognition device the time to pass both words ('rose' the noun and 'rose' the verb) to the syntactic processor, which has thrown out the verb (meaning *stand up*) and kept the noun (meaning *a flower*). So when the visual word is presented, after a delay, only the noun is now available to the mind and so only it can prime 'flower'. The verb 'rose' is unavailable to prime 'stood'.

Figure 7-3 diagrams the nature of the mental mechanisms we have discussed so far.

The picture in Figure 7-3 is controversial. I have given you one piece of evidence that the syntactic processor does not talk to and help the word recognition device. Some psycholinguists are not convinced by this evidence and offer other evidence that the syntactic processor can indeed talk to the word recognition device. I introduce the model in Figure 7-3 and the piece of evidence we have discussed not to argue that the matter is settled, but to make clear to you what the issue is. In particular, I introduce this model and this piece of evidence to make clear what the concept of *encapsulation* means, a concept we discuss below.

Encapsulation

Linguists and psycholinguists have a special way of talking about the sort of picture that is emerging in our diagrams (Figures 7-1 through 7-3) above. When one device (like the word recognition device) sends its results to another device (like the syntactic processor), but that second device (the syntactic processor) cannot talk to the first one (the word recognition device) and influence (help) its decisions, the first device is said to be **encapsulated.** It is "sealed off" from being influenced by other devices and makes its decisions on its own.

Thus, the word recognition device makes the decision that /roz/ can be either the noun or verb 'rose' without consulting the syntactic processor (which could have told it to forget considering the verb). The word recognition device is, then, "encapsulated" or "sealed off" from the syntactic processor. Psycholinguists believe that encapsulated devices are fast and efficient at doing the work they do (which is why human biology has given rise to them). But, in a sense, they are also "stupid" (for example, the word recognition device fails to use information the syntactic processor has, information that would be, in the case we looked at, helpful). On the other hand, within the word recognition device, the two subdevices, the phoneme detection device and the mental lexicon, do talk to and influence each other. So they are not encapsulated in relationship to each other, though they are encapsulated in relation to the syntactic processor.

As we consider other devices that are part of the speech-understanding system (for example, the device that gives meaning to the results of the syntactic processor), we can always ask (and try to test) whether or not the device is encapsulated.

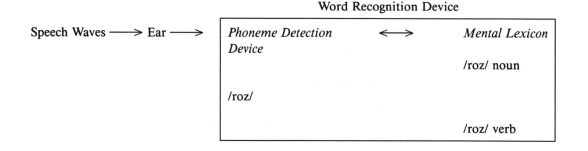

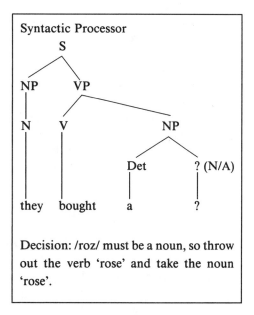

FIGURE 7-3. Upon recognizing /roz/ in the sentence 'They bought a rose', the word recognition device passes both the verb 'rose' (stand up) and the noun 'rose' (the flower) to the syntactic processor, which rejects the verb and takes the noun. The syntactic processor does not stop the word recognition device from considering both choices, though "it knows" by the time it has received 'They bought a' that it cannot use a verb.

——————————————— **E X E R C I S E** ———————————————

Exercise E. How does the discussion in the preceding two sections help explain why psycholinguists might differ on the answer to Exercise D above?

———

The Syntactic Processor: Parsing

Now we will take up the question as to how the syntactic processor carries out its work of bundling words into phrases and sentences. The operation by which the syntactic processor takes the words coming to it from the word recognition device and bundles them into phrases and sentences is called **parsing,** and the syntactic processor is said to be parsing the sentence.

Obviously, the syntactic processor must know the phrase structure rules of English, and must use them to group words into phrases. For example, confronted with the string of words 'The man loaded the boxes on the cart', the syntactic processor, knowing that English sentences are made up of an NP (the subject of the sentence) and a VP, and knowing that NPs in English often have the structure DET N ('the man'), will bundle the words 'the' and 'man' into the phrase 'the man' and label this an NP and the subject of the sentence. It will make 'loaded' the verb of the sentence.

When the mental lexicon passes the word 'loaded' to the syntactic processor, we assume it also passes the whole lexical entry of the word. This lexical entry will tell the syntactic processor that 'loaded' requires an object NP naming the thing loaded (what we called a THEME in Chapters 2 and 6, the semantic role of an NP naming an entity that moves, is located, or changes state). The entry will also tell the syntactic processor that this verb semantically assumes a prepositional phrase naming a location (what we called a LOCATION in Chapters 2 and 6) where the thing loaded was loaded (so even 'The man loaded the boxes' assumes he did it somewhere and that this has been left out because it is obvious from context or irrelevant). So the syntactic processor will look for these (an object naming the thing loaded and a prepositional phrase naming the location where it was loaded).

When it gets the words 'the cart', it will make these words an NP and the object of the verb 'loaded'. It will assign this NP the semantic role THEME in the sentence. Finding the words 'on the cart', it will assume these are the PP naming where the loading was done. It will assign these words the semantic role LOCATION. Given that loading something requires an ACTOR who has loaded them, the syntactic processor will assign the semantic role ACTOR to the subject of the sentence. Note that we are assuming that the syntactic processor does a little bit of semantic work since it assigns semantic roles like ACTOR, THEME, and LOCATION (roles it knows where to assign from consulting the lexical entry for 'loaded').

After all this work, the syntactic processor will have constructed the representation shown below:

2.

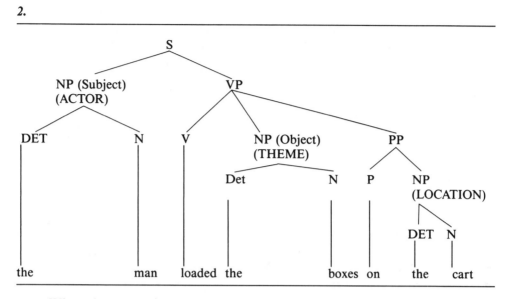

When the syntactic processor has constructed the representation shown in example 2, it has parsed the sentence (assigned the words a syntactic structure).

A Problem for the Syntactic Processor: Garden-Path Sentences

If we assume that the syntactic processor works in the way we have spelled out in the last section, it is going to run into trouble with certain sentences. Consider the two sentences below:

3a. Mary hit the man with a stick

3b. Mary hit the man with a wart

The sentence in 3a is ambiguous. It can mean that Mary (the ACTOR) hit the man (the PATIENT) with a certain INSTRUMENT, namely a stick. Or it can mean that Mary (the ACTOR) hit a man who had or was carrying a stick, where the whole phrase 'the man with a stick' names the PATIENT. In this case, we could add another phrase to the sentence, naming the INSTRUMENT (such as 'Mary hit the man with a stick with her purse'). The sentence in 3b is similarly ambiguous, being able to mean that Mary hit a man using a wart as an INSTRUMENT or that she hit a man who had a wart. Of course, in this case, the first reading is funny, because it is absurd to say that someone used a wart as an instrument to hit someone else.

When we read these sentences out of context, it is clear that the first meaning of 3a comes much more readily to mind. In fact, for many people, even 3b causes something of a "double take" as they mistakenly first consider the (inappropriate and comical) meaning where the wart is the INSTRUMENT. Thus, 3b can, at first, seem funny. Such sentences are sometimes called **garden-path sentences** because we are led down a "garden path" in considering one structure (the one appropriate to the first sort of meaning) when the structure for the second meaning is intended (as most usually in the case of 3b).

There are many types of garden-path sentences. For example, the sentence in 4 is a famous case of a garden-path sentence. This sentence so badly garden-paths us that it takes some time to figure out what the sentence really means:

4. The horse raced past the barn fell

When we are first presented with this sentence, we attempt to take the string of words 'the horse raced past the barn' as a complete sentence. When we get to the word 'fell' and realize that the preceding words cannot be a complete sentence, we are confused. We must backtrack and reparse (assign another syntactic structure) to the sentence as a whole. The appropriate meaning is *The horse (which was) raced past the barn fell.*

To see what is happening here, let us look at the syntactic structures for the two possible meanings of sentence 3a. The tree in 5a below gives the syntactic structure for the first meaning (where Mary used a stick to hit the man), and the tree in 5b gives the syntactic structure for the second meaning (where the man has the stick and there is no mention of what instrument Mary used to hit the man).

5a.

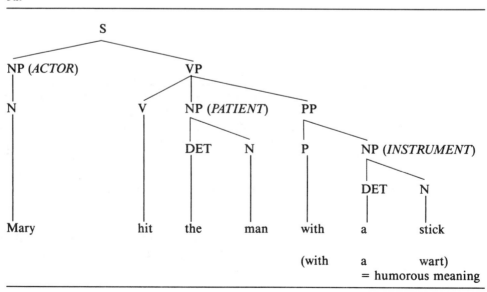

5b.

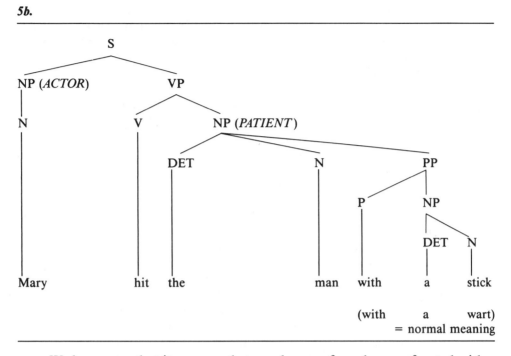

(with   a   wart)
= normal meaning

We have seen that it appears that speakers prefer, when confronted with a sentence like 'Mary hit the man with a stick' or even 'Mary hit the man with a wart' to consider first the structure in 5a (where for 3b the phrase 'with a wart' is given a humorous reading meaning that Mary hit the man using a wart). This is what garden-paths people if the meaning intended was the one represented by the tree in 5b. In this case, they will have momentarily considered the wrong analysis (as they most certainly also do in the case of a sentence like 4, 'The horse raced past the barn fell').

Of course, what is happening here cannot really be settled just by consulting our intuitions. What is happening in the mind/brain when the syntactic processor parses a sentence happens in microseconds and is, for the most part, done unconsciously. What the syntactic processor does is usually not even open to our conscious minds. Thus, psycholinguists have to use indirect measures, from laboratory experiments, to try and guess what the syntactic processor is doing.

There is evidence from studies of people's eye gaze and reading speed when reading sentences like 3a and 3b that they are indeed garden-pathed in such cases. Their syntactic processors appear first to consider the sort of structure given in 5a for both 3a and 3b and resort to the one in 5b only later (if needed, as in the case of 3b). Thus, in a sentence like 'Mary hit the man with a wart' (which only has the second reading—represented by the tree in 5b—in any meaningful sense), people will take longer to read this sentence than an equally long, but unproblematic sentence (one with no possible structural ambiguity). They will also fixate their gaze around the problematic phrase ('with a wart') longer than in a more normal case. This seems to indicate that they have momentarily assigned the wrong analysis to the sentence (the sort in 5a), and only later catch on to the right one (the one in 5b). The longer reading time seems to be caused by the syntactic processor's need to reverse analyses and give up the one in 5a and resort to the one in 5b.

So we see that people appear to be led to some parses (assignments of syntactic structure) more readily than others. Thus, they appear first to consider a tree like the one in 5a, and only later, realizing that that tree won't work (if it won't), consider a second possibility, the one in 5b.

The question is why people should favor certain syntactic structures over others. Some psychologists have proposed that there is a general parsing principle that determines such matters in a large number of cases. They call this principle **minimal attachment.** As the words of a sentence come into the syntactic processor one at a time from the word recognition device, the syntactic processor bundles them into phrases and finally into a sentence as a whole. In doing so, it first tries the least complex analysis of the sentence. Thus, in 'Mary hit the man with a stick/wart', the syntactic processor tries to place the prepositional phrase 'with the stick/wart' under the verb phrase, rather than to create a complicated NP 'the man with the stick/wart'. And in 4 ('The horse raced past the barn fell'), the syntactic processor first tries to make 'the horse raced past the barn' a simple sentence, rather than assume that it is a complex NP ('the horse (which was) raced past the barn') that is the subject of another verb ('fell').

While many psycholinguists have allegiance to such an account, in the next section I will develop a somewhat different account of what is happening in these garden-path sentences.

------------------------------- **E X E R C I S E** -------------------------------

Exercise F.   In what way would the syntactic processor be garden-pathed by the following sentences? (Why might the syntactic processor consider, however momentarily, an analysis for each sentence that is not the one the speaker intended?) Why do you think the syntactic processor prefers these unintended analyses and thus attempts to impose them? Give your view in your own words—you might propose different reasons for different cases.

1. The man loaded the boxes on the cart on the van.
2. They are loving children. (This sentence was uttered intending to mean that 'they' are children who are loving and nice, not that 'they' are engaged in the act of loving children.)
3. John said he had a date yesterday. (This sentence was uttered intending to mean, *Yesterday, John said that he had a date.*)
4. The child left alone died.

Using Lexical Entries and Argument Structures
in Parsing

We can get some feeling for what might be going on in the case of garden-path sentences if we consider the two sentences in 6a and 6b:

6a. The man examined by the attorney was unconvincing

6b. The evidence examined by the attorney was unconvincing

There is evidence (this time the evidence comes from looking at the patterns of people's brain waves as they comprehend sentences like 6a and 6b) that people are garden-pathed in a sentence like 6a. That is, when they get to 'by the attorney', they show evidence that they are putting in extra effort or extra work in processing the sentence. The reason for this is that they have assumed the sentence is going to continue as an active sentence like 'the man examined X (for example, 'the man examined the evidence'). When they get to 'by the attorney', they realize this guess is wrong and that 'the man examined' is not a subject ('the man') plus main verb ('examined'), but rather part of a complex subject ('the man (who was) examined by the attorney'—a relative clause construction).

But, it turns out, people are not garden-pathed in 6b. They show no evidence for any extra effort or extra work when they get to 'by the attorney' (they are not, in this case, subconsciously surprised by this sort of continuation). Why? When they get to the verb 'examined', they know this cannot be the active verb of a sentence like 'X examined Y', because the noun they have just heard names an inanimate thing (evidence) and only animate things can examine something. Thus, by the time they have heard 'examined' they know that they must be listening to the passive participle form of 'examine' and that 'evidence' is what got examined, not what did the examining. They are, then, not surprised to hear the ACTOR in a phrase like 'by the attorney', since this is how ACTORS are designated with passive participle forms of verbs (as in 'examined': 'The evidence was examined by the attorney').

To account for what happens in sentences like 6a and 6b, we will assume that the word recognition device sends each word it recognizes to the syntactic processor, and the syntactic processor attempts to bundle these words into phrases and sentences as it gets them; that is, it attempts to parse (assign a tree to) the sentence that is being said. This is as we have been assuming all along. We will, however, further assume that when the word recognition device sends verbs (or any other word, for that matter) to the syntactic processor, it sends not just the word but the entire lexical entry for the verb.

This lexical entry for the verb lists the pronunciation, meaning, and syntactic properties of the verb. In particular, it lists the **argument structure** of the verb. The argument structure of the verb gives information about how many noun phrases the verb requires or allows to make a grammatical and meaningful sentence, as well as the semantic roles (for example, ACTOR) these noun phrases play in the sentence. Thus, when the word recognition device recognizes the verb 'examined' in 6a and 6b and sends it to the syntactic processor, it sends the whole lexical entry for this verb. This entry contains the following information (along with much more not shown here):

> 'examine'
> verb
> argument structure: ACTOR *examines/d* PATIENT
> passive form: PATIENT *is examined* (by ACTOR)

Let's consider what happens when the syntactic processor has received from the word recognition device the words 'the man examined' and received the entry above for the word 'examined'. Remember, the syntactic processor is getting each word as the word recognition device recognizes it in the speech stream and is trying to bundle the words it is getting into phrases and sentences (that is, it is trying to parse the sentences being uttered).

When the syntactic processor gets 'the man examined' and the above entry for 'examine', it will assume (guess) that 'the man' names the ACTOR called for in the argument structure, and will then be expecting to hear an upcoming noun phrase naming a PATIENT. When it gets 'by the attorney', it realizes it was wrong, and 'the man' could not have been the ACTOR. The syntactic processor has to backtrack, making 'the man' the PATIENT, and realize that 'the man examined by the attorney' contains the passive form of 'examined' used in a reduced relative clause construction (the relative clause is reduced because 'who was' is missing: 'the man (who was) examined by the attorney'). Thus, the syntactic processor has momentarily garden-pathed, considered that 'the man' was the ACTOR (which was wrong in this case), and has required extra effort to undo this mistake and get the right analysis.

In the case of 6b, when the syntactic processor gets 'the evidence examined' and considers the lexical entry for 'examined' (see above), it knows that 'evidence' can't be an ACTOR, since it is not animate or even capable of initiating action, and so must be the PATIENT. Therefore, the syntactic processor will immediately realize that it must be listening to the passive form of the verb 'examine'. Thus, it assumes (guesses) that it may hear a "*by* phrase" with the ACTOR in it, and it does ('by the attorney'). So here everything works smoothly and there is no garden path and no extra effort required.

The reason that sentences like 3a and 3b ('Mary hit a man with a stick/wart') garden-path people, then, is as follows: When the word recognition device passes 'hit' to the syntactic processor, it gets the whole lexical entry for the verb. This entry tells it that 'hit', in the active voice, has the following argument structure: ACTOR *hits* PATIENT (with INSTRUMENT). The INSTRUMENT phrase is optional, but one always understands that some instrument is used in an act of hitting, whether it is overtly mentioned or not. Thus, the syntactic processor gets ready to hear an INSTRUMENT phrase. Upon hearing 'with a stick/with a wart', it first guesses that this is the instrument, eventually realizing in the case of 'with a wart' that this is very unlikely.

—————————————— E X E R C I S E ——————————————

Exercise G. Show how an account using argument structure and lexical entries, like the one I have given above, can explain why the syntactic processor garden-paths in the two cases below. HINT: You can consider the argument structure of 'load' to be ACTOR *load* THEME in/on-LOCATION (that is, some ACTOR loads something, a THEME, at some LOCATION that is marked by the preposition 'in' or 'on') and the argument structure of 'love' to be ACTOR *love* GOAL (that is, some ACTOR directs his or her love toward a certain person or thing as its object or GOAL).

1. The man loaded the boxes on the cart on the van.
2. They are loving children.
   (with the meaning intended in Exercise F)

7.5. PARSING SENTENCES IN DISCOURSE CONTEXT

Now let's consider what might happen when sentences like 3a and 3b ('Mary hit the man with a stick/wart') are comprehended not in isolation, but in meaningful discourse contexts. We assume that in addition to the word recognition device and the syntactic processor, there is a **semantics/discourse processor** that is attempting to figure out the meanings of words, phrases, and sentences and their connections to sentences uttered earlier in the discourse. That is, we are assuming a picture of the speech comprehension system that looks something like Figure 7-4.

Figure 7-4 shows a picture in which, as the word recognition device recognizes words, it passes them (and their entire lexical entries) to both the syntactic processor and the semantics/discourse processor. The syntactic processor attempts to bundle the words it gets into phrases and sentences and, as it does this, it passes the information about phrases and sentences it has found to the semantics/discourse processor (as it discovers this information, it immediately passes it on). The semantics/discourse processor assigns meanings to the words it gets and to the phrases and sentences it receives. It assigns these meanings based on the lexical entries of the words, the syntactic information it has gotten from the syntactic processor, and the information it has constructed from the previous sentences in the discourse.

Now consider a discourse like that in 7:

7. Two men yelled at Mary. One had a long beard and the other had a large wart on his face. Mary took a stick and *she hit the man with the wart.*

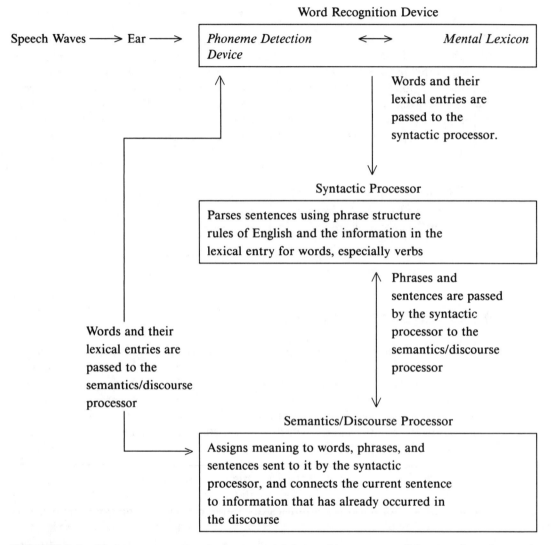

FIGURE 7-4. Various component devices or modules making up part of the speech-understanding system.

There is currently controversy among psycholinguists as to what happens in cases like that in 7. The question is this: Will the syntactic processor, when it gets to 'she hit the man with the wart', momentarily consider the wrong analysis, as it appears to do out of context? That is, will it garden-path and momentarily think that 'with a wart' names an INSTRUMENT? Or will the syntactic processor use the discourse information that the semantics/discourse processor has constructed prior to getting the words 'she hit the man with the wart' to save it from making, however momentarily, this mistake (taking this structural garden path)?

In the discourse context that precedes 'she hit the man with the wart' in 7, it is made clear that Mary has a stick, which is an excellent instrument to use in hitting people. And it is made clear that there are two men involved, one of whom has a wart. This is all information that the semantics/discourse processor knows by the time the word 'hit' has come into the syntactic processor and the semantics/discourse processor, since the semantics/discourse processor has already analyzed these previous sentences.

The syntactic processor and the semantics/discourse processor are both working on the words that the word recognition device has recognized, each doing their job. As the syntactic processor assigns words to phrases, it passes this information to the semantics/discourse processor. When the syntactic and semantics/discourse processors get to the word 'hit' in 7, the semantics/discourse processor could help the syntactic processor out by telling it that, based on the meaning of the previous sentences, an INSTRUMENT (namely the stick) has already been mentioned, and thus is not likely to be overtly mentioned again. Thus, the syntactic processor should, upon getting 'hit', not expect an overt INSTRUMENT phrase. Furthermore, the semantics/discourse processor knows that two men have been mentioned in the context, one with a beard and one with a wart. Thus, if one of these is going to be mentioned again, he will in all likelihood have to be singled out by mentioning the beard or the wart. Thus, the syntactic processor, getting 'hit', should look, in this context, not for an INSTRUMENT, but for the mention of a man with a beard or a wart.

If the semantics/discourse processor can give this information to the syntactic processor (can speak to it and help it out with its job), then, in this case, it will save the syntactic processor from garden-pathing and, upon getting 'hit', momentarily expecting to get an INSTRUMENT phrase in the upcoming speech stream. And, when the syntactic processor gets 'the man with a wart', it will be ready and willing to make this a single phrase naming the entity that got hit (the PATIENT). It will never be tempted to think that perhaps 'the man' is the PATIENT and 'with the wart' is an INSTRUMENT phrase. If this happens, that is, if the semantics/discourse processor talks to the syntactic processor and helps it out, by giving it information about the meanings of sentences from the preceding discourse, then the syntactic processor is not encapsulated from the semantics/discourse processor (but, rather, can listen to it and get help from it). Remember that what is happening here is happening unconsciously in the mind/brain and in a matter of microseconds. So the matter has to be settled by experimentation, not people's intuitions.

I will assume (the matter is, however, controversial) that the semantics/discourse processor can talk to the syntactic processor. Then, our account of the discourse in 7 will be as follows: The syntactic processor, when it gets to 'hit', will also access the argument structure of hit (ACTOR *hits* PATIENT (with INSTRUMENT)). The semantics/discourse processor knows that Mary has a stick and that sticks are good instruments for hitting and knows that a man with a wart and a man with a beard have already been mentioned. The semantics/discourse processor gives this information to the syntactic processor. Thus, on hearing 'hit' and considering the argument structure of 'hit', the syntactic processor assumes that the stick is the INSTRUMENT and that therefore the instrument need not and will not be mentioned again. Thus, when it hears 'with the wart' it is not tempted to think it is hearing the INSTRUMENT phrase and will immediately assign this phrase as part of the larger phrase 'the man with the wart', especially knowing such a man has been mentioned as one of two men in the scene (and would have to be mentioned again to distinguish the one that got hit from the one that didn't).

--------------------------- E X E R C I S E S ---------------------------

Exercise H.   If we accept that the semantic/discourse processor does talk to and help the syntactic processor, explain why in the following context the syntactic processor will not be garden-pathed by 'she hit the man with a stick', despite the fact that out of context the syntactic processor clearly prefers to parse this as 'she (ACTOR) hit the man (PATIENT) with a stick (INSTRUMENT)', which is the wrong meaning for the discourse below:

> Two men yelled at Mary. One had a big stick and the other one had a gun. Mary took her purse and *she hit the man with the stick.*

Exercise I.   When 'she hit the man with the stick' means that she took a stick and hit the man with it, it is pronounced with stress (emphasis) on 'stick' and perhaps a slight hesitation between 'man' and 'with':

> she hit the man/with the STICK

How is the sentence most naturally pronounced in the discourse in Exercise H, and in what way does this differ from the way it is pronounced out of context with the meaning 'she took the stick and hit the man with it'? How could this difference help the syntactic processor (provided it gets told about it)?

The Semantics/Discourse Processor

It would take us far afield to go into any detail about how the semantics/discourse processor works. This is a large and complicated topic and one about which psycholinguists still know less than they would like. Clearly, the semantics/

discourse processor, which is itself probably made up of a variety of subcomponents, has a lot of work to do. It must, using the lexical entry of each word, assign a meaning to each word in a sentence. These lexical entries have been passed from the word recognition device (which got them out of the mental lexicon).

But the semantics/discourse processor must also put the meanings of the words together into the meaning of the sentence as a whole. Further, the semantics/discourse processor must relate the meaning of the sentence to the context in which it has been uttered, relating it to the other sentences that have come before it and those that will come after it in the discourse (see Chapter 2). And the semantics/discourse processor must also assign the correct "speech act" to the sentence; that is, determine whether it is a promise, a statement, a threat, an offer, and so forth (see Chapter 10). This is not a matter just of surface form, since a sentence like 'I will visit your house' can be, in different situations, a claim, a promise, an offer, or a threat. Finally, the semantics/discourse processor has to compute what the sentence says about the social relations of the participants in the discourse and the various devices the sentence uses to signal politeness or formality (see Chapter 9).

One thing is fairly clear about how the semantics/discourse processor works. It takes the syntactic structure of a sentence from the syntactic processor and uses this syntactic structure and the meanings it has already constructed for previous sentences in the discourse to assign a meaning to the sentence. It then discards the syntactic structure of the sentence and keeps a record only of the meaning of the discourse as a whole. This is why people have very poor memories for the syntactic form of sentences they have heard, though they have good memories for the meanings of the sentences they have heard.

For example, psycholinguists have shown that people having heard one of the sentences below cannot remember which they have heard (and will often claim they heard the wrong one) only a few sentences later in a discourse. This is because the two sentences have the same meaning, and all people can remember is this meaning.[3]

8. The owner of the magic staff dispatched the ship

9. The dispatcher of the ship owned the magic staff

So we might conclude that people are storing the meanings of sentences, not the syntactic forms in which they have been heard. But even this is not quite correct. Consider the following situation. Subjects are presented with a passage that starts with the sentence in 10 below. Then later in the passage they see either the sentence in 11a or the sentence in 11b (some subjects see one, the others see the other):

---

[3]Examples in this section are from Alan Garnham's book *Psycholinguistics: Central Topics* (London & New York: Methuen, 1985).

10. By the window was a man with a martini

11a. The man with the martini waved to the hostess

11b. The man by the window waved to the hostess

Now, clearly, the phrase 'the man by the window' in 11b and 'the man with the martini' in 11a do not have the same *meaning* (what we called *sense* in Chapter 2), though in this particular passage they do *refer* to the same person (they have the same "reference" or "extension" in the terms we used in Chapter 2). Since they do not have the same meaning, if people store meaning, we might expect that people will remember which of 11a or 11b they have heard. At least we might expect that they will remember whether the man who waved to the hostess was described in doing that act as being by the window or as having had a martini.

However, subjects who had heard passages like this could not later remember which of 11a or 11b they had in fact heard. They could not remember how the man who had waved to the hostess was described. So, if they in fact heard a passage like 'By the window was a man with a martini . . . [other sentences] . . . The man with the martini waved to the hostess', they may well think later, if asked, that they actually heard 'the man by the window waved to the hostess'. Even though in the sentence 'The man with the martini waved to the hostess', the phrase 'the man with the martini' does not mean the same thing as 'the man by the window', subjects do not store that the man was described one way or the other, since in this passage (though not in many other cases, of course) the two phrases refer to the same person.

Thus, subjects had stored (kept a record of) neither the syntactic form they had actually heard, nor of the meaning of the phrases they had heard. If they had kept such a record of the meaning, then the phrase 'the man with the martini', having a different meaning than 'the man by the window', would have been stored (recorded) differently, and subjects would have been able to tell whether they had heard this meaning or not.

What did the subjects keep a record of, then? They kept a record of the general content of what they have heard, not the details of its syntactic form or meaning. Since the two phrases above, in this passage, refer to the same man, they only keep a record that *this man* (who has various properties, including having been by a window and having had a martini), however he was originally described, waved to the hostess. They keep a record of the general content of the discourse (passage) as a whole.

To be more precise about what the semantics/discourse processor is keeping a record of (after it has thrown away a detailed record of the syntactic form and details of meaning of the sentences it has heard), we will say that it produces a representation of what the *world* would be like if the passage were true. Such a representation is a **mental model** of a situation in the real world or an imagined world. This representation is not closely related to any linguistic description of the sentences the semantics/discourse processor has "heard," either in terms of their syntactic form or details of their literal meanings. Of course, the syntactic processor has to compute syntactic forms and the semantics/discourse processor has to use these forms and other information to compute literal meanings for the sentences. But the semantics/discourse processor does this to construct a mental model and, once having done it, keeps the mental model and dispenses with the rest.

─────────────── **E X E R C I S E** ───────────────

Exercise J. When subjects hear a short passage that contains a sentence like 1 below, they will later, when shown a list of sentences and asked which they have previously heard, falsely claim to have heard sentence 2 below.[4]

  1. Three turtles rested on a floating log and a fish swam beneath them.
  2. Three turtles rested on a floating log and a fish swam beneath it.

Why do you think this is so? However, when subjects initially hear a short passage containing a sentence like 3 below, and not 1, they do not, upon being shown 2 later, claim to have heard it. Why?

  3. Three turtles rested beside a floating log and a fish swam beneath them.

What does this sort of data suggest to you that mental models are like?

7.6. THE MEANINGS OF WORDS

One of the hardest problems in psychology is the specification of meaning. Part of the difficulty here is that different types of words have different types of meanings. In this section, we will look at some of the different types of words and the different accounts of their meanings.

  Certain concepts seem to come to human beings either because they are part of the innate endowment of human beings or because they come from the early experience of the world that any human would have to have to end up a normal human being (or a combination of these two factors). Such concepts will be given a single, simple word in all languages, such as 'see', 'have', 'own', 'become', 'not', 'alive'. Or they may be encoded directly in the morphology or

[4]Data from J. D. Bradsford, J. R. Barclay, and J. J. Franks, "Sentence Memory: A Constructive versus Interpretive Approach," *Cognitive Psychology,* 3 (1972), 193–209.

syntax of a language, as the concept of *direct causation* is in English in sentences like 'John broke the vase' (which means he *caused* the vase to break, as compared to 'The vase broke', which means it just broke, but no one necessarily caused it to break) or 'John thickened the soup' (which means he *caused* the soup to become thick, as opposed to 'the soup thickened', which means it just became thick without anyone necessarily causing this to happen).

I suggested in Chapter 2 that such basic concepts may be part of a *language of thought* that exists prior to the acquisition of any verbal language. Children seem to learn such words by direct acquaintance. Then, beyond such words, there are words that have as their meanings a combination of the meanings of these simpler concepts. So a word like 'die' seems to combine the simpler concepts 'BECOME NOT ALIVE', 'kill' to combine the simpler concepts '(directly) CAUSE TO BECOME NOT ALIVE', and 'persuade' the simpler concepts 'TO CAUSE SOMEONE TO COME TO BELIEVE OR DO SOMETHING', where the words in small capital letters stand for basic concepts in the language of thought and not English words.

Many words fall into related systems or what have been called **semantic fields** or **networks.** For example, there are many verbs of possession, like 'give', 'take', 'pay', 'trade', 'buy', 'sell', and 'spend'. Semantically, 'give' and 'take' are the simplest. Roughly speaking, both mean 'TRANSFER OF AN OBJECT FROM ONE PERSON TO ANOTHER.' If the person *with* the object initiates the transfer, one uses 'give', and if the person *without* the object initiates it, one uses 'take'. 'Pay' and 'trade' come next in complexity: They add to the basic meaning of 'give' and 'take' the notion of an obligation involving money on one side ('pay') or the notion of a mutual contract for the exchange of objects ('trade'). The most complex verbs are those that combine all these components: a transfer, an obligation involving money, and a mutual contract to exchange one object (the money) against another. These verbs include 'buy', 'sell', and 'spend'.

Besides these words that encode basic concepts or words whose meanings seem to combine these basic concepts, there are words that are defined purely in terms of other words (which themselves may be explicated through combinations of basic concepts). Words like 'repine', and many other relatively rare words, are usually acquired only through coming to know how to define them in terms of more common words ('repine' means *to mourn or complain*).

Words like 'bird' and 'tiger' (which philosophers call "natural kind terms") constitute yet another class of words. A word like 'bird' seems to have two parts to its meaning. Its meaning appears to be made up of a set of **defining features** and a set of **characteristic features.** These features are various properties that birds *must* have (= defining features) or *usually* have (= characteristic features), in terms of which we identify birds in the world. All birds possess the defining features of birds or else they wouldn't be members of the category. All birds are feathered, lay eggs, have two legs and two wings, are warm blooded, and so on. But birds also possess characteristic features. They usually have short legs, are rather small, are able to fly easily, sit in trees, have a musical call, and so on.

These features, of course, are not properties of all birds, but they are so common they are thought to be characteristic of birds in general.

Some words seem to have no defining characteristics, but the things that the word designates just have "family resemblances." The things the word can be used for do not have any one thing or set of things in common. The most famous statement about "family resemblance" terms comes from the philosopher Ludwig Wittgenstein, who uses the word 'game' as an example.[5]

> Consider for example the proceedings that we call "games". I mean board-games, card-games, ball-games, Olympic games, and so on. What is common to them all? . . . For if you look at them you will not see something that is common to *all*, but similarities, relationships, and a whole series of them at that. . . . Look for example at board-games, with their multifarious relationships. Now pass to card-games; here you find many correspondences with the first group, but many common features drop out, and others appear. When we pass next to ball-games, much that is common is retained, but much is lost.—Are they all 'amusing'? Compare chess with noughts and crosses. Or is there always winning and losing, or competition between players? Think of patience. In ball games there is winning and losing; but when a child throws his ball at the wall and catches it again, this feature has disappeared. . . . And we can go through the many, many other groups of games in the same way; and see how similarities crop up and disappear.
>
> And the result of this examination is: we see a complicated network of similarities overlapping and criss-crossing: sometimes overall similarities, sometimes similarities of detail.
>
> I can think of no better expression to characterize these similarities than "family resemblances"; for the various resemblances between members of a family: build, features, color of eyes, gait, temperament, etc., etc. overlap and criss-cross in the same way.—And I shall say: 'games' form a family.

One way to look at the meaning of a word is as a mental model (in the mind) of typical circumstances in which the word could be used. This model will have somewhat different properties depending on exactly what type of word we are concerned with. We might think of a mental model of a word's meaning as a set of "videotapes" in the mind that store typical examples of situations in which the word would be correctly used. For abstract words like 'honest' and 'justice', this approach seems to be particularly appropriate. People cannot define these words, but they can talk about typical examples of where they would apply.

There is evidence that the context in which a word is uttered encourages

---

[5] I quote the relevant passages from Wittgenstein's book *The Philosophical Investigations* (New York: Macmillan, 1958) pp. 31–32, paragraphs 66 and 67 (I suppress the paragraph numbers below).

people to focus on those parts of the mental model associated with a word that are most relevant to that context. Thus, we know that diamonds are hard, precious, shiny stones. But not all these properties are equally relevant in all contexts. If people are asked "Is a diamond brilliant?" in a context where they have just heard the sentence "The mirror dispersed the light from the diamond" (which calls to mind properties of diamonds that are relevant to the question "Is a diamond brilliant?", namely that they are shiny and bright), they respond faster than when they have been asked this question in a context where a sentence like 'The goldsmith cut the glass with a diamond' has been heard (which calls to mind an irrelevant property, namely that diamonds are hard) or 'The film showed the person with a diamond' (which doesn't call to mind any particular property). The first context ('The mirror dispersed the light from the diamond') appears to facilitate calling to mind the relevant aspect of diamonds (that they are shiny) that is needed to answer the question ('Is a diamond brilliant?').

—————————————— E X E R C I S E S ——————————————

Exercise K.   If we visited another planet and found a substance that looked and felt just like water, and that could be drunk and bathed in just like water but that turned out not to have the chemical composition of H_2O, would you call it water or not? Why? If science discovered that house cats are genetically related to foxes and not to lions and tigers, should we call them foxes? Why? If we discovered an animal in the jungles of Brazil that looked just like a deer and acted like one, but that turned out to have the same genes as a goat, should we call it a goat or a deer? Why? If your answer to the cats/foxes question is that we should keep calling cats *cats,* but your answer to the deer/goat question is that we should call them goats, why did you go with genes in the latter case, but with looks in the first? What issues about word meaning arise here?

Exercise L.   If I have an object in my house that looks like a chair and I use it to sit on, but you find out that its designer meant it to be a table, would you call it a table or a chair? Why? If I use my kitchen table to sit on, and invite guests to do so, does this make it a chair? Why or why not? How do you know when to call something a cup, a mug, a glass, a bowl, or a vase? What issues about word meaning arise here?

7.7. LANGUAGE PRODUCTION

We have discussed some of the details of the way in which humans understand speech. That is, we have traced something of the process by which sound comes in the ear and is converted to meaning by the mind. Now we will briefly discuss this process going in the other direction.

Units of Planning

In *producing* speech we go from meaning to sound. In speaking, people are planning what they are going to say and how they are going to say it, but this planning process is not conscious, and so we are not aware of it. Psycholinguists seek to understand how this unconscious planning process is carried out.

One fertile source of hypotheses about planning in speech is **speech errors.** For example, consider a speech error like the one in 12 below:

12. 'glear plue sky'   (instead of 'clear blue sky')

The speaker who made the error in 12 intended to say 'clear blue sky'. What has happened is obvious. The word 'blue' begins with the sound /b/, which is a voiced stop (that is, a stop consonant with the feature [+voice]). The word 'clear' begins with the voiceless stop /k/ (that is, a stop consonant with the feature [−voice]). The speaker, in trying to produce 'clear' (/klɛr/), with its initial voiceless stop, has anticipated the upcoming initial stop of 'blue' ((/blu/) and has switched the feature [+voice] of /b/ with the feature [−voice] of /k/. Thus, instead of producing a /k/ (a [−voice] sound) in 'clear', the speaker produces a voiced version of /k/, namely /g/; and instead of producing a /b/ (a [+voice] sound) in 'blue', the speaker produces a voiceless version of /b/, namely /p/. I diagram what has happened in 13:

13. *intended:*   klɛr   blu   skaɪ
                       | |
                    [−voice]   [+voice]

     actual: glɛr   plu   skaɪ
                       | |
                    [+voice]   [−voice]

A speech error like the one shown in 12 and 13 gives us evidence for two things: (a) the psychological reality of phonetic features (like [+voice] and [−voice], because it is these that are switching positions); and (b) the fact that people must be planning more than one word at a time. The speaker could not have anticipated 'blue' while saying 'clear' unless the speaker already had planned to say 'blue' by the time he or she had begun to utter 'clear'.

So we are not planning speech one word at a time. But how many words do we plan at once? Consider a speech error like the one in 14 below, where one whole phoneme, not just a single feature, from late in a phrase is substituted for another one that occurs early in the phrase:

14. 'The f̲iring of minority f̲aculty'   (instead of 'the hiring of minority faculty')

In this error the speaker has intended to say 'the hiring of minority faculty' but has produced 'the firing of minority faculty'. The speaker has anticipated the /f/ of 'faculty' at the end of the phrase 'the hiring of minority faculty' and replaced the /h/ of 'hiring' with /f/. In this case, then, the speaker must have planned the whole phrase as a single unit. When she then tried to get it out of her mouth, she anticipated the end of the phrase and it influenced the beginning of the phrase.

Evidence like that above leads psycholinguists to believe that speech is planned in units at least as large as a phrase, and probably often as large as a clause (simple sentences).

Stages of the Planning Process

Speech errors can also illuminate the stages through which the unconscious planning process goes as the speaker moves from thought to speech. Consider an error like that in 15 below:

15. 'a burly bird'   (instead of 'an early bird')

The speaker who said 15 intended to say 'an early bird' but said 'a burly bird' instead. The /b/ of bird was anticipated as the speaker spoke and influenced the beginning of the word 'early'. In English, the indefinite determiner 'a/an' alternates between two forms, 'a' (which occurs before consonants) and 'an' (which occurs before vowels). This is a morphophonemic alternation (see Chapter 3). Note that in the speech error in 15, the speaker, having changed 'early' to 'burly' thanks to the upcoming /b/ in 'bird', has changed the word from one beginning with a vowel ('early') to one beginning with a consonant ('burly'). The speaker then chooses 'a' (which goes with 'burly') instead of 'an' (which would have gone with 'early'). So the speaker must first have planned the words 'early' and 'bird', then switched the /b/ of 'bird' to the beginning of 'early', and only then (after making the switch) chosen 'a' instead of 'an' as the form of the indefinite determiner. We see something of the temporal stages of the production process here. It looks as if the words in a phrase or sentence are chosen prior to the application of morphophonemic rules like the rule that chooses 'an' or 'a' for the indefinite determiner.

The error in 16 shows us something about the relationship between word choice and inflections in the production process:

16. 'There are many churches in our minister'   (instead of 'There are many ministers in our church')

In this error, the speaker has exchanged the words 'church' and 'minister'. But note that the plural inflection (/s/), which 'minister' was supposed to have in the intended output, is retained in the error. The word 'church' has the plural ending that 'minister' was intended to have. Thus, the stem morphemes 'church' and 'minister' have switched, while the plural morpheme has stayed where it was intended to be. I diagram this below in 17:

17. *intended:*   there are many minister-s in our church

actual: there are many church-es in our minister

Errors like that in 16 and 17 make it look as though inflections like the plural ending are planned separately from the words that are going to be in a sentence. They can stay in place when the words that they will ultimately be attached to switch around.

Some psycholinguists have proposed on the basis of such evidence that the speaker first plans a syntactic frame for a sentence. This frame contains the syntactic categories that will be in the sentence and the function (grammatical) words it will contain. Then the speaker plans the actual content words that will fill this syntactic frame. Finally, the speaker applies morphophonemic rules (like choosing 'a' or 'an' as the pronunciation of the indefinite determiner). Figure 7-5 diagrams this proposed process.

The error in 16 and 17 above was made between Stages 3 and 4. At Stage 3, the word 'church' was inserted where the word 'minister' should have been inserted (into the position marked 'X'). However, the plural affix that was planned for this position is already sitting there. Later at Stage 4 this plural affix is phonologically spelled out as /əs/, which is the form of the plural that the word 'church' takes (since it ends in a sibilant sound). Had 'minister' gotten into this slot, it would have taken /z/, since 'minister' ends a voiced (nonsibilant) consonant.

FIGURE 7-5. Stages of the Planning Process in Speech Production (Moving from Thought to Speech)

STAGE 1: Thought generated in the mind as a set of ideas (e.g., ideas having to do with lots of ministers being in our church, though these ideas are not yet expressed as words; actual words for these ideas are not yet chosen; the ideas are represented in terms of concepts in the language of thought, not English as of yet).

STAGE 2: Syntactic frame planned, containing inflections and function words. The places where content words will eventually be are held by 'X' and 'Y', which stand for ideas that have not yet been put into words.

(cont)

Figure 7.5 (cont)

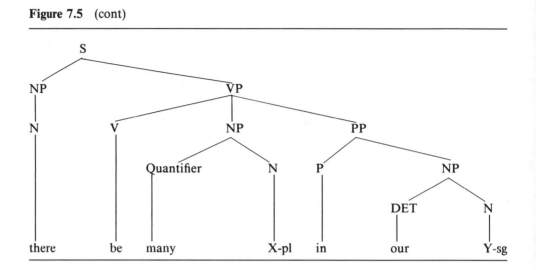

STAGE 3: Content words are chosen to symbolize the ideas that were generated in Stage 1, and are inserted into the syntactic frame planned in Stage 2.

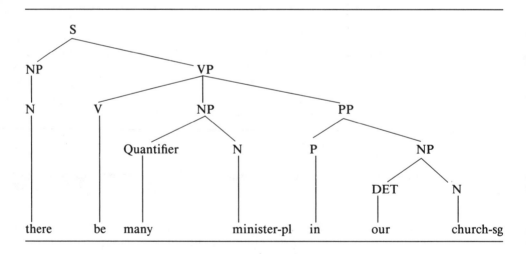

STAGE 4: Application of morphophonemic rules and other phonological rules:

there are many minister-s in our church

STAGE 5: Neuromuscular commands to articulators to produce sounds in the sentence

─────────────────── **E X E R C I S E S** ───────────────────

Exercise M.   For each of the types of speech error below, characterize clearly
what the error is. The speech errors under each number are called one of the
following: word exchanges, sound segment exchanges, shifts, anticipations,
morpheme exchanges, syllable exchanges, perseverations, malapropisms, phonetic feature exchanges, and blends. Can you match each of these terms to the
corresponding sort of error below (that is, match each label to one of the numbers
below)?

1a. . . . but a *beach* on the *bikini* is all right.
(intended: but a bikini on the beach is all right.)

1b. Other things would *expect* us to *lead* that . . .
(intended: Other things would lead us to expect . . .)

1c. Older men *choose* to *tend* younger wives.)
(intended: Older men tend to choose younger wives.)

2. He favors *push*ing *bust*ers.
(intended: He favors busting pushers.)

3. That book by Norm*el* and Rum*an*hart.
(intended: That book by Norman and Rumelhart.)

4a. Marmosets li*p* sa*ck* from trees.
(intended: Marmosets lick sap from trees.)

4b. That's what *T*omsky was *ch*alking about.
(intended: That's what Chomsky was talking about.)

4c. We will go down to the sound *r*oof *pr*oom.
(intended: We will go down to the sound proof room.)

5. . . . the *g*lear *p*lue sky . . .
(intended: the clear blue sky)

6a. They get weird ever*ier* day.
(intended: They get weirder every day.)

6b. No one quite know what*s* to do with it.
(intended: No one quite knows what to do with it.)

7a. Wnatchie is the app*ital* capital of the world.
(intended: Wnatchie is the apple capital of the world.)

7b. I'd like some smo*y*ked oysters.
(intended: I'd like some smoked oysters.)

8a. Take your feet out of the stirrups and wallop him in the ch*ollops.*
(intended: Take your feet out of the stirrups and wallop him in the chops.)

8b. I'd like a cup of co*pp*ee, please.
(intended: I'd like a cup of coffee, please.)

9a. Nobody gets very *upcited* about that.
(intended: Nobody gets upset/excited about that.)

9b. I don't like your *insinuendoes.*
(intended: I don't like your insinuations/innuendos.)

10a. We need something to break up the *monogamy* around here. (from the television show "All in the Family")
(intended: We need something to break up the monotony around here.)

10b. She went to the *groinocologist.* (from the television show "All in the Family")
(intended: She went to the gynecologist.)

Exercise N.   In terms of the theory of language planning developed earlier, why *wouldn't* we expect the following speech errors to happen?

1. an burly bird
(intended: an early bird)

2. They *on*dicted him *in* three charges of drunk driving.
(intended: They indicted him on three charges of drunk driving.)
(HINT: 'Indicted' is a single word.)

7.8. BEYOND SENTENCES: STORIES

So far we have dealt only with the understanding (comprehension) and production of sentences. But, of course, sentences occur in discourses that make up connected stretches of language. These connected stretches of language constitute things like stories (and other sorts of narratives), explanations, descriptions, arguments, excuses, and many other forms of language. As people understand sentences that occur in a story, for example, they must try to connect these sentences all together into a coherent whole. Psycholinguists are also concerned with how people understand larger stretches of language, not just isolated sentences.

To see the sorts of issues that arise here, we will consider what it takes to understand simple stories. Figure 7-6 shows a simple "folk" story about a fox and bear. I have diagramed the story in a rather odd way to bring out something of its structure as a coherent and unified piece of language.

Setting:
1. There was a fox and a bear who were friends.

2. One day they decided to catch a chicken for supper.
3. So they ran very quickly to a nearby farm where they knew that chickens lived.

    Success

4. The bear, who felt very lazy, climbed on the roof to watch.

    5. The fox then opened the door of the hen house very carefully.
    6. He grabbed a chicken and killed it.

Regrettable mistake   Loss

7. As he was carrying it out of the hen house, the weight of the bear on the roof caused the roof to crack.
8. The fox heard the noise and was frightened, but it was too late to run out.

Regrettable mistake

9. The roof and the bear fell in, killing five of the chickens.
10. The fox and the bear were trapped in the broken hen house.
11. Soon the farmer came out to see what was the matter.

FIGURE 7-6. Diagram of the "plot motifs" in a simple story

One way we can look at stories is as follows:[6] Stories are made up of little **plot motifs** or simple plot units. These plot motifs are simple happenings that we can readily recognize on the basis of our everyday experience of the world. For example, when a character has a goal (wants something), decides to do something to achieve this goal, and then does achieve this goal, we can call this a **success.** When a character is in a positive situation and something happens to make the situation negative, we can call this a **loss.** On the other hand, when a negative situation turns out to have positive results, we could call this a **hidden blessing.** When a negative situation happens and a character needs to get out of it, we could call this a **problem** for the character.

[6]See Wendy Lehnert's paper "Plot Units and Narrative Summarization," *Cognitive Science,* 4 (1981), 293–331.

There can be more complicated plot motifs that combine these simpler ones. For example, when a character does something that unintentionally causes a problem for herself or another character and this problem leads to a negative outcome (the character or characters cannot get out of the problem), we can call this a **regrettable mistake.** Or if the positive outcome of a success quickly turns into the negative outcome of a loss, we can call this a **fleeting success.**

Figure 7-6 diagrams the fox and bear story in terms of such plot motifs. Sentence 1 is just the setting for the story, an introduction to the characters. Sentences 2 and 3 state a goal and an attempt to achieve it that in sentences 5 and 6 is attained. So this is a success, and I label the arrow connecting these sentences as a success. The positive outcome stated in sentences 5 and 6 (the positive outcome of the success), however, becomes negative in sentences 7 and 8, so I have labeled the arrow connecting sentences 5, 6, 7, and 8 as a loss. Since the success led quickly to a loss, it was a fleeting success (so as not to clutter the diagram, I have left this label off). It was the bear's getting on the roof in sentence 4 that led to the problem created in sentences 7 and 8, and this problem is not resolved but leads to the negative outcome of the fox and the bear being trapped while the farmer comes to get them. Thus, I have labeled sentences 4, 7, 8, 9, 10, and 11 a regrettable mistake.

Some psycholinguists have argued that such plot motifs are reflected in the way people remember and summarize stories, as well as in the way they engage in relatively long pauses at certain points in a story. If such plot motifs capture the ways in which people understand stories, and this evidence suggests they do, then it would appear that people understand stories the way they understand actions in the world, that is, in terms of the **goal structures** of the actions of human (and human-like) characters. The goal structures of human action are the goals people have, the decisions they make about them, the series of subgoals they may break the overall task into, and the actions they take to realize these subgoals and the final larger goal they are subordinated to.

If this is correct, then people ultimately recover from a story and store in mind the plot motifs and their combinations that make up the story. They can then dispense with the details of the sentences that composed the story. It is in terms of such plot motifs that people can summarize what they have heard, or recapitulate it in full in their own words. It would then also be the case that such plot motifs and combinations of them would organize how we think about experience and would be the sorts of ideas we start from when we begin the process of unconsciously planning and then speaking a story.

--------------------------------- **E X E R C I S E** ---------------------------------

Exercise O. There are many approaches in linguistics and psychology to stories and story structure. I discuss stories further in Chapters 9 and 10. Consider the following simple story:

THE TIGER'S WHISKERS

(1) Once there was a woman who needed a tiger's whisker. (2) She was afraid of tigers but she needed a whisker to make a medicine for her husband, who had gotten very sick. (3) She thought and thought about how to get a tiger's whisker. (4) She decided to use a trick. (5) She knew that tigers loved food and music. (6) She thought that if she brought food to a lonely tiger and played soft music, the tiger would be nice to her and she could get the whisker. (7) So she did just that. (8) She went to a tiger's cave where a lonely tiger lived. (9) She put a bowl of food in front of the opening to the cave. (10) Then she sang soft music. (11) The tiger came out and ate the food. (12) He then walked over to the lady and thanked her for the delicious food and lovely music. (13) The lady then cut off one of the tiger's whiskers and ran down the hill very quickly. (14) The tiger felt lonely and sad again.

1. This story, in one sense, falls into the following parts or sections: Section 1: Sentences 1 and 2; Section 2: Sentences 3, 4, 5, and 6; Section 3: Sentence 7; Section 4: Sentences 8, 9, 10, 11, 12, 13; Section 5: Sentence 14. Describe why the story can be said to fall into these parts, and characterize each part (What is each part about, what role does it play in the story?). What linguistic features do the sentences in each of these parts or sections have in common (for example, are the verbs in each section in any way alike)?

2. Section 4 (sentences 8–13) carries the "main action" of the story. How would you further divide into parts this one section, and why?

3. What similarities are there between this story and the fox and bear story? Can you give a general characterization of what most stories have in common? (For example, some people have argued that all stories involve a lack that motivates the action of the story. How is this true of the fox and bear story? How is it true of the tiger's whisker story?)

RECOMMENDED FURTHER READING

ALLMAN, WILLIAM (1989). *Apprentices of Wonder: Inside the Neural Network Revolution.* New York: Bantam Books. (A lucid and easily accessible introduction to why the mind does not work like a digital computer.)

CLARK, HERBERT H. & CLARK, EVE, (1977). *Psychology and Language: An Introduction to Psycholinguistics.* New York: Harcourt Brace Jovanovich. (Parts are now a bit dated, but still a wealth of information and the best book on the full range of topics in the field.)

GARNHAM, ALAN (1985). *Psycholinguistics: Central Topics*. London & New York: Methuen. (A clear and readable introduction.)

HATCH, EVELYN M. (1983). *Psycholinguistics: A Second Language Perspective*. Rowley, Mass.: Newbury House. (A clear and readable introduction with the accent on issues germane to second-language use and development.)

JOHNSON-LAIRD, PHILIP N. (1983). *Mental Models*. Cambridge, Mass.: Harvard University Press. (A rigorous but lucid discussion of how humans think.)

LEVELT, WILLEM J. M. (1989). *Speaking: From Intention to Articulation*. Cambridge, Mass.: M.I.T. Press. (A masterful and fairly accessible introduction to and survey of language production.)

MANDLER, JEAN M. (1984). *Stories, Scripts, and Scenes: Aspects of Schema Theory*. Hillsdale, N.J.: Erlbaum. (A good and short introduction to psycholinguistic approaches to stories.)

OSHERSON, DANIEL N. & SMITH, EDWARD E., EDS. (1990). *Thinking: An Invitation to Cognitive Science*, vol. 3. Cambridge, Mass.: M.I.T. Press. (A set of excellent, clearly written, and accessible articles.)

ROSENFIELD, ISRAEL (1988). *The Invention of Memory: A New View of the Brain*. New York: Basic Books.

STILLINGS, NEIL, FEINSTEIN, MARK, GARFIELD, JAY, RISSLAND, EDWINA, ROSENBAUM, DAVID, WEISLER, STEVEN, & BAKER-WARD, LYNNE (1987). *Cognitive Science: An Introduction*. Cambridge, Mass.: M.I.T. Press. (An accessible and clear introduction.)

CHAPTER 8

Language Acquisition

The Growth of Language in the Child

8.1. INTRODUCTION

The question of how children acquire language is one of the most fascinating and difficult problems in linguistics. A child is faced with a rather serious problem in acquiring a language. The grammar of any language will produce an infinite number of sentences. We can prove this simply by considering the fact that there is no longest sentence in English or any other language. For any sentence I give you, no matter how long, you can add words to it and make it longer (for example, 'Mary is happy', 'Bill believes Mary is happy', 'Sue thinks Bill believes Mary is happy', etc., or 'Mary is very happy and Sue is very happy too', 'Mary is very happy and Sue is very happy too, but John is not very happy', 'Mary is very happy and Sue is very happy too, but John is not very happy, though Rose is quite happy', etc.). Since there are an infinite number of sentences in any language, and any speaker can utter sentences no one has heard or said before, rote memory or literal imitation cannot be the primary mechanism by which children acquire language.

Children have acquired a great deal of their language by age five or so. Throughout this period, children hear only a finite number of sentences but have to acquire a grammar capable of generating an infinite number. Such young children are rarely corrected when they make grammatical errors and are never given overt instruction about the rules of the language. Though some families correct children's speech more than others, there is no evidence that children pay much attention to these corrections. Further, we know that children can acquire language perfectly well with no correction at all.

Thus, children rarely or never gain any direct information about ungrammatical sentences, either through correction or overt instruction. This is called the **problem of no negative evidence.** Though it would seem to be helpful in figuring out the grammatical rules of a language to be shown some examples of ungrammatical sentences, sentences that break the rules, children in fact only get information about grammatical sentences by hearing people utter them. To make matters worse, since all real speech contains some disfluencies and speech errors, children do hear some ungrammatical sentences (for example, when someone changes midstream what they want to say), but children are not told these are ungrammatical.

Imagine that I teach you chess in the following fashion: I start playing chess with you, telling you nothing overt about the rules of the game. You watch the moves I make and assume these are acceptable moves by the rules. I purposely, however, make a few unacceptable moves, moves that break the rules of chess, but I do not tell you which these are. When you move your pieces, I never correct you if you make an unacceptable move. Would you ever learn the rules of chess this way? All children learn their first language under such conditions.

More surprisingly yet, except for extremely disordered children, all children, regardless of "intelligence," learn language under these conditions. No one fails. Furthermore, they all learn the language at a master's level; regardless of "intelligence" all children master their native language to about the same degree of mastery as all others. Little Mary Jane Smith is not better at conjunction and worse at prepositions than little Johnnie Jones. Johnnie Jones doesn't master the active–passive distinction while Mary Jane fails to.

When we think about it, this is somewhat odd. For most other things in life that involve learning—whether it is mastering a musical instrument, learning to play basketball, or mastering modern physics—some people do it better than others, and there are rather wide skill (or "intelligence") differences that seem to determine how well or poorly one will do. But everyone, unless there is something quite seriously wrong with them, masters a language to an incredible degree of sophistication. Acquiring a language is the greatest intellectual feat most of us ever pull off in our lifetimes. No animal—even a chimpanzee—has acquired anything remotely resembling the complexity of a human language. Language is truly what makes us human.

EXERCISE

Exercise A. List five activities that people master at different levels of ability (for example, learning to play the guitar) and five that we humans seem to master at comparable levels of ability (for example, walking), barring serious disabilities. In Section 8.1, I argue that language falls into this latter group. Can you see any way or ways in which the items on each list are similar to each other and differ from those on the other list?

8.2. GENERALIZATION: GOING BEYOND THE DATA

Consider the following nonlinguistic problem: I give you the word pairs below:

1a. fish, scales   cats, fur   humans, skin

Now I give you a word pair with one member left blank and ask you to fill in the blank:

1b. birds, _____

You would surely fill in the blank with the word 'feathers'. Why? Looking at the data in 1a, you have drawn a generalization that the second member of the pair is the word for the substance that covers the thing named by the first word in the pair. Since scales cover fish, and fur covers cats, and skin covers humans, you conclude that 'feathers' is the missing word in 1b, since feathers cover birds. This type of reasoning is called **analogical thinking** or **drawing an analogy** (feathers are related to birds just as skin is to humans, fur to cats, and scales to fish). It is obviously a powerful and important mode of thinking that we humans engage in all the time in our daily lives.

Of course, analogy doesn't always work. You might think that since you burned your mouth eating a certain pepper, all other peppers will burn, but that's not true—some peppers are mild. On the other hand, anyone who fails to generalize from having burned their hand on a gas stove to the realization that they will burn their hand on an electric one is in for another burn. We would not survive if we did not generalize from our past experience, regardless of the fact that sometimes such generalizations are wrong.

Children clearly generalize from the language data they are exposed to. They will say things like 'breaked' (instead of 'broken') or 'hitted' (instead of 'hit') in analogy with regular past-tense forms like 'kicked', 'loved', and 'wanted'. They say things like 'feets' (instead of 'feet') in analogy with regular plurals like 'cats', 'eyes', and 'toes'. Of course, these generalizations are wrong, but they show us that the child has learned the general rule for forming the past tense of verbs and the plural of nouns in English. The child simply has to learn further that certain forms are exceptions to the general rule.

It is through the process of generalization that the child goes beyond mere memory and imitation to acquire a language. However, generalization turns out to be a very dangerous tool in acquiring language. In fact, it is easy to show that generalization alone is not enough to acquire a language, and that if children simply used generalization the way we do in our everyday lives, they would foul up the process of language acquisition and never acquire the language.

A Problem With Generalization in Language Acquisition

Linguists are primarily interested in discovering the *unconscious knowledge* (linguistic competence) native speakers have that allows them to know what does and what does not count as a *grammatical sentence* in their language. It is this unconscious knowledge that speakers put to use when they speak and understand their language. Linguists sometimes refer to this unconscious knowledge as the *grammar* of the language, using the word 'grammar' in a somewhat novel way. The word stands not for what people have written in grammar books, but for what people have stored in their heads through the process of language acquisition, a process that is far along before people have read any books.

What does this unconscious grammatical knowledge consist of and how does the child go about acquiring it? Consider the data below, and ask yourself what generalization any reasonable person would draw from this data:

2a. John will give a book to Mary
2b. Who will give a book to Mary?   (answer: John)
2c. What will John give to Mary?   (answer: a book)
2d. Whom will John give a book to?   (answer: Mary)

The only reasonable generalization to draw from data like this is the following one: In English there is a relationship between declarative sentences, like 2a, and wh-questions, like 2b–2d (questions with wh-words in them, like 'who' and 'what'). This relationship is as follows: One can form a grammatical wh-question by placing a wh-question word ('who' or 'what') in the position of any noun phrase (for example, 'John', 'a book', 'Mary') in a declarative sentence and moving the wh-question word to the front of the sentence. You also have to invert the helping verb ('will' in 2a above) or add a form of 'do' in other cases, but we will ignore this and concentrate only on the wh-question word. (NOTE: Remember that we call any noun (for example, 'John') or set of words that functions like a noun ('a book') in a sentence a *noun phrase,* or NP for short.)

Thus, one can take a declarative sentence like 2a ('John gave a book to Mary'), place a wh-question word in the position of the NP 'a book', and get 'John gave what to Mary'. Then one can move the wh-question word to the front of the sentence (and invert the subject and helping verb) and get 2c 'What will John give to Mary?' The other cases above work the same, except that other NPs have been replaced by the question word and moved to the front of the sentence. In a question like 'What will John give to Mary?', every English speaker knows (unconsciously, at least) that 'what' is the direct object of 'give' (names the thing given), though it is placed at the front of the sentence and not after 'give' where direct objects normally occur (that is, where they occur in declarative sentences, as in 'John will give *a book* to Mary').

Call this generalization the **English wh-question generalization** (we could also call it the **English wh-question rule,** since 'rule' is just a technical term for a generalization that covers a large number of cases). This generalization is supported by everything the child ever hears, or anything any adult has ever heard, and it makes an infinite number of correct predictions. Given a new declarative sentence, any English speaker can correctly predict the various wh-questions that can be formed from it. For example, consider the cases below, which show also that the length of the sentence does not affect the operation of the rule:

3a. Kittens will eat *cookies*

3b. Kittens will eat *what?*

3c. What will kittens eat?

4a. Mary believes kittens will eat *cookies*

4b. Mary believes kittens will eat *what?*

4c. What does Mary believe kittens will eat?

5a. John claims Mary believes kittens will eat *cookies*

5b. John claims Mary believes kittens will eat *what?*

5c. What does John claim Mary believes kittens will eat?

In each case, 'cookies' is replaced by 'what' and 'what' is placed at the beginning of the sentence to form a grammatical question. Obviously, there is no longest wh-question (we can keep making longer ones), so there are an infinite number of them. Since this is true, no one could memorize them all, and thus speakers must know what is and what is not a grammatical wh-question by applying a rule or generalization like the one we have stated.

A generalization like this one, which is never disconfirmed by the data and which makes an infinite number of correct predictions, is a good one. Under such conditions, one would be irrational not to draw this generalization from such data. The surprising thing is that the generalization is wrong! Furthermore, all we adults unconsciously know that this generalization is wrong, though we have never seen a counterexample or anything to tell us that it is wrong.

Consider the declarative sentence in 6a below:

6a. Mary will kiss the kitten that eats cookies

Our English wh-question rule surely predicts that if we change 'cookies' in 6a to 'what' ('Mary will kiss the kitten that eats *what?*') and place it at the front of the sentence, we will get a grammatical question, as we have done all along. But we do not; the prediction is wrong:

6b. *What will Mary kiss the kitten that eats?

Even though it obeys the rule we have formulated, 6b is totally ungrammatical and every English speaker knows it (you know it, you clearly don't think 6b is grammatical English). Furthermore, no child ever says any such thing. That is, this is *not* a case like the situation where a child makes a mistake like 'feets' (thereby showing us he or she has drawn the generalization that noun plurals in English are marked by the ending '-s'). Children never make the sort of mistake that is represented in 6b. But why not? The only reasonable generalization they could have drawn about how wh-questions are formed in English (the one we drew above) clearly suggests that 6b ought to be grammatical.

Our knowledge that sentences like 6b are ungrammatical is, then, an example of linguistic knowledge we adults have in our heads, but for which we never had any evidence as children (or later, for that matter). In fact, all the evidence we had pointed to just the opposite conclusion. Thus, in no normal sense of the word can we be said to have "learned" it (we learn what we have evidence for), though we indeed *know* it. To make matters more mysterious, notice that a case very similar to 6b is grammatical:

7a. Mary will claim that the kitten eats cookies

7b. Mary will claim that the kitten eats *what?*

7c. What will Mary claim that the kitten eats?

It is hard to say why we should be able to question 'cookies' in 7a (by producing the grammatical 7b) and not 'cookies' in 6a (by producing the ungrammatical 6b).

Innate Knowledge and Universal Grammar

In sentence 6a above, the material 'that will eat cookies' is called a **relative clause.** This material modifies the NP 'the kitten':

6a. Mary will kiss the kitten *that eats cookies*
                             relative clause
                             modifying NP 'the kitten'

6b. *What will Mary kiss the kitten *that eats (what)?*

Notice that in 6b the question word ('what') that is in front of the sentence is actually the direct object of 'eat' (names the thing that is eaten), the verb inside the relative clause. To form 6b we have placed a question word ('what') in the position of 'cookies' in 6a and then moved it to the front of the sentence, following our wh-question rule. It turns out, as one sees in considering the ungrammaticality of 6b, that our wh-question rule fails when it operates on NPs that are inside relative clauses. More generally, no material can be moved from inside a relative clause. In other words, no sentence type, like the wh-question in 6b, can contain material outside a relative clause when in a declarative sentence this material would have been inside a relative clause. The object of 'eat', 'cookies' in 6a and 'what' in 6b, is inside the relative clause in the declarative sentence and thus cannot be outside it in the question. Relative clauses are 'islands,' and nothing inside them can be questioned since English questions NPs by placing them at the front of the sentence, thus away from their normal position in a declarative sentence.

Our question is, how do children come to know that 6b is ungrammatical, that is, how do they ever discover that relative clauses are islands? The only rational generalization they could have drawn from the data they were exposed to predicts (incorrectly) that 6b is grammatical. No one ever says things like 6b, and no one ever tells children such things are ungrammatical. So how do they gain this linguistic knowledge we all come to have?

At this point, many linguists make a very strong claim. They conclude that we all know that relative clauses are islands *not* by having *learned* it (we should have learned the opposite if we were paying attention to the data), but on the basis of *innate knowledge* that specifies that sentences such as 6b cannot be part of a human language. The claim is, then, that the course of human evolution has equipped human beings with a biological capacity for acquiring language. This biological capacity specifies the basic design properties of any human language. And one thing it specifies is that relative clauses are islands; that is, that no language can form one sentence pattern (for example, wh-questions in English) by placing material that would normally be inside a relative clause in a declarative sentence outside the relative clause (such as at the front of the sentence in the English wh-question).

If this claim were true, it would explain why children are never tempted to try things like 6b or think they are grammatical, despite the fact that all the data they are exposed to should make them think such sentences are grammatical. Since all human beings share the same biology, and thus have the same innate biological capacity for language, this claim would also predict that what is true of English here is true of all languages, that is, that this is a language universal. It would predict that a sentence like 6b would be ungrammatical in any language. If her biology tells an English-speaking child that things like 6b are ungrammatical, the same biology must tell Portuguese children the same thing when they are learning Portuguese. Of course, not all languages form questions the same way English does. But linguists have discovered that any language that has a rule like English's wh-question rule cannot apply this rule to any material inside a relative clause. In all these languages, the translation of 6b is ungrammatical. As is always the case in science, there are further subtleties to the matter, and the full account involves consideration of other aspects of the grammar of the languages concerned. But the basic facts are clear and widely agreed on.

People who do not like this appeal to innate knowledge (and many psychologists in particular do not) have the burden of explaining how anyone, given the data, could ever have discovered the facts above, and furthermore, why no child in fact fails to. Many children say 'goed' instead of 'went', but none say 6b though it is just as reasonable a conclusion.

Noam Chomsky, the founder of contemporary theoretical linguistics, has referred to the human biological capacity for language as our **language acquisition device** (**LAD** for short). He defines the central problem of linguistic theory to be giving an account of how the child acquires language based on properties of the LAD (given to each of us by our biology) and the child's exposure to data from a particular language. The LAD contributes the basic design properties that are common to all languages, what Chomsky calls **universal grammar.** The interaction of this innate knowledge with actual data from a specific language, like English, gives rise to the actually attested languages in the world, which, of course, differ from each other in a number of ways, but which at a deeper level have many abstract and complex properties in common (like the one we have investigated here, but there are many others).

Chomsky believes that the data any child is exposed to in acquiring a language is seriously insufficient to determine the grammar (rules) of the language. Left merely to consider the data and draw rational generalizations from it, the child would never discover the correct grammar (as we saw above). Furthermore, the absence of information about ungrammatical sentences (the problem of no negative evidence) and the presence in the data of speech errors that go uncorrected and unremarked on make the problem of acquiring a grammar solely on the basis of the input impossible. Thus, Chomsky argues that the child must have been supplied with rich innate knowledge about what human languages are like, knowledge that guides the child in his or her processing of the input to the correct grammar.

Many people don't like the use of the word 'unconscious knowledge' here (though I think it appropriate); another way Chomsky has put the matter is to compare the unfolding of language in the child's mind to the way in which intricate physical organs, like the eye or heart, unfold in the course of embryonic development under the control of our human genetic inheritance. Language is not learned in the normal sense of the word "learning," rather it grows in the mind. It does, of course, require exposure to data and social interaction for that growth to take place, just as cells require interaction with surrounding cells to form into an eye and not a heart, and plants require sun and earth to grow.

Chomsky believes that universal grammar, our innate knowledge of the basic or core properties of human language, often leaves open a small number of choices ("parameters"). The child innately knows what choices are available and makes the choice that is appropriate for the language he or she is learning based on exposure to the data from that language. This is one way that innate knowledge and exposure to data interact and one way we can account for the differences there are among the world's languages. For example, universal grammar allows languages to have free word order or fixed word order. Within fixed word order, universal grammar determines that prepositions and verbs occur in the same order vis-à-vis their objects (either *'in* the house' and *'eat* the meal' with the objects following as in English, or 'the house *in'* and 'the meal *eat'* with the objects preceding as we would translate many other languages). The child thus needs to pay attention to the data to determine if his or her language is fixed or free word order, and if fixed, which ordering of preposition and object or verb and object it adopts. The child is "programmed," however, to expect the same ordering for verb and object and preposition and object, and can use his or her information about one ordering to set the other. This is an overly simple example, but it gives the flavor of the approach.

───────────────────── E X E R C I S E ─────────────────────

Exercise B. The argument developed in the preceding two sections is an important one. In fact, while such arguments are controversial, they are a large part of what has made many scholars interested in linguistics. The same sort of argument can be made with many other types of data. Develop a similar argument in your own words, using the data below (note that 2b and 2c are ungrammatical, and that 1a and 2a mean much the same thing):

1a. John saw Sue with Mary.	*Answer:*	
1b. Who did John see Sue with?	Mary	
1c. Who did John see with Mary?	Sue	
1d. Who saw Sue with Mary?	John	
2a. John saw Sue and Mary.		
2b. *Who did John see Sue and?	Mary	
2c. *Who did John see and Mary?	Sue	
2d. Who saw Sue and Mary?	John	

Generalizations and U-Shaped Growth

We saw above that children learning English draw the correct generalization about how to form wh-questions in English, but do not extend this generalization to contexts disallowed by universal grammar (for example, relative clauses). Thus, children never produce incorrect forms like 6b above (*'What will Mary kiss the kitten that eats'). In many other cases, however, children do draw generalizations that lead them to produce forms and sentences that are unacceptable in the adult grammar.

For example, once they correctly form the generalization that English forms the past tense of verbs by adding '-ed', they overextend this generalization to produce forms like 'breaked' (rather than 'broke') and 'goed' (rather than 'went'). The generalization that English forms the past tense of verbs by adding '-ed' is not as general as the child thinks it is. Irregular forms like 'went' and 'broke' do not obey it. Similarly, children will overextend the regular plural ending of English ('-s') to produce forms like 'feets' (rather than 'feet') and 'mouses' (rather than 'mice').

The overgeneralization of the regular '-ed' past-tense ending and the regular '-s' plural ending exemplify a now-famous phenomena in child development (not just language development, but other aspects of development as well): **U-shaped behavioral development.** In U-shaped development the child first does something correctly (by adult norms), which constitutes the top of the left leg of the U, then appears to do the same thing incorrectly, which constitutes the bottom trough of the U, and finally returns to the correct behavior, which constitutes the top of the right leg of the U. Such behavior occurs in many aspects of child development, as well as in the development of new skills on the part of adults. It seems at first sight fairly mysterious.

In regard to the past-tense forms of English verbs and the plural forms of English nouns, U-shaped development proceeds as follows: First children produce *correct* instances of plural and past-tense forms. Some of these forms represent "regular" past and plural forms (for example, 'shoes', 'dogs', adding the ending '-s', and 'walked', 'jumped', adding the ending '-ed'), and others represent irregular forms, that is, forms not predictable by any rule (for example, 'feet', 'mice', in the case of plural forms, and 'went', 'broke' in the case of past-tense forms). At this stage, children look like they have acquired the correct adult grammar in regard to the past tense of verbs and the plural of nouns. At the next stage, the correct but irregular forms (like 'feet' and 'broke') are partially or totally eclipsed by incorrect forms that conform to the general pattern of adding '-s' for the plural and '-ed' for the past. For example, 'feet' becomes 'feets', and 'mice' becomes 'mouses'; 'went' becomes 'goed', and 'broke' becomes 'breaked'. At this point, children look like they have "lost" the correct adult grammar. Eventually, of course, the correct forms reassert themselves, and the child's grammar once again conforms to the adult's. Thus, the course of development is, like a U, up, down, and up again.

One commonly accepted interpretation of this sequence of events is as follows: The child's initial correct usage is really not the same as the adult's, despite the fact that it looks that way. The child has, in fact, learned (memorized) the relevant forms, whether regular ('dog/dogs'; 'kick/kicked') or irregular ('foot/feet' and 'break/broke'), as individual cases, in isolation from each other. The child does not realize that pairs of words like 'dog' and 'dogs', 'foot' and 'feet', or 'kick' and 'kicked', 'break' and 'broke' are related to each other, but has learned each of these words separately and in isolation from the form it is related to in the adult grammar. However, after having acquired some exemplars of the regular pattern (the forms that add '-s' for the plural and '-ed' for the past), the child comes *unconsciously* to recognize their systematicity and to *abstract rules* (like 'add -*s* for the plural of nouns'; 'add -*ed* for the past of verbs') that allow him or her to create new exemplars at will. When these new rules come into operation, the child at first applies them in a blanket fashion, as yet unaware that there are instances where the rules do not apply (namely the irregular forms). At this point, overregularized forms like 'breaked' replace irregular forms like 'broke'. Thus, the child has moved from merely memorizing isolated forms to seeing a relationship between them and abstracting rules (general statements) from the data, rules which he or she applies too generally, as if they had no exceptions.

Eventually, the correct irregular forms reenter the child's speech or regain strength, though in the case of some children overregularized forms persist for years. Once again, then, the child's grammar matches the adult grammar. But now the child's grammar is not just superficially like the adult's in that the adult and the child have the same superficial forms. Now they actually operate with the same rules; plural nouns and past-tense verbs are integrated into the same system and are no longer isolated forms.

The difference in the child's understanding of plural and past-tense forms before and after the period of overregularization is typically explained in terms of the concept of *analysis.* Initially, the plural and past forms are *unanalyzed* by the child. That is, the child is not aware that a regular form like 'shoes' is composed of two units, *'shoe'* plus plural '-s', each expressing its own meaning, or that an irregular form like 'feet' is composed of two meanings (FOOT and PLURAL) merged into one form (with PLURAL reflected by the vowel change from 'foot'). The child is not aware that a regular verb like 'jumped' is composed of two units, 'jump' plus past '-ed', each expressing its own meaning, or that an irregular verb like 'broken' is composed of two meanings (BREAK and PAST) merged into one form (with PAST reflected by the vowel change from 'break'). The child just learns these words as unanalyzed wholes with unanalyzed meanings connected to the sorts of contexts the child has heard them used in. The onset of errors of overregularization (like 'feets' and 'breaked') indicates that analysis has taken place. The child has come to realize that '-s' and '-ed' (and the semantic concepts associated with them) are separate forms, with separate meanings. The child is now freed to enter into new combinations he or she has never heard before (for example, 'foots' and 'breaked', as well as many new words that are acceptable to both children and adults).

Recovering From Overgeneralizations

When a child "catches on" to a generalization (like the fact that English adds '-ed' to form the past tense of verbs) and begins to produce incorrect forms (like 'goed'), there is a real problem as to how the child 'recovers' from this overgeneralization. How does the child "retrench" from the overgeneralization, remove the incorrect forms from his or her grammar, and finally hit on the adult grammar? Since children are not regularly corrected by adults (or at least do not need to be), the solution to this problem cannot be that the child is told or otherwise overtly signaled that he or she has gone too far.

In a case like 'breaked', it is not implausible to say that children will eventually hear the correct form, 'broke', assume that there are not two ways to form the past tense, and so give up their innovative form 'breaked'. But we will see below that this strategy is much less plausible in many other more interesting cases of overgeneralizations.

Let's take a concrete example of a more interesting case of overgeneralization and consider the problems that arise in trying to account for how and why children ever give up their incorrect forms. Consider the following pattern in English, which every child comes to notice:

8a.	The corn grew	(NP verb)
8b.	Mary grew the corn	(NP verb NP)
9a.	The vase broke	(NP verb)
9b.	Mary broke the vase	(NP verb NP)
10a.	The soup is warm	(NP is adjective)
10b.	Mary warmed the soup	(NP verb NP)
11a.	John is sad	(NP is adjective)
11b.	Mary saddened John	(NP verb NP)

The "a" sentences above have either an intransitive verb (a verb with one NP, 'grow', 'break') or they have the verb 'be' followed by an adjective ('warm', 'sad'). The "b" sentences are called **lexical causatives** (lexical = from the mental lexicon or dictionary of words the speaker/hearer of the language has stored in his or her head). They all have the meaning that the subject (for example, 'Mary' in 8b) CAUSED the direct object ('the corn' in 8b) to do something ('grow', in 8b). The generalization that one can draw from this data is clear: A causative sentence can be formed from a sentence with an intransitive verb (like 'The corn grew') or with the verb 'be' followed by an adjective (like 'The soup is warm') by placing the subject of that sentence in object position and adding a new subject, which is interpreted as an ACTOR (like 'Mary grew the corn'). The verb of this new sentence is either identical to the intransitive verb or adjective or, in some cases, has an ending like the '-en' on 'sad' above. The new sentence ('Mary grew the corn') means that the ACTOR (Mary) CAUSED the event described by the old intransitive sentence ('The corn grew').

While this pattern is quite pervasive in English, it is not, in fact, completely general. There are verbs and adjectives that will not allow themselves to be formed into lexical causatives. 'Cry' is such a verb. From 'John cried', I cannot form a lexical causative 'I cried John', meaning *I caused John to cry*. Rather, I would have to say 'I made John cry', using the separate word 'make'. Sentences like 'I made John cry', which use a separate word to signal causation ('make'), are called **analytic causatives** (to distinguish them from lexical causatives).

Lexical causatives constitute a typical case of U-shaped development. Children start by producing correct lexical causatives (by adult standards). Then they start to produce incorrect lexical causatives, like 'I cried John', or those in 12a–c below. Eventually, they return to producing just those lexical causatives that are acceptable in adult grammar (that is, they acquire the correct adult grammar).[1]

12a. Kendall fall that toy =
Kendall caused the toy to fall
(presumably from 'That toy falls')

12b. I'm singing him =
I am causing him to sing (said of a toy with a string that when pulled makes music play)
(presumably from 'he sings')

12c. Giggle me =
you cause me to giggle, with 'you' left out as understood
(presumably from 'I giggle')

These novel causatives raise, in an interesting way, the problem of how children recover from overgeneralization. How does the child ever learn that these novel causatives are unacceptable, and why does he or she give them up? Adults understand them perfectly well and do not correct children when they utter them.

In some cases the answer may be easy. In a case like 12a, the child eventually hears the word 'drop' and realizes that this word means CAUSE TO FALL. Thus, the child gives up sentences like 'Kendall falled the toy' in favor of 'Kendall dropped the toy'. Even in this "easy" case, there is a mystery. Why should the child give up causative 'fall' when he or she hears 'drop'? Why not assume that English can say CAUSE TO FALL in two different ways, that is, why not assume that causative 'fall' and 'drop' are synonymous?

Thus, to make even this easy case work, we have to assume a principle of child language development something like: Children avoid assuming that two words can have the same meaning. Unless they have overwhelming evidence to the contrary, they will give up or assign a new meaning to any word (for example, causative 'fall' in 12a) that appears to be synonymous with a new word they hear (such as 'drop'). Something like this principle may well be correct, but the evidence for it is, at this point, equivocal.

---

[1]The examples are taken from the work of Melissa Bowerman, who gives many more similar examples in a variety of papers cited subsequently. Much of my discussion in this section and in Sections 8.7 and 8.8 below is based on Bowerman's work.

The really hard cases are ones like 12b and 12c. The language offers no other word for these cases. One simply cannot say 'I'm singing him'. One has to say 'I am making him sing', using an analytic causative. So why should the child stop saying things like 'I'm singing him' when he or she never hears a word with the same meaning and this sentence (however ungrammatical it is) is perfectly understandable? The child is not corrected when he or she says it (or, at least, children who are never corrected will nonetheless also eventually give it up).

One might speculate that the child waits a certain amount of time and never hears an adult use 'sing' this way, and then gives up his or her lexical causative use of 'sing'. The problem with this solution is that the child could fail to hear perfectly acceptable causatives in the same amount of time and end up giving up many correct forms. For example, imagine a child failing to hear something like the perfectly grammatical 'The heat spoiled the milk' (related to 'The milk spoiled') in a fair amount of time, and giving up causative 'spoil', coming to think that it is ungrammatical. Only later, maybe as an adult, does the child finally hear it used and realize he or she was wrong to give it up. As far as we know, this sort of thing does not happen. Any given causative occurs, like most sentences (given there are an infinite number of possible sentences), very infrequently. Waiting around to see if any adult will say 'I sang him' or 'The heat spoiled the milk' doesn't then seem a very good strategy.

Now for the bad news: We really do not know how the child manages to retrench from the overgeneralized lexical causatives and finally hit on just the correct forms (from the adult's perspective). One possibility is the following: In general, for a lexical causative to be grammatical in the adult language, the ACTOR must *directly* cause the event, that is, the ACTOR must directly interact with the object of the verb to bring about the event. Lexical causatives cannot encode *indirect* forms of causation. Thus, consider the sentences below:

13a. The magician broke the cup

13b. The magician made the cup break

13a is a lexical causative, while 13b is an analytic causative, using the separate word 'make' to signal the causation. 13a usually implies that the magician broke the cup by directly interacting with it, but 13b implies that he used some less direct route, like a trick or a spell. In this regard, then, notice the contrast between 14a below (an unacceptable lexical causative of the sort children will use) and 14b (an analytic causative):

14a. *The magician disappeared the rabbit

14b. The magician made the rabbit disappear

Since making something disappear is an action that must be done indirectly, only 14b using the separate word 'make' is acceptable, not 14a with a lexical causative. Thus, there is a semantic constraint on lexical causatives that stipulates they can only encode *direct* causation.

While children must learn this semantic constraint on causatives, and while this will certainly help them to limit the extension of the causative construction, it cannot be the whole answer. There are cases of direct causation that still cannot be encoded in lexical causatives. For example, while I can say 'I saddened Mary' (from 'Mary was sad'), I cannot say 'I happeyed Mary' (from 'Mary was happy'). Yet it is not clear why causing people to be happy would be any more or less direct than causing them to be sad. Further, there are cases where the causation in lexical causatives doesn't look all that direct. For example, in 'That corporation grows wheat in the Midwest', it is clearly not the corporation that is directly causing the wheat to grow, but the work force they employ and especially the forces of nature. So, once again, how does the child ever discover just the set of acceptable lexical causatives (acceptable to adults)?

─────────────── E X E R C I S E S ───────────────

Exercise C. The data below shows errors made by children ranging in age from 3½ to 5½ years old. The errors all involve talking about acts of separation.[2] What are these children trying to figure out? Why do you think they make the errors they do?

1. Mother: Pull your pants up, Eva.
   Child: Somebody *unpulled*'em.
   (= someone pulled them down/off)

2. (Child wants to move an electrical humidifier, and she says:)
   I'll get it after it's *plugged out.*
   (= I'll get it after it's unplugged)

3. Mother: The end is tucked in (discussing blanket on child's bed)
   Child: Will you *tuck* it *out?*
   (= Will you untuck it?)

4. (Child trying to get out of swimsuit says:)
   Child: How do I *untake* this *off?*
   (= How do I take this off?)

5. Child: Will you *unopen* this?
   (= Will you open this?)

6. (Child trying to pull sheet of stamps apart says:)
   Child: How do you *unbreak* this?
   (= How do you break this?)

[2]The data comes from Melissa Bowerman's paper "The Child's Expression of Meaning," *Annals of the New York Academy of Sciences,* 379 (1981), 172–89.

7. (Child holding up chain of glued paper strips says:)
   Child: I know how you take these apart. *Unsplit* them and put'em on.
   (= Split them and put'em on.)

Exercise D. Very small children often say "Daddy, lift you!" when they mean "Daddy, lift *me* up" and want to be picked up. That is, they confuse the words 'I' and 'you'. Why would they do this?

Exercise E. Below is some data from children roughly between 2½ and 6 years old.[3] What pattern in English grammar could lead children to make this sort of error? What problem or problems might children face in giving up errors like those below?

1. Choose me the ones that I can have.
2. Button me the rest.
   (request to have the rest of her pajama snaps fastened)
3. Mommy, open Hadwen the door.
4. I'll brush him his hair.

8.3. LANGUAGE AS A FORMAL SYSTEM

Language is clearly used to communicate. Many scholars stress the role of communication in child language acquisition and argue that new words or new syntactic structures enter the child's language only when they have a specific communicative job to do. In this view, the child, in the course of his or her *nonlinguistic* social and mental development, comes to want or need to communicate a specific meaning. The child is then ready to learn the linguistic form (word or syntactic structure) necessary to communicate this meaning. This is no doubt correct in some cases, and we will see relevant examples later in the chapter. But, as odd as it may seem, one can overstate the role of communication as a driving force in language acquisition. We can see this if we once again consider the child's acquisition of lexical causatives.

We have seen that initially children produce correct lexical causatives and only later produce novel ones that are incorrect by the adult's standard (like 'I fell the book'). The initial correct stage is probably one where the child is learning each new causative form in isolation and has not analyzed the relationship between pairs like 'The door is open'/'John opened the door' (= John caused the

---

[3]Data from Melissa Bowerman, "Commentary," in Brian MacWhinney, ed., *Mechanisms of Language Acquisition* (Hillsdale, N.J.: Erlbaum, 1987), pp. 443–66.

door to open) or 'The cup broke'/'John broke the cup' (= John caused the cup to break). The child sees no relationship between these pairs and just learns how to use 'John opened the door' or 'John broke the cup' without realizing these are systematically related to 'The door is open' and 'The cup broke' in form and meaning.

When the child begins to make up novel causatives like 'I fell the book' or 'I am singing him', he or she has "caught on" to the systematic pattern in English that relates sentences like 'The cup broke' and 'John broke the cup'. The child then "overdoes" this pattern, failing to see that it is not fully general, producing things like 'I fell the book'. This is the same course of development we argued for in the case of the acquisition of noun plurals and the past tense of verbs discussed earlier, where children initially produce correct forms and only later produce novel forms like 'feets' and 'breaked'.

What is intriguing about the acquisition of lexical causatives is that children produce novel causatives like 'I fell the book' just as analytic causatives like 'I made that book fall' begin to flourish and are used widely in their grammars. While adults draw the distinction between lexical causatives ('I opened the door') and analytic causatives ('I made the door open') partly on the basis of the distinction between direct causation (the lexical causative) and indirect causation (the analytic causative), this distinction appears to play no role in the child's grammar at this stage. Children use both forms (the lexical causative and the analytic causative) to express the same meanings and will even use both forms side by side in the same speech context to express the same meaning, as in the examples below:[4]

15a. Saying 'giddi-up' doesn't *make* it *go* faster   [analytic causative]
      Singing *goes* it faster   [lexical causative]
        (child bouncing on spring-horse, has been singing loudly)

15b. Okay. If you want it to die.
      Eva's gonna *die* it   [lexical causative]
      She's gonna *make* it *die*   [analytic causative]
        (child upset because another child is about to touch a moth)

The analytic causative 'I made the book fall' encodes in two separate words the concepts CAUSE (through 'make') and FALL (through 'fall'). The novel lexical causative 'I fell the book' or its adult version 'I dropped the book' encode the concepts CAUSE and FALL in one word ('fell' and 'drop') in a particular syntactic pattern (the lexical causative). The child, in mastering analytic causatives like 'I made the book fall', may come to realize that the language can encode the

---

[4]From Melissa Bowerman, "Starting to Talk Worse: Clues to Language Acquisition from Children's Late Speech Errors," in S. Strauss, ed., *U-Shaped Behavioral Growth* (New York: Academic Press, 1982).

abstract concept CAUSE in a separate word ('make') or as part of a single word that also encodes another concept ('fall', 'drop'). That is, the child comes to realize that 'broke' in 'John broke the cup' does not have a unitary meaning, but is in fact complex in meaning, encoding CAUSE to BREAK, two concepts, separately in one word. The child then sees the relationship of 'John broke the cup' (CAUSE to BREAK) to 'The cup broke' (BREAK), realizing that the latter encodes the simple state of affairs that the former speaks of as CAUSED. The child is learning to analyze the way in which English encodes concepts (like CAUSE) into words and syntactic structures, and the ways in which English relates various forms to each other in intricate patterns.

The acquisition of analytic causatives like *'make* it *die'* precedes and seems to facilitate the acquisition of truly systematic lexical causatives like *'die* it' (that is, lexical causatives that the child has analyzed as systematically related to intransitives and adjectives, such as 'it dies'). When a child uses both forms ('Eva *make* it *die'* and 'Eva *die* it') to mean the same thing in the same context as in 15b above, it is hard to argue that it is the need to communicate that is driving the acquisition of the new form (the lexical causative). The new form being acquired does not seem to enter the child's language because he or she has a new communicative need. The analytic causative ('make it die') already communicates what the child wants to communicate with the lexical causative (as far as the child is concerned, since he or she ignores the distinction between direct and indirect causation).

Rather, the child, in uttering 15b, is *exploring* the communicative resources available in English. The new form (the lexical causative syntactic pattern) is learned and used not because it gives the child an immediate "payoff" in new communicative power, but because it is "there," so to speak. In using the new form and the old one (the analytic causative) in various contexts and even side by side in the same context, the child is exploring through use and observation what meaning and shades of meaning each form can communicate, which contexts it is normally used in, and what restrictions there are on various forms. The child is trying out each form to see how it sounds, how it fits the linguistic and nonlinguistic context, much as one might try out various shirts to see how they match with various pants. Thus, it is not a communicative need that drives the discovery of form here, but rather, play with forms drives the discovery of what can be communicated and how communication works in English.

The child eventually discovers that the lexical causative and the analytic causative have different shades of meaning and that there are a host of idiosyncratic restrictions on how causatives of both types work in English (for example, we say 'John dropped the ball' rather than 'John fell the ball'; we can say 'John choked' and 'Mary choked John', but while 'John sneezed' is all right, 'Mary sneezed John' is not; we can say 'Tomatoes grow' and 'Mary grows tomatoes', but though 'Children grow' is fine, 'Mary grows children' is not).

Language has significance to a child not just as a useful tool for communication. Language is also for children a complex "object" in the environment, an object whose properties children explore just as they explore the physical world and the world of mental problems (like riddles, puzzles, and games), without immediate instrumental payoff. Language is a "formal system" (an intricate pattern of forms related to each other, a set of criss-crossing and complex generalizations). Children appear to enjoy experimenting with and exploring this formal system, much as they enjoy exploring other complicated physical and mental "objects." Many adults, on the other hand, dislike exploring complicated systems (like mathematics or computers) unless there is an immediate tie to meaning or an immediate payoff in terms of what they can accomplish. In this regard, it is adults, not children, who want immediate gratification (or, put differently, children get gratification out of discovering formal properties, as is clear to anyone who has listened to how much pleasure they get out of playing with nonsense words and songs, weaving them endlessly into various repeated patterns).

8.4. LANGUAGE AND COGNITION

Limitations on Cognition as the Basis of Language

The last section raises one of the deepest questions in the study of language acquisition: What is the relationship between language and cognition? By *cognition* I mean the concepts and ways of thinking that children are born with and those that they acquire in their interaction with the physical and social world around them, before and during their acquisition of language. Many people believe that language development is driven by and is just a reflection of cognitive development, the prelinguistic and extralinguistic development of concepts and thinking. These researchers (following in many cases the lead of Piaget, one of the most influential psychologists of the twentieth century) often argue that thought is primarily the internalization of one's own actions in the physical world, and that as thought develops it is simply mapped or translated into language. Thus, the structure of thought largely determines the nature of language, and language is seen as a passive receptacle into which thought is poured.

Others (inspired by the work of Edward Sapir and Benjamin Lee Whorf in the beginning of this century) have argued that it is rather the structure of language that determines the nature of our concepts and our ways of thinking about the world. For example, Whorf argued that speakers of different languages will think about time differently based on how their language morphologically and syntactically deals with temporal meanings. Language shapes the mind; different languages shape it differently.

Of course, there are various positions in between these two extremes. Certain concepts are in all likelihood formed without assistance from language. This is likely to be true for such concepts as the nature of three-dimensional space, of enduring objects in the physical world, and of cause and effect, concepts that appear to be universal. But other concepts are more plausibly formed through observation of how fluent speakers use language, with the new words or other morphemes they hear serving for children as a "lure to cognition."[5]

An emphasis on how language shaped thought was popular in the 1950s and 1960s. But in the 1970s and 1980s, the tide has turned and many scholars have emphasized the ways in which prelinguistic perceptions and conceptions of the world determine the nature of language and language development. To these researchers, the meanings encoded by language are provided by nonlinguistic cognitive development (the child's development of ideas and ways of thinking that come about as a result of his or her interaction with the world and other people). The child simply has to discover the forms in language that encode these nonlinguistically given meanings. In this view, language acquisition is a sort of translation procedure between the concepts the child acquires as part of normal cognitive growth and the linguistic forms he or she is exposed to in the language he or she hears. The role of language itself is passive.

However, this view is too extreme. There are important differences between the way in which languages structure meaning and the way in which nonlinguistic thought does. Thus, learning language cannot solely be a procedure of translating nonlinguistic thought into language. Nonlinguistic perceptions are finely graded. People are capable of making very delicate distinctions in what they experience and think about. They can detect and respond to a vast number of similarities and differences among objects and events. For an example, consider an object inside a container. Humans can conceive of this object being contained inside this container to varying degrees. Imagine a button resting on the palm of the hand and the hand gradually closing. We can perceive a large number of degrees of containment between the two extremes of the button just resting on the flat palm and the palm fully closed around it. The extent to which the button is contained by the palm, between these two extreme states, is a matter of degree. This is by and large how human nonlinguistic perception and cognition works.

But language *does not* work this way. Language works on the basis of *categorical* oppositions, that is, a small set of distinctions that partition a finely graded scale into a small set of categories. Consider how we would *talk* about the button contained by the palm of the hand, not how we see it or think about it outside language. English speakers must decide categorically between two possibilities, not an indefinite number of them (as in perception and conception). We have to say either that the button is 'on' the palm of the hand or that it is 'in' the palm of the hand. Between the button laying on the flat hand (clearly 'on') and the button being fully grasped by a closed fist (clearly 'in'), we simply have to decide whether to call it 'on' or 'in'. There are no other choices.

No language allows continuously graded linguistic forms directly reflecting continuously graded changes in *degree* of containment. For example, no language

---

[5]This is Roger Brown's phrase, from *Words and Things* (New York: The Free Press, 1958), p. 206.

would gradually alter the vowel before /n / between 'on' and 'in' through many small alterations of the position of the tongue (producing various vowel sounds between these two) to express various degrees of containment between being on a flat surface ('on') and being fully surrounded by a container ('in').

Speakers not only must learn to make a small set of distinctions (often two) among events and relationships that vary along a continuum, but also must learn to do so on the basis of oppositions in meaning (like 'in' versus 'on') that often differ quite a bit from one language to another. For example, Dutch makes a three-way distinction between *in* ('in', the object is contained inside a surface), *op* ('on', the object lies on a horizontal surface or is attached to a vertical surface across a large part of its own surface), and *aan* (also 'on', the object is attached to the surface by only a restricted point). Thus, Dutch says that an apple is *op* ('on') the table or a sticker is glued *op* ('on') a refrigerator, but that a framed picture is *aan* ('on') a wall, a button is *aan* ('on') a sweater, or a coat is *aan* ('on') a hook.

Children learning English are just as capable as those learning Dutch of coming to notice and learn differences in the way an apple is in contact with a table and a picture with a wall. But only those learning Dutch must actually learn how to make this distinction, and only Dutch children are "lured" to make it by the linguistic forms they are exposed to. Outside of language, there are an indefinite number of distinctions one could choose to make up concerned with an object in contact with a surface, just as we are capable of perceiving and conceiving an indefinite number of such distinctions apart from language. Different languages cut up such perceptual and conceptual continua into different, and sometimes a different number of, categories. Languages do not just passively translate distinctions already given in the child's nonlinguistic perceptual and conceptual (cognitive) development.

Thus, the English speaker and the Dutch speaker must learn to make different cuts in the continuum of states between an object on a flat surface and the object being fully contained within that surface ('in' versus 'on' for the English speaker; *in* versus *op* versus *aan* for the Dutch speaker). Children must also learn which meanings can combine together into single words in their language (whether these meanings come directly from cognition or children are "lured" to them by their language). One language will encode two meanings in a single word, while another will keep these meanings quite separate. For example, the English word 'this' means *an object close to the speaker* and the word 'the' means *previously mentioned or otherwise known information.* English keeps these two meanings separate. Hausa, on the other hand, combines these two meanings into a single word (*wannan*), which means *close to the speaker and previously mentioned.* This word is opposed to three other words that mean *close to the speaker and new information; far from speaker and previously mentioned;* and *far from the speaker and new information.* Kwakwa'la, in contrast to both Hausa and English, has a single word that means *close to the speaker and visible* and contrasts this with other words that mean *close to the speaker and invisible, far from the speaker and visible,* and *far from the speaker and invisible.* And in many languages of New Guinea and Australia, distance from speaker (close versus far) is combined with still another dimension, *height* of referent relative to speaker, for a complex set of contrasts between words meaning, for example, *close to the speaker and higher, close to the speaker and lower, far from the speaker and higher,* and *far from the speaker and lower.* Nothing in the child's perceptual or cognitive development before or apart from language can tell him or her how meanings will combine in a given language.

To summarize, nonlinguistic cognition, no matter how powerful, does not directly provide children with the categories of meaning (for example, 'in' versus 'on') they need to become fluent speakers of their language. Nor does it directly provide them with information about how these categories of meaning are or are not combinable into single words that contrast with other words (for example, 'this' versus 'that'). Some categories are no doubt so salient for humans that every language has a clear and separate morpheme, word, or particular syntactic structure for them; some distinctions are no doubt so salient that every language draws them in a clear and obvious fashion. Other categories and distinctions may be so unimportant that no language encodes them in any straightforward manner. But in between are a large number of categories and distinctions, the expression of which is not predetermined by human cognition but by the nature of the language the child is exposed to. In these cases, cognition supplies only the raw materials (the continua and finely graded scales). The individual language composes its categories out of these raw materials; it makes cuts in these continua to form the distinctions it wishes. These categories and distinctions do not exist apart from the fact that some language chooses to express them, and express them in a certain way.

There is another limitation on the view that cognition is the driving force of language acquisition. There are, in a large number of languages, some linguistic categories, such as "masculine" nouns in German, that can only be described in purely formal terms (that is, as patterns of related forms that have no direct tie to meaning). There was a time in the history of German in which nouns fell into three classes—masculine, feminine, and neuter—based on whether they named a male, female, or neuter (neither male nor female) entity. These classes were distinguished by different endings on the nouns. At this stage, the grammatical distinction among the three classes of nouns related quite directly to a salient cognitive distinction that is surely learned by children before they acquire language, or at least apart from the acquisition of language (that is, 'male' versus 'female' versus 'neither'). But in the course of its history, German has changed to obscure the relationship between the three grammatical classes of nouns and the three obvious cognitive categories of male, female, and neither. Many endings on nouns have been lost, and nouns that name male, female, or neuter entities are not necessarily any longer in the class of masculine, feminine, or neuter nouns, respectively.

So German masculine, feminine, or neuter nouns do not all share any *semantic* property (for example, the German word for 'maiden' is in the neuter class, the German word for 'tomatoe' is in the feminine class, the word for 'apple' is in the masculine class). What they do share is a set of *formal* properties. That is, the only way one knows that a noun is masculine in German is that such nouns take *der* for the definite article ('the'), not *die,* which feminine nouns take, or *das,* which neuter nouns take, and they are referred to by the pronoun *er* ('he'), not *sie* ('she'), which is used to refer to feminine nouns, or *es,* which is used to refer to neuter nouns. The child learns what counts as a masculine noun not by matching its meaning to a clear and salient cognitive category (male) given in nonlinguistic experience, but by paying attention to a purely formal regularity in the data (certain nouns are preceded by *der* and referred to by *er;* these are then taken to belong to a single class).

Children must come to the task of language acquisition equipped with the ability to carry out such formal analysis or they would never fully acquire most human languages. It has been shown that in the case of some languages such arbitrary gender systems are acquired as early as two years of age. Thus, such formal systems, with little or no tie to meaning, are not, in fact, always difficult for children (though they are indeed for adults learning languages later in life).

Of course, it is an interesting question why languages keep distinctions that have lost any transparent tie to meaning (like the distinction between masculine, feminine, and neuter nouns in German). This shows us at least that the nature of language is not completely determined by its function as a communicative system (since this distinction communicates nothing). Languages may keep such systems because they are mastered more easily by children than adults and thus serve to single out people who were born into cultures as the true insiders, and to render everyone else always in some sense an outsider. Getting the gender distinctions wrong on a German or French noun may not in any way damage communication, but it often signals that one was not born a German or a French person.

The Role of Cognition in Language Acquisition

The last section discussed the limitations of the view that human cognition determines the structure of human language. However, one should certainly not conclude from this that cognition has nothing to do with the shape of language. While language partially shapes the nature of human thought in terms of what categories and distinctions one will pay attention to, human cognition also helps shape the course of language acquisition and ultimately the nature of language. Cognition and language interact in complex ways. This section will discuss some of the ways in which cognition affects language development.

Children certainly do bring to the task of language acquisition some concepts that they have either been born with as part of their innate endowment as human beings or that they have attained in the course of their prelinguistic development as they explore the physical world and interact with other people. Children invent forms to encode these concepts if they do not find them in their language. These invented forms do not occur in their language, but often similar forms occur in other languages the child has never been exposed to. Children usually give up their inventions eventually, as they see more and more evidence that these forms really do not occur in the language to which they are exposed; though of course sometimes they do not give them up and they thereby change the language.

One particularly interesting example of children inventing a distinction that appears to exist in their thought about the world, but not in their language, is the following. To a superficial view, children seem to switch randomly between uninflected proper names (for example, 'Laura') and possessive pronouns (such as, 'my') to indicate possession. For example, a child named 'Eve' says on one occasion 'Play with Eve broom', using 'Eve broom' to signal possession, and on another occasion says 'That my bottle', using 'my bottle' to signal possession.

W. Deutsch and N. Budwig,[6] however, found that children mean different things by these different forms. The pronominal forms ('my bottle') were used when the child wished to control or claim an object to carry out an action. On the other hand, the proper name forms ('Eve broom') were used simply to indicate possession when the fact of possession was not in question. For example, when an adult wanted a little boy named 'Adam' to give up a toy car that he was playing with, Adam asserted control by saying 'my car'. However, when Adam was noting a comparison between a picture in a book and his own possession, he said, 'Just like Adam horsie shirt'.

This distinction between proper names and pronouns is used yet more generally by some children. N. Budwig[7] has gone on to find that nominal ('Laura') and pronominal ('I') forms are contrasted in a similar way when used as subjects of sentences. Children use a pronoun subject to refer to themselves with verbs expressing desires and intentions (for example, 'I want it Mommy', 'I like something else for me', 'I need toast after breakfast'). On the other hand, children use a nominal subject to refer to themselves when simply describing objects belonging to them (for example, 'Laura has a green car', 'Carol has a life belt'). Nominal forms also tend to be followed by action verbs, as in 'Carol do it', 'Sally read'. The proper name forms tend to be used when children describe themselves and their actions from the outside, so to speak, and the pronominal ones when they view themselves from the inside as a source of desire and control.

This distinction between the use of pronouns in sentences connected with desire and intention (for example, 'my shirt' or 'I need toast') and full nouns in sentences that are more descriptive and merely information-giving appears then to be one that the child has invented. It certainly does not exist in English. It is motivated by a view the child has on the way in which linguistic forms (pronouns and full nouns) hook up (or should hook up) to various contexts in which

[6]"Form and Function in the Development of Possessives," *Papers and Reports on Child Language Development*, Stanford University, Department of Linguistics, 22 (1983), 36–42.

[7]*Agentivity and Control in Early Child Language*, doctoral dissertation, University of California at Berkeley, 1986.

language is used (seeking to get or control something versus giving information). This viewpoint appears to have been formed out of the child's nonlinguistic cognitive and social development, that is, out of the child's physical and mental exploration of the world of action and interaction.

Dan Slobin,[8] one of the most influential of contemporary students of child language development, has argued that children come to language acquisition expecting certain prototypical "scenes" to be clearly encoded. These scenes are characteristic and salient events or relationships that the child has experienced in his or her own prelinguistic actions and perceptions of the world. One such scene he calls the **manipulative action scene,** which is as follows: An agent carries out a physical and perceptible change in a patient by means of direct body contact or with an instrument under the agent's control. Children are very impressed early on by their own ability to manipulate, move, destroy, or otherwise affect objects in their environments. This activity is one they expect to find clearly encoded in their language, and they appear to actively search for how it is encoded as they enter the task of language acquisition.

Children will attempt to force a direct reflection of the manipulative action scene on their language, even if their language does not as directly encode it as they might wish. For example, in Russian, the direct object of all transitive verbs is placed in the accusative case (by a special ending on the noun). However, some children acquiring Russian will at first apply the accusative ending only to nouns that are the objects of verbs of direct, physical manipulation, such as 'give', 'carry', 'put', and 'throw', omitting the accusative for less manipulative verbs such as 'read' and 'see'. These children are attempting to interpret the accusative ending as a marker of the entity affected in the manipulative action scene, rather than just a marker of grammatical direct objects.

In Kaluli there is a special marker for the subject of transitive verbs. Children often restrict this marker to subjects of verbs that fit the manipulative action scene such as 'give', 'grab', 'take', and 'hit', and omit it with verbs like 'see', 'say', and 'call', where adult Kaluli uses it also. These children are attempting to interpret this marker as expressing the agent of the manipulative action scene, rather than just a marker of the subjects of transitive verbs.

Looking for a direct expression of the manipulative action scene in English, Russian, and Kaluli, which do not so directly encode it, may seem wasted effort. But it is not. By this effort, children correctly identify some *transitive* sentences (sentences with subjects and objects) in these languages (sentences like 'I grabbed it') and learn the grammar of these sentences. Later they come to realize that this grammar applies to a wider set of transitive sentences that do not express direct manipulative action (sentences like 'I saw it'). In this sense, their initial search for

---

[8]"Universal and Particular in the Acquisition of Language," in E. Wanner and L. R. Gleitman, ed., *Language Acquisition: The State of the Art* (New York: Cambridge University Press, 1982); see also *The Crosslinguistic Study of Language Acquisition,* two volumes, edited by Slobin (Hillsdale, N.J.: Erlbaum, 1985).

a direct encoding of the manipulative action scene can serve as an entry point into language acquisition.

Finally, in English, we can note that some two-year-olds use 'my' for the subject of a sentence when the subject is a prototypical agent, with a highly action-oriented verb and a direct effect on an object (for example, 'My blew the candles out', 'My take it home'). They use 'I' for subjects that are less agentive and where the sentences express experiences ('I like peas'). Thus, these children appear to be trying to make a distinction between the subjects of sentences that express the manipulative action scene and subjects of sentences that do not, a distinction that English does not make.

So children do not just passively wait to see what concepts the language to which they are exposed will express. They actively look for some concepts and conceptual distinctions, concepts and distinctions that they must have attained either as part of their innate cognitive endowment as humans or from their nonlinguistic experience in interacting with the physical and social world.

In summary, this section and the previous one argue that the following lesson can be drawn from the novel forms children use and the errors they make: *Both* the structure of the language to which children are exposed (in terms of the categories and distinctions that language has forms for) *and* the child's own nonlinguistic cognitive predispositions for certain concepts and distinctions contribute to the language learner's organization of meaning.

8.5.   STAGES OF LANGUAGE ACQUISITION

In our discussion thus far, we have yet to do justice to the fact that language is acquired over time, one stage at a time. In this section we will gain some feeling for the course of language development through the child's first few years of life.

There is a great deal of variability among children in the course of language development. Children do not all reach the same milestones at the same time. This variability does not relate to any differences in intelligence or even to any differences in linguistic skills among children, as long as it is within normal ranges (which are quite wide). It does, perhaps, relate to differences of personality and family setting. Because there is so much variability in the ages at which different children reach various stages of language development, it is best to discuss language acquisition in terms of the *tasks* the child must accomplish and the ways in which children go about these tasks, not in terms of the *ages* at which children accomplish them.

The Beginnings

The first task facing any child is making a start, that is, breaking into the language in the first place. How do children begin to use a communication system (language) they do not know? Part of the answer to this question, as we have seen, is that children are given help by their biology. The human biological endowment for language specifies within fairly narrow limits what a human language will look like and guides the child in the hypotheses he or she draws about what forms and rules exist in the language he or she is exposed to.

For example, all languages in the world have nouns and verbs, even though they may have few or no other categories of words. It is thus a plausible hypothesis that the child comes to the job of language acquisition (unconsciously) knowing that the language he or she is exposed to will have nouns and verbs, and actively looks for the instantiations of these categories. However, the child is initially confronted with a stream of sounds which he or she cannot yet identify and has no idea which sounds constitute nouns and which constitute verbs (the child doesn't even yet know which sounds constitute words!). Furthermore, the child has no idea what any of these sounds *mean,* whether they are nouns of verbs or anything else for that matter. Having figured out the meanings of a few sentences, the child's innate knowledge about nouns and verbs will be useful. But it is not of much use until the child has figured out these initial meanings. And the question is, how does the child do this?

We will get nowhere in answering this question if we just concentrate on the child. At the outset, what is happening is that a *linguistic communication system* is being established between the child and the adult. In adult language, the meaning of a word, phrase, or sentence is ultimately what the speaker has in mind (that is, what the speaker *intends* to communicate). We hearers "guess" or decode what the speaker has in mind through our knowledge of words and grammar and through what we know about the speaker. In this sense, meaning is mental, psychological, and internal. Furthermore, we adults spend a good deal of our time talking about our beliefs and thoughts, which are not visible. None of this will do for the child. The child's problem is that he or she does not yet know the language and so has no access to these internal meanings, to what is in people's minds. Thus, meaning must be made social, public, and overt for the child.

First of all, children have a communication system before they are able to communicate in language. Their first communication system is one of cries and gestures signaling the child's own desires and emotions. Eventually, the child (usually somewhere near the end of the first year of life) adds vocalizations to these gestures. Sometimes these vocalizations are just "general want expressers" with no apparent content of their own. For example, a child may make an open-handed reaching gesture toward an object while uttering an [m]-initial monosyllable that varies somewhat from occasion to occasion, or may utter something like 'na' whenever he or she wants something. These combinations of gesture and sound have something like the meaning *I request of you,* where the actual request is left to be guessed from context. Sometimes the request has a bit more content, as the child says something like 'up' or names an object (for example, 'ball'). The accompanying gesture (reaching or pointing) is necessary at this point to provide "backup" (redundancy) for the child, who is trying to use sounds as part of a communication system that is still under construction.

These single "word" utterances are called **holophrases.** While they often look like words (such as 'up'), they are not really words since they cannot combine with other words to form phrases or sentences. Further, holophrases have *uses* that are comparable to those of *sentences* (not words) in adult language. They are used to perform linguistic acts like requesting or greeting. The holophrase period (which used to be called "the single word stage") spans the age range roughly between 9 and 18 months. While gestures originally co-occur with holophrases (and precede them in development), they gradually lose their dominant role (before the end of the holophrase period).

There is another way in which talking of these holophrases as "words" is misleading. In the last few years, we have come to realize that not all children proceed in exactly the same manner in acquiring language. There are two important early strategies, the *bottom-up* and *top-down* approaches. When using the bottom-up approach, the learner tries to work with chunks that are as small as possible—often only single (usually stressed) syllables of the adult language (extracted from, and taken by observers to correspond to, whole adult words). These small chunks are eventually filled out (unstressed syllables are added) and combined to produce longer utterances (see below).

By contrast, users of the top-down approach seem to feel comfortable working with much longer chunks of language (often referred to as *formulae*) that correspond to whole words or phrases of the adult language. The child memorizes and uses these large chunks without knowing what their parts are (for example, 'look at that!'), that is, the child uses them as unanalyzed wholes. These longer chunks are eventually analyzed into their constituent parts, which can then used in new combinations to form new utterances (see below).

Most learners use both these approaches, although particular learners may prefer one approach to the other. I will use the term 'holophrase' to refer to any chunk (a single syllable, a word, or a whole phrase) that functions as an unanalyzed whole for the child.

Before and during this holophrase period, the child is involved in an immense amount of social interaction, much of which has the character of fixed routines or rituals. Initially, a routine may be as simple as the parent responding to a child's sound or action as if it was meaningful. The child smiles and the parent says "Oh, what a nice smile!" The child burps and the parent says "There's a nice little burp!" The child makes a noise and the parent says, "There's a nice noise!" The parent is making the child a conversational partner when the child cannot yet talk. Or the parent places the child on his or her knee and says "giddy up!" and bounces the child. The parent stops and says "giddy up!" again and bounces the child again. Eventually the child makes a sound when the parent stops, and the parent treats it as "giddy up!" and bounces the child. The child has here come to fill a slot in the interaction, a slot originally supplied by the parent, and then interpreted by the parent to be the appropriate response. Or the child makes an indecipherable sound when the refrigerator opens and he or she sees milk. The parent takes the sound to mean *milk* and says "Oh, you want some milk?"

In all these cases the child is *inserted* into social interaction *as if* carrying out his or her part. The child is given a place in the interaction by the parent and supported in the interaction before the child could ever carry his or her own weight. As the child develops, the parent demands more and expects the child to take a more responsible part in the interaction. But the parent only withdraws support gradually as the child is able to take on more and more responsibility for his or her own role. Children have to learn both what the words and sentence patterns of their language are and how to use them appropriately in social interaction. Early routines, by combining words and supported social interaction, accomplish both simultaneously.

Early communications often require an *act* as a response, usually a highly specific act, and one which has been repeated on numerous occasions. For example, the parent says "Where's the baby?" and the child turns toward a particular picture of herself; the parent says "How big are you?" and the child smiles and places her hand on top of her head; the parent says "clap, clap!" and the child plays a game of clapping the palm of her hand with the parent's; or the parent says "High, high" and the child raises her arms to facilitate dressing. These specific and often repeated acts overtly *show* what the words mean. Further, the repeated and fixed character of these interactions support the child in interaction, inserting the child in a secure place in the interaction with a part (or "role") he or she can readily play.

As the child's language develops, this overt tie to objects in the physical world and to social interaction continues. For example, requests play a large role in the initial development of language. Holophrases like 'door', 'on', 'off', and 'open' are (for the most part) first used as requests (for example, 'door' used to mean *I request that you open the door*) and only later as statements ('door' used to mean *that is a door* or *I open the door*). Requests involve the child and adult in an interaction, often one that has been "practiced" before. Further, requests may emerge first because it is easier for the child to guess the meaning of a form when it used to make a request, since the effect is then acted out visibly by the addressee. In this sense, meaning is made visible for the child.

For the child, words, actions, and social interaction are integrally intertwined. Meaning is originally then a matter of this public intermixture of words, actions, and social interaction. Only subsequent to this intermixture does meaning become internalized in the mind, as something psychological (though we will argue later that it always keeps something of its interactional character). For the child meaning is public, overt, acted out socially in the world.

Combining Words

The child's next task is to be able to produce combinations of words (two-word and multiword utterances). To do this, the child first has to realize that *one* utterance can have separate components of meaning, that is, that different parts of the utterance can communicate different things. There are two early ways in which children accomplish this. First, they begin to use the intonation pattern of an utterance to communicate different information than the actual word or words uttered. Starting at 15 months, one child may utter 'Mama', 'Anna', or 'Dada' with a rising intonation to mean *Where are you?*, but with a falling intonation contour for greeting someone. Second, at about the same time, children often combine a gesture and an utterance, where the gesture is not redundant with the word uttered but itself communicates something separate. For example, one child uses a headshake simultaneously with an utterance to negate the utterance (rather than using a separate word to do this). This is quite different than the earlier use of gesture and speech, where both communicated the same information.

The child makes the transition to two-word and multiword utterances gradually. There are two major routes to true two-word and multiword combinations, and we will look at each of these in turn. These two routes take place simultaneously. Most children use both of them, though each child uses them in somewhat different ways and emphasizes each somewhat more or less strongly. A few children specialize in one or the other.

Before we discuss these two routes to true two-word utterances, I will mention a phenomenon that often accompanies them. Children often extend a holophrase by adding extra, meaningless phonological material. This allows the child to practice articulatory skills prerequisite to more sophisticated combinations without requiring him or her to have to process two different words in the same utterance.

Now on to the two routes to true two-word utterances. In the first route, the child comes to chain related holophrases together. In the first half (or longer) of the holophrase period, the child communicates for the most part by using only one holophrase, which may be repeated. When the child switches to a different holophrase, the previous communicational interaction is over and done with, and the child has turned to a new interest. In the later part of the holophrase period, however, unifying threads begin to connect successions of holophrases. While they are still holophrases in that they are set apart from each other by their own separate intonation contours and usually by a pause, they have a thematic unity in that they appear to be about one topic.

These chained holophrases usually appear when the child has acquired between fifteen and forty individual holophrases (around 17 to 20 months). The child usually has been speaking only a few holophrases for a number of months (three to twelve) and within the space of a month or so—at around 17 to 20 months—accelerates the rate of acquisition of new words from a rate of around three or four per month to between thirty and fifty per month (however, individual differences are common here; some children spurt early and for some the rate of vocabulary development is more uniform).

When the child first begins to chain related holophrases together, each holophrase is related to an event in a sequence of actions in which the child is engaged: What happens first gets talked about first and the next holophrase relates to what comes next in the temporal sequence of events. The number of holophrases thus "chained" might be as large as six. The structure of the outside action supports the child's developing ability to chain several related items together. However, these holophrase chains tied to action soon give way to successions of holophrases about a situation that has been defined in advance of speaking, and where the individual holophrases are not tied to particular movements or shifts in context.

It is a common phenomenon in child development that when a child is working on developing a new skill, old ones temporarily deteriorate. This is often true in the case of these successions of related holophrases. Since the child must expend effort to relate holophrases to each other and chain them together, the individual holophrases in the chain often suffer phonetic regression to earlier, more baby-like forms. For instance, when one child pretended to step on a researcher's tape recorder she said 'tay' for 'tape' and then 'te' for 'step', but on the same day she was able to pronounce these forms more fully as 'tape' and 'tep' when they occurred as isolated holophrases.[9]

These chained holophrases are not acquired in social isolation. Not only are they originally supported by the structure of actions the child is involved in, but they are also often supported by the social interaction the child is a part of. For example, consider the social interaction below between a child named Brenda and her mother:

Child: Kimby
Mother: What about Kimby?
Child: Close

The child says something ('Kimby', a name). The mother asks what about it and the child says something further ('close', an action that Kimby performed). The child's first holophrase can be seen as a *topic* statement, the mother's question as a request for a *comment,* and the child's answer as giving a *comment.* Through such interaction the child is learning the discourse notions of topic and comment. Further, the child is also coming to understand the relationship between an argument/noun ('Kimby') and a predicate/verb ('close'). As the child develops, she begins to take over both roles, and no longer needs a push from her parent—that is, she can say both the topic and comment by herself, in a succession of chained holophrases.

When these chained holophrases become fluently combined by being placed under a single unitary intonation contour and by having little or no pause between them, the interactional process shown above can go yet a step further. The parent takes for granted that the child can give a whole topic-comment pair and seeks from the child another comment, as in the example below, another instance of communicative interaction between Brenda and an adult:

[9]See Ronald Scollon, *Conversations With a One-Year Old.* (Honolulu: University Press of Hawaii, 1976).

Child:	Tape recorder	(pause)
	use it	(pause)
	use it	
Adult:	Use it for what?	
Child:	talk	(pause)
	corder talk	(pause)
	Brenda talk	

The second major route to true two-word and multiword utterances is based on those cases where the child has memorized and produces adult multiword utterances as a whole, without being aware of the individual parts of the utterance. These are the holophrases we referred to above as *formulae* in the preceding section. The child produces forms like 'all done', 'all gone', 'look it', 'my turn', 'what's that', 'look at that' without having analyzed their constituent parts (to the child they are just one form with a unitary meaning that he or she has picked up from observing their contexts of use). Later the child learns to analyze these formulae into their parts and to recombine these parts to form new utterances.

The way in which the child goes about this analysis is something like the following: The child initially memorizes a set of related expressions like 'all clean', 'all done', 'all dressed', 'all dry', or 'more pen', 'more coke', 'more cook', 'more doggie' (meant *give more coke to doggie*), or 'no pen', 'no night night', 'no go out', 'no change', where each combination is learned individually. The child eventually comes to realize that these combinations have parts and that there is a pattern apparent in the set of related expressions (all the 'all' expressions, or all the 'more' expressions, or all the 'no' expressions). At this time, the child realizes that a pattern like '*more* + x', for instance, which means RECURRENCE OF X, can be abstracted from the set of forms involving 'more'. At this point, the child will begin to produce novel combinations he or she has never heard before, such as 'more car' meaning *drive around some more*.

At first, each such pattern is tied to the particular constant word involved (for example, 'all' or 'more' or 'no') and expresses only a narrow semantic relationship (like "recurrence"). Further, these early patterns tend to exist independently of each other. Thus, the child does not have general rules, but specific patterns tied to individual words and narrow meanings. Eventually, however, these limited scope patterns are combined into more general ones. For example, two formulae like '*little* + x' (which combines various words with 'little') and '*hot* + x' (which combines various words with 'hot') will be combined into a more general pattern 'PROPERTY + x', where PROPERTY stands for any word that names a property or attribute that things can have. The child will then be able to produce new combinations freely, like 'old doggie', when he or she learns new property terms such as 'old'. Or the specific pattern '*little* + x' could be combined with the specific pattern '*see* + x' to produce '*see* + *little* + x', a three-word combination. Eventually, of course, the child will generalize 'PROPERTY

+ x' to the yet more general 'ADJECTIVE + NOUN', and patterns like '*see + little* + x' to 'VERB + OBJECT NP' (where OBJECT NP can = adjective + noun).

Through rote memorization followed by the extraction of specific patterns, and their subsequent generalization, the child comes eventually to abstract word classes (for example, all the words that can fill x in the pattern 'PROPERTY + x', or that can occur after '*more*'—these and other such "privileges of occurrence" constitute the class of *nouns*). The child also comes to recognize the syntactic structures in language, such as 'NP-subject verb NP-object'.

Through various combinations of these two routes, children eventually produce fluent, connected two-word utterances, where there is little or no pause between the words, both words are covered by one unitary intonational contour, and the child clearly knows the utterance is made up of two separate words functioning together. The child's speech at this stage can sound "telegraphic" (like a telegram), since most of his or her word combinations are content words (for example, 'go car') with no function words in between (not 'go in the car').

Roger Brown, in many respects the founder of the modern study of child language, examined transcripts of children's two-word utterances from a number of languages.[10] Brown found that children everywhere expressed the same small group of semantic relations (meanings) in their speech. Table 8-1 lists the eight most prevalent semantic relations found by Brown (pp. 193–97), with examples of each (I have slightly changed Brown's terminology).

Notice that at this stage the identical utterance spoken on different occasions can convey two quite different meanings. 'Mommy sock' can mean on one occasion *Mother's sock* (possessor + possession) and on another occasion *Mommy, put my sock on* (agent + object). The context in which the child utters

[10]*A First Language: The Early Stages* (Cambridge, Mass.: Harvard University Press, 1973).

TABLE 8-1

SEMANTIC RELATION	EXAMPLES
Agent + action	mommy come; daddy sit
Action + object*	drive car; eat grape
Agent + object	mommy sock; baby book
Action + location	go park; sit chair
Entity + location	cup table; toy floor
Possessor + possession	my teddy; mommy dress
Object + attribute	box shiny; crayon big
Demonstrative + object	dat money; dis telephone

*'Object' means *word that names a physical object*, not *grammatical direct object*.

Adapted from Table 5.2, p. 147 in Helen Tager-Flusberg, "Putting Words Together: Morphology and Syntax in the Preschool Years," in Jean Berko Gleason, ed. *The Development of Langauge* (Columbus, Ohio: Charles E. Merrill, 1985), pp. 137–71.

these (that is, the physical and social setting) must determine which the child means. We can raise the interesting question as to how the child represents these different utterances of 'Mommy sock' in his or her own head—how does the child tell them apart?

We do not, in fact, know how the child represents these two-word utterances in his or her own head. Does the child represent something like 'eat grape' when it means *I am eating a grape* as AN UNMENTIONED NOUN NAMING AN AGENT (myself) + A VERB NAMING AN ACTION ('eat') + A NOUN NAMING AN OBJECT THAT IS ACTED ON BY THE AGENT ('grape'), with unconscious knowledge of both syntactic categories like noun and verb and semantic relations like AGENT, ACTION, and PATIENT (= being acted on)? Or does the child just represent it in semantic terms like AGENT (unmentioned) ACTS ON OBJECT? Or is the child's representation even poorer than this? What the child produces (that is, 'eat grape') must surely represent much less than he or she actually knows, since children at this stage can comprehend much longer utterances than they can produce. But what exactly children know (unconsciously) about their two-word utterances is still a mystery.

────────────────────── **E X E R C I S E S** ──────────────────────

Exercise F.   Tape record a child of around three years of age. Ask the child questions and play with the child (using various toys as available). Try to get the child to engage in as much talk as possible. Transcribe at least 100 "utterances" of the child. Describe how you knew what an utterance was (that is, how did you define it in order to carry out this assignment?). Then (a) describe clearly and explicitly how the child's language (grammar) differs from adult English, and (b) discuss the role context plays in the child's communication and in how the hearer understands it.

Exercise G.   Observe a mother or father (whichever appears to be the primary care giver) interacting with an infant under one year of age. Take notes and then describe the communication system that exists between parent and child. (How does the parent talk to, gesture to, and interact with the child? How does the child respond; how does the child initiate interaction? Look not just at words, but at gestures, body positions, eye gaze, cries and other noises, and anything else you find important.)

──

8.6.   NOMINALS AND MEANING

We have argued that the early linguistic system of the child is centered around actions and social interaction that render meaning visible and that support the child's place in social and linguistic interaction. Somewhat paradoxically, vocabulary counts extending into the second year have shown that **nominals** (words that tend to name objects, not actions) constitute more than half of the child's vocabulary and that action words are fewer. However, while it is true that children usually have more nominals in their vocabularies early on, these nouns (except for the names of common interlocutors) are not used as often as other types of expressions, which either name actions (such as 'go') or are used for social-expressive purposes ('bye-bye').

Further support for the centrality of action comes from the frequent observation that words such as 'in', which have both a dynamic directional sense (*to move into the inside of something*) and a static locative one (*to be inside something*) in the adult language (for example, 'he went *in* the room' versus 'he is *in* the room') enter the holophrastic child's speech first in their dynamic sense (for example, 'in' is used to mean *go or move in*) and only later come to bear the static meaning too.

The past decade has seen a great deal of literature on children's acquisition of nominals. This research has raised interesting questions about the nature of children's mental representations, and, ultimately, about the nature of meaning in language. The literature has proposed two rival hypotheses about the nature of children's mental representations for nominals: a *criterial attributes* account and a *prototypes* account.

The criterial attributes view in its strongest form holds that the meaning of a noun (like 'bird') for a child is a list of attributes or properties (for example, feathers, two feet, a beak, etc.) that objects must have for the word to be applied to them (each feature must be present, and when they are all present, that is enough to ensure that the word correctly applies). Prototype theories, on the other hand, hold that the child stores in his or her head an internal representation of "best examples" as the basis for applying nominals. Thus, in the case of 'bird', the child stores an internal representation, perhaps in terms of images or sketches, of the best examples of birds (birds like robins, sparrows, and pigeons, probably not ones like turkeys, penguins, and ostriches, which are less prototypical birds). Objects are candidates for being labeled with a word ('bird') if they are sufficiently similar to the stored prototype(s) for that word (so canaries clearly make it, penguins probably slide by, but flying squirrels and flying fish do not).

One phenomenon that was intensively studied, and that was at first taken as evidence for the *criterial attributes* view, was children's **overextensions.** Children starting in their second year often use a word to refer to things that an adult would not use it for, that is, they extend its coverage beyond what the adult would allow. For example, a child might use 'dog' not just for dogs, but for all furry animals, or may use 'moon' not just for the moon, but for all round or shiny objects. One child used 'shoe' not only in situations where shoes were involved, but also while handling her teddy bear's shoeless feet, passing a doll's arm to an adult to be refitted on the doll, putting a sock on a doll, and when looking at a picture of a brown beetle. It looks as if the child has a smaller set of criterial attributes for a word like 'dog' (perhaps just 'animal' and 'furry'), for instance, than the adult (who includes features like 'canine').

Overextension is, of course, an advance on children's earliest uses of words. For younger children, referents of a word are very tightly circumscribed: 'baby' might initially relate to a unique picture; 'ticktack' might at first signify only father's watch; 'Papa' might initially only be the child's father, though later it is used "indiscriminately" for any man in the street. The characteristic pattern is for nominals to be underextended first and only later to apply to a wider range of entities (perhaps then going as far as an overextension). For instance, for one child, at eight months, only shoes in his mother's closet counted as 'shoes'. He would even crawl past a pair of his mother's shoes placed near him on the floor when responding to 'Where's the shoes?' Overextensions first appear in the beginning of the second year and represent an attempt to generalize the meanings of words beyond the specific contexts they were learned in (usually as part of rituals or routines).

However, various versions of prototype theory can account for overextensions as well. Consider the child above who used 'shoe' for shoes, a doll's arms, a teddy bear's feet, and a brown beetle. One version of prototype theory[11] would attribute to the child's mind something like videotape recordings of one or more shoe-involving episodes from her life, filed in the child's mind in association with a representation of the pronunciation of the word 'shoe'. Other nominals in the child's vocabulary would have had their own episodic recordings. When the child wanted a label for the beetle (or the doll's arm or socks, or indeed for a shoe), she compared what she was currently experiencing with episodes in her mental "video" library and found that the current input was closer to something in the 'shoe' collection than to anything else. For the beetle, the similarity was probably visual appearance (the beetle in the picture did somewhat resemble a shiny brown shoe); for the arm, the relevant similarity was probably the action of being fitted on to a body; for the doll's socks and shoes, it was probably similarity in both appearance and action. As soon as the child learns a more appropriate word (for example, 'sock' or 'beetle'), the overextension ceases.

In this view, we assume that children start with mental representations ("videotapes") that are too specific, too closely tied to the original occasions of use or the rituals/routines that the words first appeared in. The noun is originally treated almost as if it is a proper name ('baby' names just one specific picture or 'shoe' means just the shoes in mother's closet). Eventually, the child learns to match objects to the videotape more flexibly (the child interprets the videotape less literally, if you like). Before the child has lots of words, however, this can lead the child to matching objects to the videotape too generally, because he or she has no videotapes that match it better.

This idea of a "videotape" library would work as well for the meanings of verbs (for example, 'take a bath', 'go night night', 'drive', 'eat'), and brings out the way in which meaning, whether for nouns or verbs, is originally and ultimately

[11]Patrick Griffiths, "Early Vocabulary," in P. Fletcher and M. Garman, eds., *Language Acquisition,* 2nd ed. (New York: Cambridge University Press, 1986), pp. 279–306.

tied to the social contexts and interactions words are used in. There is no reason to believe that meaning works differently for adults. Adults just have more and more sophisticated tapes and match objects and actions to them in a perhaps more sophisticated fashion. In this view, the meaning of a word like 'bachelor' is not ADULT UNMARRIED MALE (a set of necessary and sufficient properties something must have to be called a "bachelor"). Rather it is a videotape or "script" of a typical scenario or scenarios involving bachelors (namely, men who have gone a bit beyond marriageable age and who are thus highly "available"). This would explain why people have trouble when asked whether the Pope is a bachelor: He just isn't in the script, since he is out of the marriage game altogether.

——————————— E X E R C I S E ———————————

Exercise H. Below are some verbs children from 2 to nearly 6 years old made up. All of these verbs are related to nouns (thus, they are called *denominal verbs;* 'denominal' means *from a noun*). These examples are taken from Eve Clark's paper, "Lexical Innovations: How Children Learn to Create New Words."[12] Eve Clark says of these examples: "Children are much slower in mastering well-established verb meanings than they are in mastering noun meanings. . . . As a result, they have few verbs available early on for talking about a large range of actions. To communicate about particular actions, many children take up the option of coining new verbs from nouns where the noun in question designates one of the objects involved in the particular action being talked about. . . . The importance of such innovative verbs is that they allow small children—as young as 2—to be very precise, in context, about the actions they are talking about" (p. 322). Considering what we have said over the last several sections about how the child acquires language (for example, the role of action, context, making meaning visible), why might the child find the sorts of sentences below more appealing than their more adult-like versions (in parentheses)? How would such "errors" relate to the view of meaning as "videotapes" of salient actions and interactions stored in the mind?

1. You have to scale it.
   (= You have to weigh it.)
2. It's trucking.
   (= A truck is passing.)
3. String me up, Mommy.
   (= Tie my hat—hat is fastened with a bead and string.)

[12]In W. Deutsch, ed., *The Child's Construction of Language* (New York: Academic Press, 1981), pp. 299–328.

4. I'm crackering my soup.
(= I'm putting crackers in my soup.)

5. We're gonna cast it.
(= We are going to put it in a cast—role playing a doctor dealing with a broken arm.)

6. I'm sticking it and that makes it go really fast.
(= I'm hitting the ball with a stick and that makes it go really fast.)

8.7. ACQUISITION OF MORE COMPLEX STRUCTURES: PASSIVES

As children move past the two-word stage, they must begin to learn to control the full syntax of English, including the patterns necessary to ask questions ('Can I help you?', 'Who(m) can I help?'), embed sentences ('I think I can help', 'I want to help', 'I want Mary to help'), form a variety of other types of subordinate clauses ('When I wake up, I'll help you', 'I'll help you, because I like you'), form relative clauses ('The boy who gave me the sticker . . .') and passives ('The puppy was hurt by the baby'), and so on through many quite complex structures. This all demands mastering the syntactic rules of the language (for example, inverting helping verbs in questions—'I can help', 'Can I help?'). The child must also learn the full range of uses and meanings of function words and other grammatical morphemes in English (for example, 'the' in 'the dog', the plural endings on nouns and the past-tense endings on verbs, the possessive ending '-s' in 'John's book', 'that' in 'I think *that* I can help', 'to' in 'I want *to* help', the full range of helping verbs, prepositions, and adverbs, and so on).

These matters constitute a whole branch of the study of child language development and would take us too far afield if we discussed them in any depth. I will discuss the acquisition of one complex structure—passive sentences—to give you the flavor of the issues that arise.

Most English active, declarative sentences with a transitive verb ('The baby helped the mother') have passive variants ('The mother was helped by the baby'). Before the age of three or four, children do not understand passive sentences. To understand what happens after that age, we have to make a distinction between semantically "reversible" and semantically "irreversible" sentences. Semantically reversible sentences are sentences where both NPs in the sentence could plausibly act as ACTOR or PATIENT. For example, in 'The car hit the truck' (active) or 'The truck was hit by the car' (passive), the car is the ACTOR and the truck the PATIENT, but it is just as plausible that a truck hits a car as that a car hits a truck. Only the syntax of these sentences tells you what is the ACTOR and what the PATIENT. Semantically irreversible sentences are sentences where only one NP could plausibly act as ACTOR. For example, in 'The boy ate the hot dog' (active) or

'The hot dog was eaten by the boy' (passive), not only the syntax tells us that the boy is the ACTOR and the hot dog the PATIENT. Our knowledge of how the world works tells us that boys can eat hot dogs, but hot dogs cannot eat boys.

By three or four, children can understand irreversible passives (like 'The hot dog was eaten by the boy'), but not reversible ones (like 'The truck was hit by the car'). In fact, if asked to act out a reversible passive like 'The truck was hit by the car', children will have the truck push the car (which is the wrong interpretation). What appears to be going on is this: The children interpret the irreversible passive ('The hot dog was eaten by the boy') on the basis of their real-world knowledge (that boys eat hot dogs and hot dogs don't eat boys), not their knowledge of syntax. Faced with a reversible passive like 'The truck was hit by the car', they cannot fall back on real-world knowledge, since cars can hit trucks and trucks can hit cars. In this case they use a word-order strategy (which, in fact, leads to wrong results). They know that English uses predominantly NP verb NP sequences that, in active sentences, mean 'ACTOR action PATIENT'. Consequently, when they hear a reversible passive sentence like 'The truck was hit by the car' that they cannot figure out by real-world knowledge, they ignore 'was' and 'by' and treat the sentence as if it was an active sentence.

By four or five, children properly understand both reversible and irreversible passives. They now use the syntax of the sentence to decode it, not just their real-world knowledge or a word-order strategy that takes any sequence of NP verb NP to be 'ACTOR action PATIENT'. However, for some reason, this is true only of sentences with action verbs (like 'hit', 'push', or 'kiss'). If the passive has a nonaction verb (like 'love' in 'John was loved by Mary'), then many five-year-olds still do not understand it. Only by middle childhood do they completely understand, and productively use, passive sentences.

The acquisition of the passive demonstrates many of our basic themes in this chapter. Children faced with a structure they do not know (like the passive) first try to figure out what it means from the context of action and social interaction around them. Thus, they can figure out 'The cat ate the hot dog' because they can probably see the cat eating the hot dog and because they know cats eat and hot dogs don't. If they cannot rely on the setting to help them figure out the meaning of a sentence, they rely on fairly specific patterns that they have generalized from the data. In the case of 'The truck was hit by the car' they rely on the pattern that says that any NP verb NP sequence is 'ACTOR action PATIENT', a generalization that is wrong here, but, of course, right in many other cases (for most active sentences).

Eventually, children have to move beyond using real-world knowledge and specific and simple patterns. They have to learn that the helping verb 'was' in 'The truck was hit by the car' signals that the verb is passive and thus its subject, which is normally an ACTOR, is in this case a PATIENT. They also have to learn that the little word 'by' marks the NP 'the truck' as the ACTOR, despite the fact that it is not where ACTORS usually are (in English). But action continues to play a significant role for some time in children's language, since they understand passives with nonactional verbs still later (like 'Mary was loved by John'), perhaps because they "act out" sentences in their heads as a backup to their understanding of their syntax.

EXERCISES

Exercise I. Why would young children have trouble understanding a sentence like 'John received a gift from Mary'?

Exercise J. Why do you think that children often interpret a sentence like 1a below as 1b, which is the correct interpretation, but interpret a sentence like 2a below as 2b, which is the wrong interpretation? (We can tell how they interpret such sentences by asking them to act them out with toys and puppets.)[13]

1a. The cat that bit the dog ate the rat.

1b. The cat bit the dog and the cat ate the rat.

2a. The cat bit the dog that chased the rat.

2b. The cat bit the dog and the cat chased the rat.

8.8.   CHILD-DIRECTED SPEECH

In many cultures, and, in particular, in the middle-class American homes that have been until recently the focus of most research on child language development, parents do not talk to their small children the way they talk to their adult peers. They "simplify" their speech to their children. And many investigators have argued that this sort of simplified speech plays a role in how the child acquires language. In middle-class American homes, for the most part, it was mothers who spent the most time talking and interacting with small children, so this sort of simplified speech to children (sometimes called "baby talk") used to be called "motherese." However, we now realize that it is not just mothers, but all adults and even children as young as 4 and 5 years of age, who produce simplified, redundant speech when addressing 16- to 36-month-olds. Thus, I will call such speech **child-directed speech.**[14]

---

[13]This data is based on work by Susan L. Tavakolian, *Structure and Function in Child Language,* doctoral dissertation, University of Massachusetts at Amherst, 1977.

[14]Following Catherine Snow in her paper "Conversations with Children," in P. Fletcher and M. Garman, eds., *Language Acquisition,* 2nd ed. (New York: Cambridge University Press, 1986), pp. 69–89. Much of the discussion below is based on Snow's work.

Child-directed speech is simpler in terms of the length of individual utterances and in terms of its grammatical complexity (for example, less subordinate clauses are used in speech to children). It is also more fluent and contains less false starts, disfluencies, and hesitations than speech to adults. Furthermore, child-directed speech is highly redundant; adults frequently repeat themselves and paraphrase their utterances. Some adults use certain "sentence frames" quite frequently (for example, '*That's* NP'; '*Where's* NP'; '*See* NP').

It is possible that child-directed speech is partly an adjustment made in response to cues from the child. If adult speech is too complex for them, children can become inattentive and fail to comply with requests or respond to questions. These cues may cause adults to simplify their speech until it reaches a level of complexity at which the child is optimally attentive.

We have seen above that in the initial stages of language learning, meaning must be rendered visible for the child through overt actions and clear and repeated social interactions (rituals/routines). When the children are faced with a word or syntactic pattern they do not understand, they use the meaning they do understand from overt actions and clear social contexts to decode and eventually learn the new word or new syntactic pattern.

As part of this overall process of rendering meaning clear and accessible, adults limit their utterances to the present tense, to concrete nouns, to comments on what the child is doing and on what is happening around the child. Adults make statements and ask questions about what things are called, what noises things make, what color they are, what actions they are engaging in, who they belong to, where they are located, and very little else. This is a very restricted set of things to talk about when one considers that older children and adults also discuss past and future events, necessity, possibility, probability, consequence, implication, comparison, and many other abstract topics. This limitation on the semantic content of child-directed speech can, to a large extent, explain its syntactic simplicity. Such concrete and simple content can be easily expressed in short utterances without subordination or other syntactic complexities.

The most interesting and significant finding in the literature on child-directed speech is that children's language development is facilitated when adults and older peers engage in certain practices that are often part of child-directed speech. These practices include situations where the adult takes the telegraphic utterances of the young child and expands them into full and correct sentences. Investigators used to think that this worked because the adult was giving "grammar lessons" to the child in showing the child the whole adult sentences he or she was "aiming" at. However, we now know that if the adult merely provides extra conversation with the child built around the child's utterances, this will facilitate language acquisition just as well.

In fact, it turns out that the most facilitative practice an adult can engage in is what has been called *semantic expansions* of the child's language. Such expansions don't just fill out the structure of what the child has said, rather they incorporate the child's topic into the adult utterances and then add new information to it. Research has shown that the percentage of adult utterances that are *semantically related* to preceding child utterances is the best predictor of the child's linguistic ability and that there is a high correlation between the percentage of adult speech related to child activities and the size of the child's vocabulary. This implies that children who learn to talk quickly and well have considerable, if not constant, access to semantically related adult utterances.

The following breakfast-table conversation between a 29-month-old and his parents is a good example of adults expanding a child's language and in particular engaging in semantic expansions.[15]

Child: pancakes away
duh duh stomach
Mother: pancakes away in the stomach, yes, that's right
Child: eat apples
Mother: eating apples on our pancakes, aren't we?
Child: on our pancakes
Mother: you like apples on your pancakes?
Child: eating apples
hard
Mother: what?
hard to do the apples, isn't it?
Child: more pancakes
Father: you want more pancakes?
Child: those are daddy's
Father: daddy's gonna have his pancakes now
Child: ne ne one a daddy's
ne ne one in the plate
right there
Father: you want some more on your plate?

We do not know exactly how such semantically contingent expansions work to promote language development. However, it appears that information about the structure of language is more useful to the child if it is presented in utterances that express the child's own intentions or that are related to topics of the child's choice.

The role of such semantically contingent expansions has been called into question by the discovery that many non-Western cultures, and many non-middle-class social groups in the U.S., do not engage in such practices. And, of course, their children acquire a native language with all the skill and mastery that any child does.

Not all cultures are willing to adapt adult speech to children, and not all cultures have the high regard for verbal precocity that middle-class Americans

[15]From Catherine Snow's paper cited above, p. 82.

often do. In some societies, for example among the Kipsigis of Kenya and rural Blacks of Louisiana, children's comprehension skills are valued more highly than their verbal production. Most speech addressed to children in these cultures consists of directives and explanations, rather than questions or comments on their activity. Among some cultures, for a variety of cultural reasons, semantically contingent expansions of children's language is not only rare, but culturally inappropriate (for example, among the Kaluli of Papua, New Guinea, and among Samoans).

However, in these cultures there may well be social facilitators other than semantic expansion, facilitators that work just as well. Although Kaluli mothers, for instance, do not provide their children with semantically contingent speech, it would be incorrect to conclude that they pay no attention to language learning. In fact, the Kaluli believe that quite explicit help and teaching is required if children are to develop beyond their immature language forms into competent speakers. Their techniques for teaching involve a considerable amount of direct modeling, with instructions to imitate. The utterances presented for imitation are meant to be used by the child for carrying out effective social interaction, and they are not simplified or otherwise adapted to the child's language level. The parent insists only that the child utter such models, not that he or she necessarily comprehend them.

For example, when a five-year-old Kaluli child named Beinalia took too much food, her mother said to her 27-month-old brother Wanu, "Whose is it? Say like that," and Wanu then said "Whose is it?". The mother then said "Is it yours? Say like that" and Wanu said "Is it yours?", and so on for several more turns. Wanu may not have fully understood what he was saying, but—as in our examples of rituals and routines above—he was being inserted into a social interaction in a way that supported him and rendered him successful beyond his abilities on his own.[16]

Here we get to the heart of the matter, perhaps. The actual type of interactional support, whether semantic expansion or direct modeling or something else, that a culture gives its children is not important. But that children get some social support is crucial. Think of the child as an apprentice, apprenticed to the language mastery of the adults and older peers. There are many ways for the master carpenter to pass on his or her skills to an apprentice, but they all involve letting the apprentice practice those skills in tandem with the master, supported by the master, and in ways that allow the apprentice to carry out tasks that he or she could not accomplish alone. The situation appears to be no different in language development, and, indeed, no different in the later development of literacy.

The master places the apprentice in recurrent situations, whose context and structure of action and interaction is clear and well known, allowing the apprentice to practice the subskills of a larger skill over and over again in a

---

[16]See Snow's paper cited earlier, pp. 85–86, and references therein.

supportive environment. This is what we saw when we discussed rituals and routines above, and what we are seeing when we look at semantic expansions in middle-class American homes, or direct modeling and imitation in Kaluli homes.[17]

Semantically contingent adult speech, rituals and routines, direct modeling and imitations all constitute instances of highly predictable situation-specific adult speech. They occur in different cultural and social settings but all have one thing in common: They allow speech to be highly comprehensible even without a complete grammatical analysis. The child can understand the meanings of sentences whose structure he or she does not yet fully understand, and this semantic understanding ultimately leads to understanding the new syntactic structure.

However, we are left with a deep paradox. We argued at the beginning of this chapter that there is a human biological capacity for language that guides the course of language acquisition. The fact that language acquisition occurs successfully in such a wide variety of cultural settings would seem to show that it is biologically programmed and indifferent to the nature of the different social environments in which it is acquired. This would lead us to believe that it would show no facilitative effects based on how parents talk to their children, since this is an aspect of the social environment and varies across cultures. But it does indeed show such social facilitative effects. That it does show these effects paradoxically suggests, then, that it is sensitive to environmental effects. This seems to conflict with the earlier claims about biological programming (and the empirical fact that language is successfully acquired in such diverse settings across the world).

We certainly have not as of yet resolved this paradox. But our discussion clearly indicates that language acquisition requires both a rich lead from biology and certain socializing experiences. These experiences differ across cultures but have in common that they ultimately insert the child into a social world that renders language meaningful.

EXERCISE

Exercise K.   Record yourself or a friend telling the story below to a fellow adult and then to a six- or seven-year-old child (read the story several times, then put it aside and tell it in your own words). If you cannot get a hold of a child, have your friend or yourself role play talking to a six- or seven-year-old child (if you are

---

[17]The view of learning as based on apprenticeship is developed, in somewhat different terms but brilliantly, in the Soviet psychologist Lev Vygotsky's work. Vygotsky is one of the major developmental psychologists of the twentieth century—his work is available in English translation: for example, see L. S. Vygotsky, *Mind in Society: The Development of Higher Psychological Processes* (Cambridge, Mass.: Harvard University Press, 1978).

recording a friend, do not stay in the room when he or she is role playing talk to a child; just leave the recorder running). Discuss the differences between the way the story was told to the adult and the way it was told to the child. Why do you think that these specific differences occurred?

THE FOX AND THE BEAR

There once was a fox and bear who were friends. One day they decided to catch a chicken for supper. They decided to go together because neither one wanted to be left alone and they both liked fried chicken. They waited until night time. Then they ran very quickly to a nearby farm where they knew chickens lived. The bear, who felt very lazy, climbed up on the roof to watch. The fox then opened the door to the hen house very carefully. He grabbed a chicken and killed it. As he was carrying it out of the hen house the weight of the bear on the roof caused the roof to crack. The fox heard the noise and was frightened, but it was too late to run out. The roof and the bear fell in, killing five of the chickens. The fox and the bear were trapped in the broken hen house. Soon the farmer came out to see what was the matter.

RECOMMENDED FURTHER READING

BEEBE, LESLIE M., ED. (1988). *Issues in Second Language Acquisition: Multiple Perspectives.* New York: Newbury House. (A good introduction to issues in second-language acquisition; deals with psycholinguistics, sociolinguistics, neurolinguistics, bilingualism, and education.)

FLETCHER, PAUL & GARMAN, MICHAEL, EDS. (1986). *Language Acquisition,* 2nd ed. New York: Cambridge University Press. (Excellent readings on current issues.)

FRANKLIN, MARGERY B. & BARTEN, SYBIL S., EDS. (1988). *Child Language: A Reader.* Oxford & New York: Oxford University Press. (A collection of classic papers.)

GLEASON, JEAN BERKO, ED. (1989). *The Development of Language,* 2nd ed. Columbus, Ohio: Merrill. (An introduction to language development, each chapter dealing with a different aspect.)

GOODLUCK, HELEN (1991). *Language Acquisition: A Linguistic Introduction.* Oxford: Basil Blackwell. (A good introduction to various aspects of language acquisition, including phonology, morphology, syntax, semantics, and cognition, with an emphasis on ties to aspects of linguistic theory.)

KESSEL, FRANK S., ED. (1988). *The Development of Language and Language Researchers: Essays in Honor of Roger Brown.* Hillsdale, N.J.: Erlbaum. (A readable set of papers by Roger Brown's students from over the years—

many of whom are now leaders in the field—about their work and the development of the field.)

OCHS, ELINOR (1988). *Culture and Language Development: Language Acquisition and Language Socialization in a Samoan Village.* New York: Cambridge University Press. (Excellent and accessible study of the interaction between language acquisition and socialization.)

ROMAINE, SUZANNE (1984). *The Language of Children and Adolescents: The Acquisition of Communicative Competence.* Oxford & New York: Blackwell. (A good introduction to language development after early childhood, especially in its social setting.)

CHAPTER 9

Language, History, and Society

9.1. DIALECTS AND STANDARD LANGUAGE

It is clear that not everyone in the United States speaks alike. We are all aware that President John Kennedy from Massachusetts spoke differently than President Lyndon Johnson from Texas. When two people speak the same language, but vary in aspects of grammar, vocabulary, and pronunciation, they speak different **dialects** of that language. When they share the same grammar and vocabulary, but differ only in their pronunciation of the language, they have different **accents.** This distinction between dialects and accents is not always relevant to my discussion, and when it isn't, I will use the term 'dialect' to refer to both.

In many societies, certain ways of pronouncing the language become prestigious, while other ways are looked down on. It is often assumed by nonlinguists that prestigious pronunciations are inherently better or more pleasing. However, other factors in society, having nothing to do with sound or language, determine what will be considered prestigious and what not. This is clear if we note that the prestige form of one language area can turn out to be the stigmatized form of another. In the prestige form of English in New York City, there is a clearly audible [r] sound after the vowel in words like 'car', 'north', and 'guard'. But in Great Britain the audible inclusion of this [r] sound in this position is not prestigious, and sounds "rustic" or even comic, being primarily associated with patterns of pronunciation in rural southwest England. Even in New York, there has been a reversal in social evaluation in the history of the /r/ sound. Before the Second World War, failing to pronounce an [r] after the vowel in words like 'car', 'card', and 'guard' had high status and was used by members of all social classes. However, by at least the 1960s, failing to pronounce [r] after vowels had become associated with casual style and lower social status. Thus, whether a certain feature in a dialect is prestigious or not is determined only by the prestige the speakers of that dialect have in the society based on their influence, wealth, or power, for instance.

We have concentrated so far on matters of pronunciation, but the same point can be made for grammar: The prestige of particular variants is socially motivated and linguistically arbitrary. To use 'what' as a relative pronoun, as in 'the house what I saw', is neither more nor less efficient, neither better nor worse in any objective sense, than to use the more prestigious form 'the house which I saw'. It is simply that some dialects of English use the item 'what' as a part of their relative pronoun system, while others do not.

Standard Language

There is a variety of English in the U.S. used widely on the public media (movies, radio, television) and in schools and other public institutions. This variety is called **Standard English.** It is the most prestigious form of English in the U.S. (though it differs from the standard and prestigious form in Great Britain, for instance). Because people across the country hear this dialect and are influenced by it, their own local dialects tend not to vary too much from this standard. Thus, in comparison to other times and places, the dialects of American English are not all that different from each other.

Why should a society—as many do—have one dialect that is singled out as standard and prestigious, especially since there is no objective linguistic reason why this dialect is any better than the others spoken in the society? Standardization is motivated by social, political, and commercial needs. A large, pluralistic society like the U.S. needs to standardize its units of money and its weights and measures. It would create chaos if every city or state had its own money, for instance. Language is also a medium of exchange, although a much more complex system than money, and the aim of language standardization is the same: to ensure fixed values for the counters (whether dollars or words) in a system. In language, this means preventing variability in spelling and pronunciation by selecting certain forms to count as "correct." It means establishing "correct" meanings of words ('aggravate', for example, is determined to mean *make more serious,* not *annoy,* despite the fact that most people use it also to mean the latter) and uniquely acceptable word forms ('he does' is acceptable, but 'he do' is not). It means fixing certain sentence forms as "acceptable" (for example, 'the house which I saw') and others as "unacceptable" ('the house what I saw'). These "decisions" are not usually made by a body of people sitting down and deciding such matters. Rather, as a society gets complex enough to require a standard dialect, the dialect associated with the influential and powerful in the society is gradually adopted as the standard or correct form. We should note, however, that there are various regionally defined variations in how English that counts as "standard" and prestigious is pronounced. For simplicity's sake I will ignore these for now.

There is, in a sense, no one who actually speaks what we have been calling standard English. While one can come close to obtaining uniformity in the written language, this is much harder in spoken language. Even so-called standard English incorporates variability and change. What Standard English actually is thought to be depends on the acceptance (mainly by the most influential people in the society) of a common core of linguistic conventions. There will always remain a good deal of fuzziness around the edges. All of us deviate in some ways from what is considered (even, in some instances, by ourselves) Standard English. Therefore, it may be more appropriate to speak of a standard language as an idea in the mind rather than a reality. It is in fact a set of abstract norms to which actual usage may conform to a greater or lesser extent.

The historical process by which a dialect becomes standard often runs something like the following: A variety of the language is selected as a standard through the course of time, usually a variety used by an influential group or used in a powerful and influential part of the country. This variety is then spread geographically and socially by various means (official newspapers, the educational system, the writing system, discrimination of various kinds against nonstandard speakers). As this variety is diffused across the society as a whole, it becomes necessary to use it in writing and as much as possible in speech to attain power, influence, and prestige in the society. It also gains more uses or functions than more local dialects (for example, its functions to speak and write about technology and science) and thus expands in vocabulary and to some extent in structure to serve these new functions. It is also eventually codified by being put into grammar books and dictionaries, and these books become regarded as "authorities." People come to believe that the language is enshrined in these books (no matter how many mistakes and omissions they may contain), rather than in the linguistic and communicative competence of the people who use the language every day. However, these books rarely keep pace with the inevitable changes that occur in even a standard dialect as society and technology changes.

While the existence of a standard dialect can make for efficiency and bind a society together, it can also be used to discriminate against people and to uphold an unjust social hierarchy. Ultimately, schools are the guardians of standard language, the place where it is originally transmitted and thereafter maintained. Families who over time have access to good schools and long-term schooling (college) eventually adopt standard English as the language of the home. Their children go to school already equipped with the foundations of the variety of language the school uses and rewards. These children further expand that language at school, and usually succeed in school.

On the other hand, families that over time do not have access to good schools or to long-term schooling retain their own local and community-based dialects (though they are, of course, inevitably influenced by school-based language to some degree). Their children do not go to school with the foundations of school-based language, and they face a somewhat harder task than the children discussed in the preceding paragraph. Their children succeed in school less often and get less quality schooling. They are thus less influenced by standard, school-based language practices, and tend to get less good, less powerful, and less influential positions in society.

However, it is not just dialect differences at the grammatical level that matter here. Even more crucial are differences in the way that language is organized at the discourse level (in conversations, descriptions, arguments, narratives, and so forth). Discourse differences are intimately tied to how people make sense of the world and each other. We will discuss these matters in Chapter 10.

Black Vernacular English

All dialects of a language are rule governed and reflect the mastery that all children achieve when they learn their native language. Nonetheless, because of social prejudice, some people in the U.S. believe that some dialects of English are inferior to others. The dialect that is, perhaps, the victim of the most social prejudice is that spoken by many lower-socioeconomic black Americans. This dialect is often referred to by linguists as **black vernacular English** (**BVE** for short).

We will see below that any dialect is spoken in several different forms, depending on the degree of informality or formality the speaker wishes to achieve. Furthermore, black Americans who speak BVE usually can "shift" their dialect toward standard English depending on whether they are talking to a fellow black who speaks BVE or to a white or black who does not.

Many people confuse BVE, which white people rarely if ever hear in its form most distinctive from standard English, with "black slang." This is wholly inaccurate. Slang exists in almost all groups as a distinctive vocabulary used to mark oneself as an insider. BVE is a dialect with its own distinctive set of grammatical rules, not just a distinctive vocabulary. BVE is probably the dialect of English that is most different from standard English. However, it is nonetheless very similar to standard English and in almost all respects mutually intelligible with standard English. There are only a few places where its difference from standard English can cause real miscommunication and confusion.

Black people who speak BVE do not do so because they are poor, though poverty helps the dialect to survive. BVE survives in urban ghettos and in the rural South because of patterns of segregation. This causes black people to talk much more often to each other than to blacks and whites from middle- and upper-class communities. This allows them to keep a distinctive dialect. BVE has its origins in a dialect of English spoken by the slaves in early America. While it has changed a great deal over the years under the influence of standard English, it remains a separate and distinctive dialect of English.

Relation of Black Vernacular English to Standard English

BVE, like many languages around the world, often leaves out the copula (the verb 'to be') when it would occur in the present tense in standard English. Thus, where standard English would say 'She is hungry' or 'She's hungry', BVE says 'She hungry'. In the past tense, both dialects say 'She was hungry'.

This difference makes BVE appear more different from standard English than it actually is. We can see this if we consider the data below, where an asterisk (*) in front of a sentence indicates that that sentence is ungrammatical in the dialect concerned. This data will allow us to understand the way in which dialects of languages tend to be related to each other.

	BVE		Standard English
1a.	She hungry	*1b.*	She's hungry
2a.	I leaving	*2b.*	I'm leaving
3a.	I know who he is	*3b.*	I know who he is
4a.	*I know who he	*4b.*	*I know who he's
5a.	That where he is	*5b.*	That's where he is
6a.	*That where he	*6b.*	*That's where he's

In standard English most sentences with a copula in the present tense can occur in two forms. The verb 'to be' can be kept as a separate word (as in 'She is hungry') or it can be contracted (as in 'She's hungry'). When it is contracted, the copula (for example, 'is' in 1b or 'am' in 2b) is phonologically reduced and said as part of the subject (represented in spelling as 'she's' or 'I'm'). However, there are cases where standard English does not allow the copula to contract. Though one can say 3b 'I know who he is' with 'is' uncontracted, one cannot contract it in this position and say 4b *'I know who he's'. This is simply ungrammatical. Similarly, while one can say 5b 'That's where he is' with uncontracted 'is' at the end of the sentence, one cannot contract this 'is' and get 6b *'That's where he's'.

The data above clearly shows a generalization about the relation between BVE and standard English: Wherever standard English allows the copula to contact (as in 1b and 2b), BVE allows the copula to be absent (as in 1a and 2a). Wherever standard English does not allow the copula to contract (as in 4b and 6b), BVE will not allow the copula to be absent (as in 4a and 6a). In these latter cases, both standard English and BVE use the full form of the copula (as in 3a and b 'I know who he is').

We see here a deep similarity between the two dialects, but a similarity that is not apparent by a mere superficial view of the data. The absent copula in BVE corresponds exactly to the contracted copula in standard English. The difference is relatively trivial, and in fact the BVE way of doing things here is at least as common, if not more so, across the world's languages as is the standard English way of doing it.

——————————————— E X E R C I S E ———————————————

Exercise A. The data below is from two varieties of English spoken in Singapore. The variety labeled "acrolect" is the most prestigious and formal variety of Singapore English. It is very similar to standard English in the U.S. and Great Britain. The variety labeled "basilect" is the variety of Singapore English that is most different from standard English. For each set of sentences below, state clearly and explicitly what the difference is between these two varieties of English. Can you make any generalizations about how the basilect differs from the acrolect? (NOTE: The basilect looks more different from standard English because basilect speakers have less contact with native speakers of standard English. Thus, they are freer to introduce changes into the language, changes that resemble the sorts of linguistic features that creole speakers introduce into their languages—we will discuss creoles below.)[1]

ACROLECT:

1a. You can't (or cannot) smoke here.
You can't (or cannot) wear shoes here.
This one you can't (or cannot) borrow.

BASILECT:

1b. Here cannot smoke.
Here cannot wear shoe.
This one cannot borrow.

ACROLECT:

2a. He lost his job because of his age.
I cannot buy it because I haven't got enough money.
The child was scolded for being late.

BASILECT:

2b. He old so lose his job.
Money not enough so cannot buy.
The child late so got scolded.

---

[1]The data for this problem is adapted from J. C. Richards, "Form and Function in Second Language Learning: An Example from Singapore," in R. Andersen, ed., *New Dimensions in Second Language Acquisition Research* (Rowley, Mass.: Newbury House, 1981).

ACROLECT:

3a. I have been working for six months.
I left school three months ago.
My father has passed away.

BASILECT:

3b. I worked six months already.
I left school already three months.
My father already pass away.

ACROLECT

4a. Your wife is Margaret, isn't she?
You are staying in the hotel, aren't you?
You want another coffee, don't you?

BASILECT

4b. Your wife Margaret, isn't it?
You staying hotel, isn't it?
You want one more coffee, isn't it?

Black Vernacular English, Language Change, and Language Design

Many rules in BVE are like the one we looked at above: BVE takes a tendency that exists in standard English (for example, to reduce the copula by contraction) and carries it farther (have no copula at all). Many phonological differences are like this as well. For example, standard English has a tendency to reduce consonant clusters at the ends of words in fast speech. Therefore, words like 'past', 'lost', and 'desk' are often said in fast speech as [paes], [las], and [dɛs], respectively. BVE carries this tendency further, pronouncing these words without the final consonant, yet more commonly (and in the case of some black children) using a form like /dɛs/ as the normal and regular pronunciation.

However, there are some areas where standard English and BVE differ more significantly. In these areas, BVE can teach us something important about the relationship between the dialects of a language and the way that language changes through time. BVE uses a form of the verb 'to be' that is not used in standard English—it is "bare," in that it is not inflected for tense (as 'am/is/are' are for the present tense or 'was/were' are for the past are). The BVE bare 'be' is seen in an example like 'My puppy, he always *be* following me'. Since this form does not exist in standard English, many speakers of standard English assume it is a mistake, or "poor English," and go on to draw the ridiculous conclusion that black children do not speak English well. However, the form has a meaning in BVE and is governed by rules, like any form in any dialect or language.

To understand how this bare 'be' form is used and to grasp its significance for language change, we must first explicate a part of the English ASPECT system. 'Aspect' is a term that stands for how a language signals the viewpoint it takes on the way in which an action is situated in time. Almost all languages make a primary distinction between the PERFECTIVE ASPECT and the IMPERFECTIVE ASPECT. The imperfective aspect is used when the action is viewed as ongoing or repeated. English uses the PROGRESSIVE (the verb 'to be' plus the ending '-ing' on the following verb) to mark the imperfective, as in 'John is working' or 'Mary is jumping'. In the first of these sentences, John's working is viewed as ongoing, still in progress; in the second, Mary's jumping is viewed as having being repeated over and over again. In 'John was working' or 'Mary was jumping', John's working is viewed as something that was extended in time or ongoing in the past, and Mary's jumping as something that was repeated over and over in the past.

The perfective, on the other hand, is used when an action is viewed as a discrete whole, treated as if it is a point in time (whether or not in reality the act took a significant amount of time). English uses the simple present or past for the perfective, as in 'Boggs dives for the ball!' (sports cast), in the present, or 'Boggs dived for the ball', in the past. The imperfective of these sentences would be 'Boggs is diving for the ball' and 'Boggs was diving for the ball'.

BVE and standard English do not differ in the perfective, though an older form of BVE used to distinguish between a simple perfective ('John drank the milk') and a COMPLETIVE that stressed that the action was finished, complete, and done with ('John done drank the milk up'). However, BVE and standard English do differ in the imperfective. Young black speakers make a distinction between ongoing or repeated events that are of *limited* duration and ongoing or repeated events that are of *extended duration*. For limited duration events they use the absent copula we saw above, and for extended events they use the bare 'be' we have discussed here. Thus, note the following contrast in BVE:[2]

Limited Duration Events

7a. In health class, we talking about the eye
    (standard English: 'In health class, we are talking about the eye')

7b. He trying to scare us
    (standard English: 'He is trying to scare us')

---

[2]Examples are based on those given in Guy Bailey and Natalie Maynor, "Decreolization?", *Language in Society,* 16 (1987), 449–73.

Extended Duration Events

8a. He always be fighting
  (standard English: 'He is always fighting')

8b. Sometimes them big boys be throwing the ball, and . . .
  (standard English: 'Sometimes those big boys are throwing the ball, and . . .')

In 7a, the talk about the eye in health class will go on only for a short while compared to the duration of the whole class. Thus, the speaker uses the absent 'be' form ('we talking'). In 7b, his trying to scare us neither lasts a long time nor is a regular, repeated occurrence, so once again the speaker uses the absent 'be' ('he trying'). On the other hand, in 8a, the fighting is always taking place, is something that 'he' characteristically does; thus the speaker uses the bare 'be' form ('he be fighting'). And in 8b, the speaker is talking about a situation that has happened often and will in all likelihood continue to happen. Thus, she uses the bare 'be' ('big boys be throwing'). Standard English makes no such contrast.

Two things are particularly interesting about this contrast made in BVE. First, it is one that is made in many languages. Second, older black speakers did not use bare 'be' in this way, but somewhat differently. The current generation of young black people is redrawing their dialect to make this distinction, using forms that existed in BVE (the absent 'be' and the bare 'be'), but with somewhat different uses. That is, they are changing their language, as all children have done through all the time language has been around. It is as if they have (unconsciously) seen a gap or hole in the English system (the failure to mark clearly in the imperfective a distinction between limited and extended duration) and filled it in.

This is one of the major ways languages change through time. Children invent distinctions that they think (unconsciously) should be in the language. Languages are changing all the time, losing and gaining various contrasts. If a language loses the ability to draw a certain contrast, and it seems to be an important one from the point of view of humans looking at the world, children may well replace it.

But one might ask, why has the nonstandard dialect introduced this distinction, and not also the standard dialect? A standard dialect changes more slowly—this dialect is the one used in writing and public media, and this puts something of a brake on change. This is good in that the dialect remains relatively constant across time, thus serving the purposes of standardization (much as a uniform money system does). However, since nonstandard dialects are freer to change on the basis of the human child's linguistic and cognitive systems, nonstandard dialects are, in a sense, often "more logical" or "more elegant" from a linguistic point of view (from the view of what is typical across languages or from the view of what seems to be the basic design of the human linguistic system).

9.2. VARIATION IN LANGUAGE AND THE SOCIAL HIERARCHY

In every dialect there exist alternative ways to say the same thing. We saw above that both BVE and standard English can pronounce a word like 'desk' as [dɛsk] or [dɛs], in the latter case dropping the final consonant. Or, to take another example, all English dialects allow the speaker to pronounce the progressive as 'I'm *going* to work' with a full 'ing', or as 'I'm *goin'* to work', with 'ing' reduced to 'in'. Though many nonlinguists assume that such variation is either trivial or reflects "sloppiness" in pronunciation, neither is true. Rather, it is meaningful and functional.

There are two primary *social motivations* behind any use of language. Speakers are either seeking *status,* that is, seeking to identify with those they see as influential or powerful or otherwise high in status. Or they are seeking to signal *solidarity* with those people whom they see as their peers, their reference group, or otherwise like themselves. In reality, however, this is an oversimplification, since many uses of speech are a compromise between these two.

If I am speaking to my boss, who is worried that I will fail to do a certain job well, I might say "I assure you I will accomplish this task successfully." If I am speaking to my friend under the same circumstances, I might say "I'll get it done, don't sweat it." To say the latter to the boss would sound flippant and out of place. It would seem as if I were presuming to be her equal or intimate. To say the former to my friend would sound rude and distant. It would sound as if I was "putting on airs" and presuming to be better than my friend.

The first response ("I assure you I will accomplish this task successfully") is an attempt to assure the boss that I am a respectable and reputable person, worthy of her respect. It is an attempt to say "I belong in your world, a public world of prestige and power." I will call this a *status-seeking* use of language, with no denigration implied. The latter response ("I'll get it done, don't sweat it") is an attempt to assure my friend that I am "a good guy," a person who comfortably fits into the peer group, who belongs in the local community of friends. I will call this a *solidarity* use of language, where I bind myself to my local group. Since in reality all of us belong to several different groups, we must use our language in quite complex and subtle ways to signal our solidarity with, and membership in, various groups.

The distinction between status uses of language and solidarity ones can also be put in terms of a continuum ranging from *formal* uses of language to *informal* uses, with various mixtures in between. We use more formal language when we are using language to strangers, in public forums (like banks and schools), or when otherwise seeking to identify with the wider society and its centers of power and influence. We use less formal language with friends and intimates, and members of our local community, when we seek to identify with more local and community-based values.

If speakers are to signal various types of status and solidarity (various degrees of formality), they must have a language that gives them options between equivalent ways of saying the same thing (referentially speaking), but ways that differ in terms of their prestige value in the community, levels of formality, or associations with various socially defined groups. For example, as we mentioned above, English speakers can pronounce the '-ing' affix of the progressive either as 'ing' or 'in' (for example, 'I am looking into it', 'I'm lookin' into it'; note also the options with the contraction of 'am'). The 'ing' pronunciation is more formal and "standard language"; it notates that one is taking on a more formal, more public identity. The 'in' pronunciation, less formal and more colloquial, notates that one is taking on a more local, casual, intimate, "just one of the group" sort of identity.

There are literally hundreds of such variable elements in English pronunciation, morphology, and syntax. The use that English speakers make of this variability is a subtle indicator of their social class and social aspirations. Table 9-1 contains data on the use of 'ing' versus 'in' in Norwich, England.[3] The data in this table indicates a typical way in which such variability patterns in a speech community, a pattern that has been replicated many times over for a number of variables in a wide variety of speech communities in Great Britain and the United States.

Table 9-1 shows the percentage of 'in' forms used by speakers from different socioeconomic classes in various speech styles defined by differences in how formal or informal they are. The styles include (a) reading word lists (= WLS), where one carefully monitors one's speech; (b) reading a whole connected passage of prose (= RPS), which is also a fairly careful style; (c) answering direct questions in an interview with a stranger, that is, the researcher, where one uses

[3]From J. K. Chambers and P. J. Trudgill, *Dialectology* (New York: Cambridge University Press, 1980), p. 71; also reprinted in J. Milroy and L. Milroy, *Authority in Language* (London: Routledge, 1985), p. 95.

TABLE 9-1.   Percentage of '–in'' in Norwich, Shown According to Style and Class

	WLS	RPS	FS	CS
Middle middle class	0	0	3	28
Lower middle class	0	10	15	42
Upper working class	5	15	74	87
Middle working class	23	44	88	95
Lower working class	29	66	98	100

WLS = word list style
RPS = reading passage style
FS = formal style (direct questions in interview)
CS = casual style (attention diverted away from recording)

From *Dialectology* (p. 71), by J. K. Chambers and P. J. Trudgill, 1980 (New York: Cambridge University Press). Copyright 1980 by Cambridge University Press. Reprinted by permission.

fairly formal language (= FS), since the stranger is not a friend or member of one's group, but less formal language than in reading; and (d) free talk, where the speaker has gotten caught up in a story and is not paying attention to the fact that he or she is being recorded (= CS). In this latter casual style the speaker does not carefully monitor his or her speech, but speaks in a manner fairly close to local community norms.

The social classes are divided into two groups of middle-class people (middle middle and lower middle) and three groups of working-class people (upper, middle, and working). Social class can be computed in several ways, based on employment, amount of education, income, or parent's employment, education or income, or various combinations of these. I will use the term 'social class' fairly vaguely here, since an explication of this complicated notion is beyond the scope this book. Let me point out only that a society like the U.S. (or any other modern, technological, pluralistic society, for that matter) falls into groups of people who differ in how much power, influence, or wealth they have (all of which represent access to prestige in our society). Furthermore, these different groups tend to communicate more and share more background knowledge and experience with each other than they do with members of other groups. It turns out that however we define social class, the sorts of linguistic facts stated below remain true.

What we see in data like that in Table 9-1 is that every social class uses more 'ing' forms in more formal styles, and more 'in' forms in less formal styles. Thus, the highest class uses no 'in' forms in the most formal style (WPS), but 28% of the time uses 'in' in the least formal style (casual style). The lowest class uses fewer 'in' forms in the most formal style (29% in word list style) than in the least formal style (100% in casual style). This is a *style* difference, showing us that 'ing' is the formal (and prestigeful) form and 'in' the informal (and less prestigious) form. This is true for all members of the community. The fact that all members of the community, regardless of their social class, view 'ing' (formal) and 'in' (informal) in the same way, along with hundreds or thousands of other such variable items, is what makes them members of one wider *speech community,* regardless of their dialect differences.

But we can also clearly see from Table 9-1 that in addition to a style difference, there is a *social class* difference. The lower one's social class, the more one uses 'in' forms regardless of style (degree of formality). Thus, the lowest social class uses more 'in' forms (29%) in their most formal style (word list style) than the highest class does in their most casual, informal style (28% in casual style). The fact that members of all social classes shift toward 'ing' in more formal styles shows they are one speech community. The *amount* of 'in' versus 'ing' they use in any single style subtly marks their membership in a particular social class. The sort of data in Table 9-1 can be repeated for many other linguistic variables.

One way to think of the data we have seen is as follows: Every member of a speech community, regardless of social class, has a set of *public norms* that represents his or her *norms* or standards for what counts as prestigious language in his or her speech community. These public norms reflect much more closely the way people from the middle and upper social classes actually speak (in any given style) than the way members of the lower social classes speak, though no one's speech ever perfectly reflects the public norms. In highly formal styles, where the speaker wants to seek status (to identify with the wider society and the people who have power and influence in it), the speaker runs his or her speech through the public norms, almost as if they were a *filter,* replacing unprestigious forms (such as 'in' or [dɛs] for 'desk') with more prestigious ones ('ing' or [dɛs]). Since the actual informal day-to-day pronunciation of the higher classes is closer to public norms, they have less to replace than the lower classes (in psychological term, less cognitive "work" to do). Inevitably then, the lower classes will still have more of the low-prestige forms, since they have more to filter out.

Each speaker also has a *vernacular community-based norm.* When speaking to members of his or her own group in comfortable ("private") settings, the speaker does not run his or her language through the above filter representing public norms, and thus allows the community's norm for the balance between 'ing' and 'in' to be achieved (which for some groups is nearly all 'in', for others nearly all 'ing', for still others more of a mixture between them). This reflects the speaker's desire to identify with, and show solidarity with, his or her own group.

But there are many cases in between, situations between the most formal and least formal contexts. These are cases where one wants to balance status seeking in the wider public world, on the one hand, and solidarity with one's own group, on the other—cases where one wants to balance the public norms and the vernacular community-based norms. In these cases, the speaker runs his or her language through the "public norm filter" to lesser degrees (or, if you like, uses a filter with a wider mesh, one that doesn't strain the soup so thin) than in the most formal cases. We thus get varieties that have less 'in' than the vernacular community-based norm (due to the public norm filter) but more than the most formal, public style (due to the lesser use of the filter). We see, then, a compromise, one that is balanced more toward the public norm or more toward the speaker's vernacular community-based norm, depending on his or her assessment of the situation and its place on a continuum between highly formal and highly informal uses of language.

We should remember that there is nothing at all inherently or logically better about 'ing' for the progressive than 'in'. It is just that one has historically arisen as the prestige norm, the other hasn't (the system would work the same if the values of 'ing' and 'in' were reversed, and the higher classes said 'in' more often).

This picture of language variation argues that each member of each social class in the society has internalized a set of *public norms* about what counts as "correct" speech. These norms represent what each member of the society *thinks* the middle- and upper-class groups speak like. For example, each person of a

TABLE 9-2. **Percentage of *'in''* in Norwich, According to Sex and Social Class of Speaker**

	Total	Male	Female
Middle middle class	3	4	0
Lower middle class	15	27	3
Upper working class	74	81	68
Middle working class	88	91	81
Lower working class	98	100	97

Adapted from a table in James Milroy and Lesley Milroy, *Authority in Language* (London: Routledge, 1985), p. 96, and in J. K. Chambers and P. J. Trudgill, *Dialectology* (New York: Cambridge University Press, 1980), p. 71.

society thinks that it is correct to say 'ing' and not 'in', and further they believe that "educated" (powerful or influential) people always say 'ing'. Of course, as we saw, "educated" (influential, powerful, or wealthy) people do *not* always say 'ing'.

These internal public norms inside the heads of members of a hierarchical society have an interesting consequence. People *judge* others' speech, as well as their own speech, by these norms, not by what is actually said (by themselves or others). Furthermore, it turns out that most people *hear* themselves as if they spoke according to their norms and do not actually realize what they really say. Thus, people lower in the social hierarchy often will condemn the speech of people who speak much like themselves as "incorrect" and will even say that such people are not fit for responsible jobs. At the same time, they hear their own speech as "correct," when in reality they are actually condemning their own speech and themselves as well (unbeknownst to themselves).

The subtlety with which social variables signal social identity can be seen if we compare Table 9-1 with Table 9-2. Table 9-2 shows the percentage of use of 'in' by males and females from the various social classes, in all styles lumped together.

Clearly, for all classes, males use the low-prestige form 'in' more often than females. Thus, how one uses this social variable is determined by the style in which one is speaking (that is, what one takes the context to be—the degree to which one wants to identify with the local peer group or the wider society), one's social class, and one's gender. There are many other social determinants of one's speech.

———————————— E X E R C I S E ————————————

Exercise B. Below I reprint an oral story told by a high school girl and below it a written version of the story. In reprinting the oral story I have made no attempt to represent the way in which the text was actually pronounced. Written language is often, but not always, more formal than spoken language (especially school-based written language; the written text below was produced for a school project). While certain forms of writing (for example, personal letters and diaries) may be less formal than some forms of spoken language (such as lectures), the written text below is considerably more formal than the oral one. Compare the two texts, pointing out informal features of the oral text and formal features of the written text. While there were many features of the pronunciation of the oral text that signaled its relative informality, these are not reproduced here and you can ignore features of pronunciation. By the way, the oral text was privately told to the girl's teacher. Since the teacher is a status figure to the girl, her oral text is more formal than it would have been to her high school peers. Nonetheless, it is less formal than the written version.

In the oral text, dots represent pauses, with three dots being a longer pause than two dots, and two being longer than one dot. I number the segments in the oral text that were said with one intonational contour.[4]

INTRUDER: ORAL VERSION

1. . . . OK . um . when I was about . . five years old
2. . . and John . he's my brother . he was about eleven
3. . . we got up real early one Saturday
4. . to make some orange juice and watch cartoons
5. . . . and . we were standing in between . . . the kitchen . . . and the dining room
6. . . . and we were . stirring up the orange juice
7. . . and just kidding around and
8. . I looked over to the front door
9. . and there was this . man
10. . standing there looking into our house
11. . . . and I didn't know who he was
12. he wasn't knocking on the door
13. . . he wasn't trying to open it
14. . . he was just looking in
15. he had this . . . brimmed hat on
16. . . looked real suspicious
17. . . and . and I said to John
18. . you know . who is this guy
19. . he's . . you know . I'm scared

[4]This data is from Stephen Gordon, *Oral Discourse and Literate Prose: An Analysis,* doctoral dissertation, Boston University School of Education, 1986.

20. what's he doing there
21. . . and John of course . he is older than me
22. . he tried to act real cool
23. . . he said . oh I don't know
24. . well . why don't we just go up and get mom
25. . and see what she says
26. . . so he told me . to run up . the stairs by the front door
27. . . . and he'd go up the back stairs
28. so we would both get up the stairs about the same time
29. and get my mother
30. . . I was real stupid
31. I ran up the stairs in the front
32. by where the guy was
33. . . . and so we woke my mother
34. . . . and she came downstairs with us real fast
35. . and he wasn't there anymore
36. . . . and . . now we're back in the house
37. . . and . and I always look at the door
38. cause I keep expecting him to come back
39. . and . . it's real weird

INTRUDER: WRITTEN VERSION

It happened early one Saturday morning when John and I got up to make some orange juice and watch the Saturday morning cartoons. I was about five; he around eleven. As we stood between the kitchen and the dining room, the early morning sun peeking out over the housetops, I glanced at the front door ahead of me. A dark, shadowed, mysterious figure stood spying into our front door window! He didn't knock or even rattle the knob. He just stared in as if he were seeking someone out.

All I could see of him was that he appeared to be wearing one of those brimmed hats of the 30's and a black overcoat.

I said to John, who I thought knew everything because he was older, "Who's that guy? What's he want? John . . . I'm scared!"

He pretended to be "big and bad." At the time, I hadn't the slightest knowledge of his fear. Looking back now, he was just as petrified as I was.

John replied cooly, "Oh . . . I dunno. Maybe he wants Ma; let's go get her. You run up the front stairs and I'll go up the back. Okay?"

Being young, naive and doing everything that would please my older, wiser brother, I stupidly ran up the front stairs nearest the stranger, while John took the safety of the back stairs!

We ran to our mother like a couple of scared chickens, both trying to explain that there was a weird man standing at the front door peering in the window downstairs. She quickly followed us down. The man had disappeared—without a trace.

We still don't know who he was or what he wanted. I can still see that dark, hovering figure looking through my front door, silently searching someone out.

9.3. COMMUNICATION AND SOCIETY

Communicative Competence

The capacity of people to select and recognize the language variety appropriate to the occasion is known as their **communicative competence.** A large part of communicative competence is controlling the sorts of social variables we have looked at above. But there is more to it than that. When we speak we try to say the minimum we can, but yet get the hearer to draw a rich set of inferences that will fill out our meaning. Thus, much of what we say merely constitutes "cues" or "clues" to guide the hearer in drawing the right inferences. What I communicate goes far beyond what I have literally said.

Different languages, and different social groups speaking a single language, differ in how they handle these cues. This fact gives rise to a great deal of miscommunication between people. For example, the sociolinguist John Gumperz[5] points out, in a discussion of conversations between speaks of American English and Indian English (from India), that speakers of Indian English formulate their turns at talk rather differently than speakers of American English. In a single turn at talk in a conversation, Indians tend to take a good deal of time to formulate background information for their main point, and they use increased stress (higher pitch and increased loudness) to mark this background information. Then they shift to low pitch and low amplitude on their main point. However, Americans hear their background information, given its length and its increased stress, as their main point, assume they are finished when this background information is done, and go on to make their own contribution, feeling that the Indian has said nothing original. The Indian feels he is always interrupted and never allowed to make his or her point.

For an example of miscommunication between members of the same social group, consider the following conversation between a husband and wife:[6]

[5]In *Discourse Strategies* (New York: Cambridge University Press, 1982).

[6]From Deborah Tannen's book *That's Not What I Meant!* (New York: William Morrow, 1986).

A husband and wife are talking about whether they should accept an invitation to visit the wife's sister:

WIFE: Do you want to go to my sister's?
HUSBAND: Okay
WIFE: Do you really want to go?
HUSBAND (angry): You're driving me crazy! Why don't you make up your mind what you want?

What is going on here is this: The wife assumes she can say outright what she wants and that her husband will say outright what he wants. The wife feels she is perfectly willing to do what the husband wishes, and, in fact, feels confident in her kindness in being willing to do so. When she asks her question, "Do you want to go to my sister's?", she means the question literally; she is asking for information about the husband's preferences so that she can accommodate them.

The husband wants to be accommodating as well. But he assumes that people—even married people—don't *directly* say outright what they want. To him, such direct statements are coercive because he finds it hard to deny direct requests. So he assumes that people *hint* at what they want and in turn pick up hints from others. And a good way to hint is to ask a question, rather than making a statement. Thus, when his wife asked her question ("Do you want to go to my sister's?"), he assumed that his wife was not really asking a question, but hinting that she wanted to go to her sister's. Wishing to be accommodating, he gives in to her wishes, as he perceives them, and says "Okay."

But the wife follows up with a second question ("Are you sure you want to go?"). The husband hears this equally as a hint about what the wife wants, rather than a genuine question. He now assumes she *doesn't* want to go and is asking him to let her off the hook. He sees his wife as irrational. First she lets him know that she wants to go, and then when he gives her what she wants, she changes her mind and lets him know that she doesn't want to go.

However, from the wife's perspective, the husband's answer ("Okay") to her initial question ("Do you want to go to my sister's?") does not sound enough like an answer to the question. It seemed to her to indicate that he was going along with something, not really saying what he wanted. Since she simply wanted to please him by doing what he wanted to do, she presses him further with her second question, "Do you really want to go?". When he explodes with "You're driving me crazy! Why don't you make up your mind what you want?", she finds him totally irrational.

Because of their different backgrounds, these two people have different ways of signaling what they mean (the wife is an American native New Yorker of East European Jewish extraction; the husband is Greek). And they each misjudge the other's signals. However, they are not aware that they have a *language* problem, since people are rarely consciously aware of their linguistic practices, and have, in fact, great difficulty bringing them to consciousness. Since they are not aware of their linguistic practices, they tend to blame linguistic problems not on the other person's language, but on the person's character, personality, or intentions.

A final example of differences in contextualization cues illuminates gender differences in language. Many men and women in the U.S. differ in how they use "minimal responses" like 'yes' and 'mm hmm' in conversational interaction (these are sometimes called "channel feedback cues"). Women tend to mean by these responses *I'm listening to you; please continue.* For men, however, these minimal responses have a somewhat stronger meaning, such as *I agree with you* or at least *I follow your argument so far.* The fact that women use these minimal responses more often than men is, in part, due simply to the fact that women are listening more often than men are agreeing. This difference, which is not one that men and women are consciously aware of, can lead to repeated misunderstandings. Since the woman is sending more minimal responses than the man would in the same circumstance, he assumes she agrees with everything he says. Since the man is sending fewer such responses than the woman would in the same circumstances, she assumes the man is not listening.

─────────────── **E X E R C I S E** ───────────────

Exercise C. "Contextualization cues" are all the aspects of a sentence by which we attempt to signal to the hearer how the sentence is to be taken (in what spirit, and what attitude it is meant to express—for example, such cues tell the hearer whether the speaker is telling a joke or being serious, whether the speaker is being rude or polite, whether the speaker is trying to be close to or distant from the hearer, whether the speaker is trying to be direct or indirect with the hearer, and many other such messages). Such cues are subtle and can differ across different social groups using the same language, thus leading to miscommunication. Below I give two scenarios involving contextualization cues. In each case, two people fail to be on the "same wavelength" because they do not understand, or at least do not respond to, certain contextualization cues in the same way. Answer the questions connected with each one:

1. A rising young executive was interviewing a prospective recruit for her firm over an informal lunch. The restaurant had a serve-yourself setup for coffee. The executive was pouring coffee for herself when a man approached and asked her to pour some for him. She obliged, gladly. He said, "Thanks, honey. I'll do the same for you sometime." The woman was insulted, and the man was surprised. They understood the contextualization cue or cues he had used differently. How might he have understood them and how might she such that a misunderstanding ensued?[7]

---

[7]Scenario based on an example from Deborah Tannen's *That's Not What I Meant!,* cited above.

2. A black graduate student has been sent to interview a black housewife in a low-income, inner-city neighborhood for a research study. The interview has been arranged over the phone by an office back at the university. The student arrives, rings the bell, and is met by the husband, who opens the door, smiles in a friendly way, and says with a laugh "So you're gonna check out ma ol lady, hah?" The graduate student replies: "Ah, no. I only came to get some information. They called from the office." The husband drops his smile, calls his wife and disappears, obviously hurt and unhappy. What contextualization cues has the husband used and how does he want his utterance taken? What has the graduate student done to make him unhappy? How could the graduate student have replied so as to accept the invitation implicit in the husband's utterance?[8]

Discourse Patterns, Literacy, and World Views

Beyond the ways in which people construct their conversation or use social variation, there are more global differences in regard to language and social interaction between different cultures and different social groups in a single society. These more global differences are rooted in the different perspectives cultures take of the world and their different ways of making sense of the world.

This can be seen clearly in the work of Ronald and Suzanne Scollon on the differences in communicative patterns and values between Athabaskan Indians, on the one hand, and Anglo-Canadians and Americans, on the other, in Canada and Alaska (differences that do not necessarily disappear when bilingual Athabaskans speak English, since such culturally specific ways of interacting and using language can be carried over from one language to another).[9]

The Scollons believe that culturally different ways of using language (whether in speech or writing) reflect different "reality sets" or "world views" adopted by the culture and are among the strongest expressions of personal and cultural identity. They argue that changes in a person's culturally specific ways of using language (what they call "discourse patterns") involve a change in identity. In particular, they argue that this happens when Athabaskans acquire Western school-based literacy, a form of language that the Scollons see as tied to a characteristically Western set of culturally specific values and beliefs. Literacy as it is practiced in European-based education is connected to a reality set or world view the Scollons term "modern consciousness." This reality set is consonant with ("goes with", "fits with", "encourages") particular ways of using oral

---

[8]Scenario based on an example from John Gumperz's *Discourse Strategies,* cited above.

[9]The Scollons' work is summarized in their book *Narrative, Literacy and Face in Interethnic Communication* (Norwood, N.J.: Ablex, 1981).

language and ways of interacting in language that are quite different from the discourse patterns used by the Athabaskans.

Athabaskans differ at various points from mainstream Canadian and American English speakers in how they engage in discourse. A few examples: (a) Athabaskans have a high degree of respect for the individuality of others and a careful guarding of their own individuality. Thus, they prefer to avoid conversation except when the point of view of all participants is well known. On the other hand, English speakers feel that the main way to get to know the point of view of people is through conversation with them. (b) For Athabaskans, a person in a subordinate position does not display, rather he or she observes the person in the superordinate position. For instance, adults as either parents or teachers are supposed to display abilities and qualities for the child to learn. However, in mainstream American society, children are supposed to show off their abilities for teachers and other adults. (c) The English idea of "putting your best foot forward" conflicts directly with an Athabaskan taboo. It is normal in situations of unequal status relations, for an English speaker, to display oneself in the best light possible. One will speak highly of the future, as well. It is normal to present a career or life trajectory of success and planning. This English system is very different from the Athabaskan system, in which it is considered inappropriate and bad luck to anticipate good luck, to display oneself in a good light, to predict the future, or to speak unfavorably of another's luck.

The Scollons list many other differences, including differences in systems of pausing that ensure that English speakers select most of the topics and do most of the talking in an interethnic encounter. Since Athabaskans typically pause longer at the end of a sentence than Canadians and Americans, their Anglo hearers assume they are finished speaking and speak themselves. The Athabaskan thinks he or she has been interrupted and the Anglo thinks the Athabaskan speaks cryptically and never fills out or finishes his or her thought. The net result of these communication problems is that each group ethnically stereotypes the other. The English speaker comes to believe that the Athabaskan is unsure, aimless, incompetent, and withdrawn. The Athabaskan comes to believe that the English speaker is boastful of his or her abilities, sure he or she can predict the future, careless with luck, and far too talkative.

The Scollons characterize the different discourse practices of Athabaskans and English speakers in terms of two different world views or "forms of consciousness": bush consciousness (connected with survival values in the bush or wilderness in which Athabaskans historically lived) and modern consciousness. These forms of consciousness are "reality sets" in the sense that they are cognitive orientations toward the everyday world, including how learning should take place in that world.

Anglo-Canadian and American mainstream culture has adopted a model of literacy, based on the values of essayist prose style, that is highly compatible with modern consciousness. In essayist, school-based prose (the sort in this book, for instance, or the sort one is asked to write in school), the important relationships to be signaled are those between sentence and sentence, not those between speakers, nor those between sentence and speaker. For a reader, this requires a constant monitoring of grammatical and lexical information. With the heightened emphasis on truth value rather than social or rhetorical conditions comes the necessity to be explicit about logical implications. Such writing is quite different than that often found in personal letters, for instance, where the relationship between writer and reader is often more important than the actual content of the text.

A significant aspect of essayist prose style is the **fictionalization** of both the audience and the author. The "reader" of an essayist text is not an ordinary human being (not *you* personally, for instance, whatever your name may be), but an idealization, a rational mind formed by the rational body of knowledge of which the essay is a part. By the same token, the author of an essayist text is a fiction, not an ordinary human being (not *me,* Jim Gee, for instance) since the process of writing and editing essayist texts leads to an effacement of individual and idiosyncratic identity. The author adopts the impersonal "authority" (note the word play "author-ity") of the "expert."

For the Athabaskan, writing in this essayist mode can constitute a crisis in ethnic identity. To produce an essay would require the Athabaskan to produce a major display, which would be appropriate only if the Athabaskan was in a position of dominance in relation to the audience. But the audience and the author are fictionalized and impersonal in essayist prose and the text becomes decontextualized (not tied closely to any specific real-world context of mutually known communicators). This means that a contextualized, social relationship of dominance is obscured. Where the relationship of the communicants is unknown, the Athabaskan prefers silence. The paradox of prose for the Athabaskan then is that if it is communication between known author and audience it is *contextualized* (in a real world of real people) and compatible with Athabaskan values, but not good essayist prose. To the extent that it becomes decontextualized and thus good essayist prose, it becomes uncharacteristic of Athabaskans to seek to communicate.

E X E R C I S E

Exercise D. Below is a story by a high school girl ("Stiff Neck") written for a school assignment. This story does not show full mastery of what I have called essayist (school-based) prose. On the other hand, the written version of the "Intruder" story in Exercise B does show such mastery. Comparing the two stories, detail how the first fails to show mastery of essayist, school-based prose style and how "Intruder" does show such mastery (to a certain level, at least). In particular, do you see any ways in which the "Stiff Neck" story shows a style that is not impersonal and decontextualized enough for essayist prose?

STIFF NECK

When I was in the tenth grade I wasn't never absent until the ending of the year. I woke up one morning and got a sharp pain in my neck. I told my sister I don't think I will be going to school so tell Dianne so she can tell Mom. My sister said I shouldn't go even though I wasn't absent. I went back to bed because I kept on getting the pain. When I woke up I couldn't get out of bed, so I heard my sister get up and told her to tell my mother, but she forgot. So I had to wait for about one hour until 10:00 A.M. I was screaming and crying calling my mother. She came up to my room and asked "what is the matter?" I told her I couldn't get out of bed that I was in pain. She tried to help me out, but I couldn't get up. I was really in pain. She told me to jump out the bed and don't think about the pain, and it worked. I still couldn't move my neck and arm it became stiff. So my mother rubbed Ben Gay on my neck and arm. I stayed home from school a couple of days. I am glad I have parents who care so much.

9.4. SOCIAL VARIATION AND HISTORICAL CHANGE

Above we discussed the way in which social variables (like varying between 'ing' or 'in') are distributed in society in terms of different styles (formal versus informal) and different social classes (upper, middle, and lower). We will see in this section that such social variation is intimately tied to the ways in which languages change through time, and, in fact, helps to explain how and why languages change.

To see this, we will consider three features from black vernacular English (BVE) that have been changing for some time now. The three features are the following: (a) pronouncing words that end in two consonants with the final one missing, thus saying [mɪs], instead of [mɪst], for the word spelled 'mist'; (b) not pronouncing [r] after a vowel, thus saying [ka], instead of [kar] for the word spelled 'car'; and (c) pronouncing the sound [θ] as [f], thus saying [fɪn] instead of [θɪn] for the word spelled 'thin'.

The data we will look at comes from a study done in Detroit by Walt Wolfram.[10] All three of the above pronunciations are variable in BVE (that is, sometimes speakers will say [mɪs], sometimes [mɪst], and so on for the others). The [mɪs] pronunciation of 'mist' is stigmatized (looked down on in the wider community) and is the less prestigious and more informal pronunciation. So also for the r-less pronunciation of 'car' ([ka]), and the pronunciation of 'thin' with an [f] as [fɪn].

[10]*A Sociolinguistic Description of Detroit Negro Speech* (Washington, D.C.: Center for Applied Linguistics, 1969).

Table 9-3 shows how different social classes in the black community in Detroit used these features around 1969. It shows the percentage of the *prestigious* pronunciations ([mɪst], [kar], and [θɪn]), that is, the pronunciations that represent standard English, for a large sample of black speech in various styles.

If we look closely at Table 9-3, we can learn something about the way in which BVE (at least in Detroit) has been changing, and, more generally, about how languages change in general. First, notice that in all social classes in the black community, people use the [θ] version of the θ/f variable more frequently than they use [r] version of the r/zero variable. This means that they are more standard-language-like in their use of [θ] than of [r]. And in turn they use the [r] version of the r/zero variable more frequently than they use both consonants in a word like 'mist' (the standard-language version of this variable). Thus, for all classes, their pronunciation of a word like 'thin' (which they are likely to say with a [θ]) is more standard than their pronunciation of a word like 'car' (which they are somewhat less likely to say with an [r]), and this, in turn, is more standard than their pronunciation of 'mist'. At the same time, as we would expect, the more prestigious pronunciation for each variable is more common in the higher classes.

Table 9-3 tells us that at one time in the past the stigmatized pronunciations ([f], no [r], and no final consonant in words ending in two consonants) were the *normal* pronunciations in BVE, perhaps even the only ones used. That means, for BVE speakers in the past, a word like 'mist' was always pronounced as [mɪs], a word like 'car' was always pronounced as [ka], and a word like 'thin' as [fɪn]. These speakers were not necessarily literate, and thus not influenced by how the words were spelled in standard English.

As black speakers left slavery and eventually interacted more with the wider white society, they gained more access to speakers of standard English. Because of their poverty and lack of power and influence, their own pronunciations were looked down on by the wider society (by the normal principle that people extend their social prejudices toward a group to that group's language). At the same time, the black speakers began to change their pronunciations to the standard English versions ([θ], [r], and final consonants). They did this both because they began to

TABLE 9-3. Percentage of Standard English Features in Detroit Black Speech

Social Class	θ instead of f in words like 'thin'	r present in words like 'car'	Both consonants present in words like 'mist'
Lower class	55	29	16
Lower working	62	39	21
Upper working	89	59	34
Upper middle	94	79	49

internalize the negative view of their own pronunciations that the wider society held, and because they looked on the wider white society as prestigious.

The higher the black speaker's own social class, the more social mobility he or she had and the greater opportunity to interact with speakers of standard English. Lower-class black speakers were restricted more narrowly to black ghettos, and thus to speaking only to other blacks (who spoke BVE). Thus, blacks from the higher classes had a much greater opportunity to switch to standard pronunciations. They would have done so at first variably, using their own stigmatized versions more frequently in communicating in informal contexts and with other blacks with whom they wanted to signal solidarity. They would have used the prestigious (more standard English pronunciations) more frequently in communicating with strangers, in formal contexts, and when interacting in the wider society.

Thus, the change from stigmatized pronunciations ([f] in 'thin', no [r] in 'car' and no final consonant in 'mist') to standard ones started in the upper classes, thanks to their greater access to the wider society. That is why in 1969 the higher classes show, in Table 9-3, the greatest percentage of standard-language pronunciations. Furthermore, if we look at Table 9-3 we see that this change is furthest along in the case of [θ] (instead of [f]); that is, everyone, regardless of social class, uses the standard pronunciation here more than in the case of the other two features. This is, then, in all likelihood, the feature that changed first (and has been therefore undergoing change the longest). The second feature to change was probably [r], since it is now the second most common standard pronunciation in the speech of all classes. Pronouncing both consonants in words like 'mist' is changing last.

The upper classes started the change, but thanks to their prestige and influence in the black community, they influenced the classes below them, who themselves then began to change. These lower classes use the standard pronunciations less often than the upper classes because they started to change later and are thus behind the upper classes in the change. Each change ([f] to [θ], no [r] to [r], and no final consonant in words that end with two consonants to final consonant) spreads to the lowest class last, and the change to having a final consonant in words like 'mist' comes last to each class. Thus, with the lowest class, the final consonant feature was, in 1969, just beginning to change (they used the standard pronunciation only 16% of the time, as Table 9-3 shows).

Table 9-3 shows that the change we are talking about was still in progress in 1969, thus the standard and nonstandard pronunciations still alternated for all social classes. If they alternate, they can be used as social variables to distinguish formal from informal styles, status seeking from solidarity. Eventually, however, if the change goes to completion, all classes would use the standard features all or most of the time. Thus, these features could no longer be used as social variables (but others would remain and new ones would take their place).

I should also point out that the nonstandard features we have been discussing here occur also in many nonstandard white dialects, and the absence of a final consonant in words spelled with two consonants at the end of the word is not uncommon in the fast and informal speech of many middle-class whites. We are talking about tendencies and trends. In all styles, middle-class speakers will use more final consonants in words like 'mist' than speakers of lower classes. The pronunciation of the final consonant is the "norm" or target for all speakers in the speech community now.

Table 9-3 can be read then not as if it is about a single time (which it actually is), but as if it is about change across time. Read this way, the upper middle class represents a way of using language that has been undergoing the changes we have talked about longer than the other classes. The other classes are all moving in the same direction as the upper middle class, but they started later and thus are less far along. The lowest class represents the last to change, thus *their pronunciation most represents what the dialect looked like in the past.* That is, we can use the way the lowest class speaks to guess about what a language looked like in the past, if the changes that a language is undergoing are of the type we are studying here.

Not all language change works the way these changes do, and sometimes change starts with the lower classes and moves to the higher (just the reverse of what we have seen here). In this latter case, if the higher classes ever become *consciously* aware that is where the change is coming from, the change will usually stop and even reverse. Because change can come from below, just as from above, lower-class speakers, and BVE speakers in particular, have also influenced the way middle-class white speakers speak.

Finally, I should point out that it is not uncommon for a group of usually younger speakers to become consciously aware that their nonstandard pronunciations are stigmatized by the wider society, but to retain them purposely as a sign of resistance to that wider society and to the social inequalities it represents. Of course, the nonstandard pronunciations can also regain ground if segregation increases and younger black speakers get less and less opportunity to interact with middle-class blacks and whites (and thus interact for the most part only with the lowest class, which retains the most nonstandard pronunciation).

--- **E X E R C I S E** ---

Exercise E.   Table 9-4 below shows the pattern of "dropping" initial [h] sounds in two English cities, Bradford and Norwich. The data comes from a relatively formal style, namely, the relatively careful style of speech used during tape-recorded interviews. We are talking about [h]-dropping in *stressed* syllables only (saying 'hot' as ''ot', for example)—all speakers of English drop [h] regularly in unstressed positions (as in 'Mary likes 'im' for 'Mary likes him').

What language change would you hypothesize is in progress in these two cities? That is, is the change one of having more initial [h] or less? Which is the more prestigious form? What class began the change first? Which class began it last? Which city began the change first? If the change went to completion, would

TABLE 9-4. Percentage of [h]-Dropping in Bradford and Norwich (Formal Style Only)

	BRADFORD	NORWICH
Middle middle class	12	6
Lower middle class	28	14
Upper working class	67	40
Middle working class	89	60
Lower working class	93	60

Based on Chambers and Trudgill, 1980, p. 69 (cited in footnote to Table 9-1) and K. M. Petyt, *Dialect and Accent in the Industrial West Riding,* Ph.D. thesis, University of Reading, 1977. Reprinted in Milroy & Milroy, 1985, p. 94 (cited in footnote to Table 9-2).

everyone say 'hot' or ''ot' for 'hot'? Language changes never need to go to completion, and a community could show the pattern in Table 9-4 for some time. We would need additional evidence to gauge how fast the change is taking place.

9.5. PIDGINS AND CREOLES

Many scholars have argued that BVE had its origins in a *creole.* In coming to understand what this term means, we will understand another important piece of the answer to the question of how and why languages change. When people come together who speak many different languages, and few of them have any one language in common, they must find some mode of communication with each other. Usually, of course, they will just learn the language of one of the groups and use this as a *lingua franca* (= a common language for groups who do not share a single native language). However, in some cases this cannot happen.

Sometimes groups come together and need to communicate only about a limited array of things. For example, sailors from different countries may meet in fishing grounds on the open sea and need to talk only about trade and fishing, or traders of various goods may visit far away countries and need to talk to the native populations only about trade. In these cases, very simple **trade jargons** arise, simplified languages used for simplified purposes. The trade jargon will have words from each language in it and be spoken rather differently by speakers from the different native language groups. The context will be rich and obvious enough (for example, a fish held up and waved in one's face) to render communication successful.

Languages like trade jargons can also arise under much more unfortunate circumstances. Large-scale social disruption like slavery and the emigration of indentured or impoverished workers may lead to large numbers of speakers of a variety of languages coming together outside their homelands. These groups, like workers from around the world coming to Hawaii to cut sugar cane in the nineteenth and early twentieth centuries, or African slaves in the various colonies, will not share one language. They will, however, need to use some of the language of the culture they are in. But because of their low status and segregation, they will have little or no access to learning the language of that culture (for example, English).

In this case—like the trade jargon case above—a simplified language will arise for restricted communication between the *dominated* groups and the *dominating* one (for example, the dominating group was English speakers in Hawaii and in U.S. slave plantations; it was French speakers in the slave colony of Haiti), as well among the dominated groups themselves when they are communicating to people outside their own language group. We can call such simplified languages **jargons.**

Such jargons are spoken rather differently by each speaker depending on his or her own native language. The jargon will be made up of some words from the dominant language, but each speaker will occasionally use words, structures, and sounds from his or her native language. For instance, below I give an example from the speech of a Japanese woman in her seventies, who came to Hawaii when she was eighteen. She spent most of her life working on a small plantation, and like other isolated individuals, her jargon never developed beyond a very rudimentary stage.[11]

1. Me   wa   niku ga   no   riku
    I   topic   meat object   no   like
    'I don't like meat'

Here the subject 'me' ('I') is followed by the Japanese particle *wa* (marking something as a topic—so 'I' is marked as the topic). *Niku* is based on the Japanese word for 'meat' and is followed by another Japanese particle (*ga,* which marks the direct object of a verb). *No* is the English word 'no', used for negation, and *riku* is from English 'like', with /l/ changed to /r/ and a vowel added after /k/ to make it fit better Japanese ways of pronouncing words. This speaker uses Japanese word order (subject object verb). She could only be understood by close friends.

Pidgins

The jargon, however, while it may last a long time or die out if it is no longer needed, can "expand." That is, if it is needed for a wider range of purposes, it will

---

[11]See Suzanne Romaine, *Pidgin and Creole Languages* (London: Longman, 1988), from which the examples in this section are taken.

begin to "conventionalize." Speakers will begin to pronounce it more alike, and they will settle on pretty much the same words and sentence forms. Most of its words will come from the language of the dominant group in the situation (for example, English). When a jargon has settled into a more agreed-on and somewhat more complicated form, we refer to it as a **pidgin.** Below is an example of another Japanese speaker using Hawaiian Pidgin English, a language with socially sanctioned norms:

2. Go bark bark bark. All right. He go . . . He stop see. Go for the dog. Go for the dog. He no go for you, the man. He no care for man. He go for the dog.

> *Translation:* The dog started barking. Alright. He's looking. (The pig) goes after the dog. He goes for the dog. He doesn't go after the man. He's not interested in the man. He goes for the dog.

Pidgins use simple sentence structures and a good deal of repetition. They heavily trade on the hearer making inferences from context to fill in much of the meaning. The words in a pidgin have no complexity (for example, compare English 'he goes', where 'goes' = 'go' + 'es', 'es' being the third-person singular agreement marker, with Hawaiian Pidgin 'he go'). Pidgins, at least in their early stages of development, are simpler than other languages. They are used for only a fairly restricted range of communication and they are no one's native language—everyone learns the pidgin as a second language. Everyone in the situation where a pidgin is used usually has a native language in which to discuss things he or she cannot well or easily discuss in the pidgin.

When a pidgin develops, one language in the mix of languages supplies the words to the pidgin, usually the language spoken by the dominant or otherwise most influential group (for example, the language of the colonizer). This language is called the **lexifier** language or the **superstrate** language for the pidgin ('lexifier language' = the language that supplies a *lexicon*—dictionary—of words to the pidgin). The people acquiring the pidgin do not have enough contact with speakers of the lexifier language to acquire it fully. Rather, they use words from that language in a simplified structure greatly influenced by their own languages. If English is the lexifier language, the pidgin is called *an English pidgin;* if it is Portuguese, it is called *a Portuguese pidgin,* and so on. The other languages in the mix of groups are called the **substrate** languages (for example, the languages of the "natives" or native populations being colonized).

Linguists are interested in pidgins because they show us the solutions to communicational problems that adults will hit on under conditions of communicational stress and need. And there are some similarities in pidgins across the world, despite differences as well. Pidgin speakers can try anything they like, based perhaps on transfer from their native language, or some other language they know, but it will not end up part of the pidgin unless it works (communicates). Since the people using the pidgin do not know each other's other languages, anything the speaker tries will work only if it is so basic to communication that all languages do something similar (it is a universal) or it is something that all the substrate languages in the particular language mix involved in the birth of the pidgin happen to do (which is less likely, but does happen). That is, the community of pidgin speakers, using for the most part words from the superstrate language, settles on a simplified grammar that contains patterns and rules that either reflect universals of language or are common to all or most of the substrate languages.

So, for example, all languages draw a distinction between a first-person pronoun ('I/me') and a third-person pronoun ('he/him', 'she/her', 'it'), but not all distinguish between a subject and object form ('he' versus 'him') or among masculine, feminine, and neuter forms ('he' versus 'she' versus 'it'). Thus, the pidgin Tok Pisin (spoken in Papua, New Guinea) drops these latter language-particular forms and has only the universal first- versus third-person distinction (thus, Tok Pisin uses only the forms *me* = 'I/me' as subject or object and *em* = 'he/him', 'she/her', or 'it', as subject or object).

Another example of a commonalty found in a great many pidgins is seen in the Hawaiian Pidgin negative sentence form, 'He no go for you', which places a simple negative word right before the verb. This is a common way of making negative sentences in many pidgins, regardless of how such sentences are made in the dominant language or the native languages of the groups using the pidgin.

While pidgins are usually used for a fairly restricted range of purposes and eventually die out when these purposes no longer exist, sometimes they eventually take on a much wider range of functions in a society. For example, they may come to serve as the national language of a society containing speakers with many different native languages, and where, for various social or political reasons, no one of these native languages can be used as a *lingua franca*. In various parts of Africa and the South Pacific various pidgins, which originally arose in some cases out of the sorts of disruption we have pointed to above, or which arose as trade languages, have come to serve as languages used for wide purposes among large groups of people—including in newspapers and in political speeches. Just as the jargon grew into an early, simplified pidgin under communicational pressure, as the functions for which the language is used grow further, the language will, generation by generation, get more complex. Such pidgins, which we can call **expanded pidgins,** while they remain second languages, are not simple languages.

Creoles

In a situation where a pidgin is used, it sometimes happens that a generation of children arises, who, for some reason, does not learn (or does not only learn) the parents' native language(s). This could happen because the parents do not both speak the same language or their native language is not useful any longer in the society. For example, children of American slaves did not long need the African languages of their parents (though African languages did remain in the U.S. for quite some time). They surely needed to use a common language among themselves for the full range of uses any human needs a native language for. They had no real access to the English of the masters, who didn't engage in extended communication with them. Thus, they had to learn the English-based pidgin of their parents as a native language.

If this pidgin was still simple, as it often was, it would hardly serve for all the purposes for which a child needs a language. In this case, a remarkable thing happens. Though this generation of children receives the pidgin as input to the process of first (or native) language acquisition, they eventually "create" out of it a language that is much more complex. This language is not called a pidgin, but a **creole**. The creole is a native language (pidgins are always second languages). Creoles are truly new languages for the world. They themselves will develop through history, and after many hundreds or thousands of years, no one may know this was how they arose.

How does the child do this, create a creole? Many linguists believe that the only plausible answer is that the child draws on his or her innate (unconscious) knowledge of what the basic design of a human language must be, an innate knowledge that has arisen in the human species through the course of human evolution. All children draw on this innate linguistic capacity in acquiring a language, but in more normal cases (such as the child acquiring English in the U.S. today) children also learn the more idiosyncratic parts of their languages that are the products of culture and historical change. They can do this because the languages they are exposed to (for example, English) are complicated enough for all their purposes and the data to which they are exposed is much fuller than the data the creole speaking child is exposed to.

But when creole-speaking children are exposed to a simplified pidgin and have little access to the dominant language, they must fall back more fully on their innate linguistic capacity. If this is true, we would expect creoles across the world to bear deep resemblance to each other no matter where they arise or what the pidgin on which they were based looks like (whether, for example, it was a pidgin that drew most of its words from French, or English, or Portuguese, or what have you), since human biology is everywhere the same. And, indeed, creoles appear to have such deep similarities.

Below I give an example of a creole spoken by an eleven-year-old boy. This is a creolized version of the pidgin Tok Pisin—this creole actually is currently arising through children acquiring the expanded pidgin, Tok Pisin, as a native language. Since this pidgin was already fairly expanded, these children had less to "create," having had a better base—an expanded pidgin—to work from. Nonetheless, they speak their creole somewhat differently than the adults speak the expanded pidgin. The child is looking at a sequence of pictures, and the sentence below is his description of the first one:

4. Fes   tru,   disla man   na   meri   blem,
First   one,   this man   and   wife   his

ol   sa   lukautim   pikinini   blol   gutpla
they   are   caring for   child   theirs well

> *Translation:* In the first one, this man and his wife, they are taking good care of their child

The child's creole *disla* is a version of what the adult would say as pidgin *dispela* (based on English 'this fellow'). The child's *blem* is a version of what the adult would say as *bilong en* (based on English 'belong him'). The child's *blol* is a version of what the adult would say as *bilong ol* (based on English 'belong all'). It is typical that children creolizing a pidgin will reduce its words to speed up the pidgin. Children demand that their native language be both efficient and fast.

In introducing such fast-speech styles, children not only speed up the language, they introduce stylistic and social variation. They use slower speech styles, with more expanded words, for more formal styles and to mark respect and deference, reserving the faster styles for more informal contexts and to mark solidarity with peers. Children also demand that a language have such stylistic and social flexibility.

When a creole is created on the basis of an undeveloped pidgin like the early Hawaiian pidgin we saw above, the creole is, of course, massively different from the pidgin. When it is created on the basis of a more developed pidgin, like Tok Pisin, it is less different, since the pidgin has already become fairly elaborated. Even here, as we have just seen, there are differences that show the work of the child's mind over and above the constructions that have been carried out, unconsciously, by generations of adults (learning the pidgin as a second language).

EXERCISES

Exercise F. The data below is from Cameroon Pidgin English from West Africa, a fairly elaborated pidgin (I have spelled the pidgin like English to make it easier to read; it is normally spelled in a more phonetic system). After the Cameroon Pidgin sentences, I have given an English translation of each. How does the word 'sweet' function in this pidgin? (HINT: Consider the following English sentences: 'He is a *lovable* man; My *love* is great; I have begun to *love* her; He spoke to her *lovingly'*.) The way 'sweet' functions in this pidgin is fairly typical of pidgins and creoles.

Cameroon Pidgin English		English
1. some sweet soup	=	delicious stew
2. dis sweet go bring palava	=	these sweet things (i.e., pieces of unexpected good luck) will cause trouble
3. di soup done begin sweet	=	the stew has begun to get tasty
4. I sabi talk sweet sweet so	=	He knows how to flatter (i.e., talk very sweetly) [sabi = know]

Exercise G. Given the data shown below, how would you characterize the uses of reduplication in Cameroon Pidgin English?

1.	some fain pikin	a lovely child
	some fainfain pikin	a really lovely child
2.	ben	bend
	benben	crooked
3.	pikin di krai	The child is crying
	pikin di soso kraikrai	The child is always crying

Exercise H. Given the data below, how would you characterize the way Cameroon Pidgin English expresses meaning in relation to individual words of English?

hos	horse
man hos	stallion
wuman hos	mare
man pikin hos	foal (male)
wuman pikin hos	filly
get bele	be pregnant
get flawa	mature, have one's period for first time
see mun	have one's period (literally: see moon)
man han	right (literally: man hand)
wuman han	left (literally: woman hand)
good hat	generous, generosity (literally: good heart)
long ai	greedy (for possessions) (literally: long eye)
long trot	greedy (for food) (literally: long throat)
wumani ee bele	a holdall bag (literally: woman she belly)
drai ai	brave (of a man) (literally: dry eye)
drai ai	brazen (of a woman)
tao han	mean, meanness (literally: tie hand)

Decreolization and the Origins
of Black Vernacular English

In a society where a creole has developed, normally the creole is looked down on by its own speakers and by the wider society in which the creole is spoken. For example, in the Cape Verde Islands in Africa, a former colony of Portugal, a Portuguese pidgin, and eventually a Portuguese-based creole, developed among the slaves. Portuguese, of course, was used by the masters. After slavery, Portuguese continued to be used in the society by the former masters and other elites in the society. It was the prestigious language. The creole was stigmatized and looked down on.

The same thing happened in the American slave states. Slaves developed a pidgin and eventually a creole for communication among themselves (they continued to use the pidgin to communicate with the whites). When they were freed, they retained the creole, but it was stigmatized by the wider society. Even the freed slaves themselves often accepted this evaluation (internalizing the negative judgment of their language, their culture, and themselves that the wider society held).

Because of the low prestige of the creole and the high prestige of the accompanying superstrate language (for example, English in the U.S., Portuguese in the Cape Verde Islands), the creole will, through time, become more and more affected by the superstrate language. As creole speakers gain more access to superstrate speakers (for example, when slaves are free and gradually attain more contact with the wider society), they change their creole more and more to resemble the superstrate language. Eventually, the creole looks not like a separate language, but rather like a dialect of the superstrate. Eventually, if the former creole speakers gain full contact with the superstrate speakers (segregation is broken down), the creole will collapse with the superstrate altogether. This process where the creole changes in stages to come to resemble the superstrate language is called **decreolization.** Thus, creolization represents a process whereby the world gains new languages (created *de novo* by children), and decreolization represents a process whereby the world loses a language (as it can when all the speakers of a language die, as has happened with many American Indian languages).

However, if in a creole-speaking society the superstrate language is removed (its speakers leave), or the superstrate language loses its prestige (because the creole speakers come to value the creole as the sign of their own worth and identity), the creole will not decreolize, but rather just change through time the way any language does. Eventually, its speakers and the rest of the world (sometimes including linguists) may not know the language ever had its origins as a creole. Swahili is a good example of such a language.

When a creole is in the midst of the decreolization process, speakers have available to them several varieties of their language, including versions that are more like the original creole, which they use to signal solidarity with the local community, and versions more like the standard version of the superstrate, which they use with outsiders and for public purposes, when seeking to identify with what counts as prestigious in the wider society.

9.6. LANGUAGE CHANGE

All languages change through time. English as it is spoken today is very different from English spoken around the end of the first millennium, what we now call "Old English." Below I give samples of English from various periods (I give a Modern English transliteration under each word from the older texts, except for Early Modern English).[12]

Old English (*Caedmon's Hymn*, 7th century C.E.)

Nu	*sculon*	*herigean*	*heofonrices*		*Weard*
Now	we-must	praise	heaven-kingdom's		Guardian

Middle English (Chaucer, *The Canterbury Tales*, 14th century)

Whan	*that*	*Aprille*	*with*	*his*	*shoures*	*soote*
When	the	April	with	its	showers	sweet

The	*droghte*	*of*	*March*	*hath*	*perced*	*to*	*the roote . . .*
The	drought	of	March	has	pierced	to	the root . . .

Early Modern English (Shakespeare, *Hamlet*, 16th century)

A man may fish with the worm that hath eat of a king,
and eat of the fish that hath fed of that worm.

One reason languages change is because they come into contact with other languages, by which they are influenced and from which they borrow words, structures, and meanings (via bilinguals who speak both languages). Thus, when the Normans invaded England in 1066 C.E., the English language was vastly influenced by the version of French the Normans spoke. Since the Normans became the powerful and elite in the society, English speakers began to consider the language of the Normans as more prestigious than English. Thus, they learned Norman French and heavily borrowed from it into their English (changing English in some ways like a creole decreolizing toward its superstrate language). This is not unlike one dialect of a language (for example, BVE saying [ka] for 'car') switching to a more prestigious pronunciation, eventually across all styles (for example, to [kar] for 'car').

But languages will change even if they are uninfluenced by other languages.

---

[12]See Victoria Fromkin and Robert Rodman, *An Introduction to Language,* 3rd ed. (New York: Holt, Rinehart and Winston, 1983).

Dan Slobin, one of the leading contemporary scholars of child language development, has argued that children place several somewhat contradictory "demands" on what they will accept as a human language in the language acquisition process.[13] These demands, of course, follow not from their conscious knowledge, but from the human biological endowment for language. These demands ultimately are what cause the child to reject a pidgin as a natural language and change it into a creole.

If we ignore for the time being the changes in language caused by adult bilinguals, children are the major force behind language change. Children are confronted with linguistic data that is based on the speech of adults, but they have to induce (guess) this grammar based on that data and their innate language capacity. In the process, they often come up with a slightly different grammar than the adult grammar, and through generations these small changes add up to major differences. Slobin's "demands" shape how children go about this process of inducing the grammar and also predicts that they will in some instances reshape the language they are faced with to make it better fit these demands. Thus, Slobin's demands are also a major force in language change.

Two of the key demands that children place on what they are (unconsciously) willing to accept as a native (first) language are as follows: First, the language must be *clear*. It must express its meanings in as straightforward a manner as possible, ideally with one clear form (morpheme) for each separate meaning. Second, the language must be *quick and easy*. Following a "principle of least effort," humans want to achieve as much as they can with the least effort. They also need to communicate as much as they can before the listener gets bored or takes over the conversation. There are, in addition, short-term memory constraints to get a message across before the speaker or listener loses track of what is going on. Thus, contrary to the demand to be clear, there is a demand to "cut corners."

These two demands are contradictory. Children learning Tok Pisin as a creole will say instead of the adult's *mi go long haus* (literally 'I go to house/home'), *mi go l:aus*. When they reduce *long* ('to') and collapse it with *haus* ('home'), they speed up the language (as they do also by placing primary stress only on *l:aus*, whereas adults place stress on both *go* and *haus*—stressing a word, which amounts to saying it with a change in pitch and amplitude, lengthens the word). This causes the language to better honor the second demand (to be quick and easy), but at the same time the language honors less well the first demand (to be clear). The adults have a clearly separate form for each separate meaning (*long* = to, *haus* = home), while the children give less material to each meaning and collapse this material into something approaching a single form.

These contradictory forces are what keeps language change going forever. If

---

[13]"Cognitive Prerequisites for the Development of Grammar," in C. A. Ferguson and D. I. Slobin, eds., *Studies of Child Language Development* (New York: Holt, Rinehart and Winston, 1973); "Language Change in Childhood and History," in J. Macnamara, ed., *Language Learning and Thought* (New York: Academic Press, 1977).

children go too far in making their language quick and easy, they make it less clear. As they correct this and make it clearer, they make it less quick and easy. If this goes too far, children begin once again to make it quick and easy, at the expense of clarity.

We can see these demands at work throughout language change. Consider for example, the change from Old English, which had a case system on its nouns, to Modern English, which does not. Each English noun had a different ending ("case marker") to signal whether the noun was functioning as a subject (nominative ending), object (accusative ending), possessor (genitive ending), or a goal of motion (dative ending). For one class of nouns the endings were as follows (I leave out length marks):

CASE	SINGULAR	PLURAL
Nominative	stan, 'stone'	stanas, 'stones'
Genitive	stanes	stana
Dative	stane	stanum
Accusative	stan	stanas

Old English underwent a change, in certain classes of words, that "reduced" the suffix vowel (the vowel in the case ending); that is, the suffix vowel received less stress and was pronounced as the 'neutral' schwa vowel [ə]. This change is part of a larger process that concentrates speech energy early in the word and reduces the material after the first vowel with stress. This change had the effect that the final vowel of the dative singular (*stane*) and the genitive plural (*stana*) both because the schwa vowel [ə], while forms like *stanes* (genitive singular) and *stanas* (nominative and accusative plural) became the same (in actual pronunciation, rather than spelling: [stɔ:nəs], Modern English 'stones'). This would give us a case system like the one below (where what is spelled as 'e' is the schwa vowel [ə]):

CASE	SINGULAR	PLURAL
Nominative	stan, 'stone'	stanes, 'stones'
Genitive	stanes	stane
Dative	stane	stanem
Accusative	stan	stanes

Case endings are now too similar to do much of a job of distinguishing the different cases. Eventually, the weak final vowels are dropped altogether and we get, after a change in the [a] vowel as well, a simple contrast between singular 'stone' [ston] and plural 'stones' [stonz]. The net result of these changes is to make the language quick and easy, thus honoring the second demand. But they erode a case system that contained information (what function the noun was playing in the sentence), and this, in turn, endangers the first demand for the language to be clear. To honor these latter demands, English came to use prepositions more widely to make up for the reduction in case markings (saying *'to* the stone*,'* rather than just the dative *stane*), and rigidified its word order to SVO (subject verb object) to use the position before the verb to mark subjects and the position after the verb to mark objects. This recovered the clarity and expressiveness of the language, but now at the cost of some speed and ease. It also meant that word-order variations (deviations from SVO order) that early forms of English could use for rhetorical expressiveness (which is, in fact, yet another of the demands children place on a language) disappeared.

The process goes on forever. There are no ideal languages; all languages are in flux as they attempt to achieve a balance among these competing forces. The introduction of a writing system for the language, and the presence of widely seen and influential public media (television and radio, for instance) can cause change to slow down by serving as a constant model of the status quo, but it cannot stop change altogether.

——————————————— **E X E R C I S E** ———————————————

Exercise I. Considering the data on BVE in Sections 9.4 (on absence of the verb 'to be') and 9.5 (on the absence of the verb 'to be' and the bare 'be' form), how do these changes from standard English reflect the two demands placed on language by children (to be clear, and to be quick and easy) that we have discussed in the section above?

9.7. LANGUAGE RECONSTRUCTION AND THE LANGUAGES OF THE WORLD

The concept that languages change through time and that two languages can be historically related to each other is an important one. To see this, consider several examples of the opening line of "The Lord's Prayer" written in several different languages over long stretches of time. The texts below come from English as it was at the time of Shakespeare (1611), of Chaucer (late fourteenth century), and of King Aelfric (about 1000 C.E.); current German and Old High German (around 850 C.E.); Welsh of the sixteenth century; and Hungarian.

The texts are spelled as in the originals, except that I have substituted the letter combination 'th' for the spelled 'þ' that occurred in the Old English and fourteenth-century English texts. This substitution makes clearer the relationship of the older English texts to the newer ones, as well as to the modern and older German texts. I give transliterations for only the Welsh and the Hungarian.

English (1611)

Our father which art in heauen, hallowed be thy name.

English (late 14th century)

Oure fadir that art in heuenes, halwid be thi name;

Old English (West Saxon, around 1000 C.E.)

Faeder ure thu the eart on heofonum, si thin nama gehalgod;

Modern German

Unser Vater in dem Himmel. Dein Name werde geheiligt.

Old High German (East Frankish, Tatian's version, around 830 C.E.)

Fater unser thu thar bist in himile, si giheilagot thin namo,

Welsh (standard version, 16th century)

Ein	tad,	yr	hwn	wyt	yn	y	nefoedd:
Our	father	that	who	are	in	the	heaven

sancteiddier	dy	enw.
be-hallowed	thy	name.

Modern Hungarian

Mi	Atyank,	ki	vagy	a	mennyekben,
Our	father,	who	art	the	heavens-in

szenteltessek meg	a	te	neved;
hallowed-be	the	thy	name;

Several things are obvious from looking at these texts. First, English today is not identical to even the English that was used in 1611, let alone the earlier versions given. We would no longer (except in church, perhaps) say "Our father which art in heauen, hallowed by thy name." To translate this line into contemporary English, we would have to write something like 'Our father (or, to avoid sexist terms, *our parent*), who is in heaven, may your name be considered holy and sacred'.

Even if we do not recognize or know how to pronounce all the words in these different texts, some look or feel more familiar than others. All the English versions and the two German versions seem somehow recognizable, even if we do not really understand them. The older English texts and the German texts look like a science fiction writer was trying to make up a new language out of one we already knew. However, we have no such experience of recognition when considering the Welsh and Hungarian texts.

We see a large number of similarities between all the English and German texts, but many less between these and the Welsh and Hungarian. For example, the words for 'father' in all the English and German texts are similar ('father', 'fadir', 'faeder', 'vater', 'fater'), and they are quite different from the words for 'father' in Welsh and Hungarian ('tad', 'atyank').

Imagine a community of people who said *fater* for 'father' (as they did in Old High German). As time went on, imagine people separated from this community, going their own way. As these people ceased to communicate with the original group and communicated only with themselves, they might change *fater* to *vater* (/f/ and /v/ are very similar sounds). No one from the original community is around to care. Perhaps the new community was influenced by speakers of some other language they had come into contact with, perhaps the change "just" happened. As time goes on, new changes might happen, either in this group, or by a new group separating off, or through influence from another language. Imagine, for instance, that two groups split off from the original group, each going separate ways. Over time, one group changes *fater* to *vater* and the other changes *fater* to *faeder,* changing the vowel sound a bit and changing the middle /t/ to /d/ (/t/ and /d/ are also very similar sounds), perhaps doing these changes one at a time over a considerable amount of time. And then, after a time, the group that says *faeder* itself splits and one subgroup continues to say *faeder* and the other starts saying *fadir.*

As time goes on, all these groups will come to speak different dialects of one language and, as more time goes on, different languages. But such similarities will tell us they once spoke the same one. In this case, we will say that these languages are historically related to each other.

Languages do not just change over time in the words they use. The way in which they form their sentences (the syntax of the language) also changes. So we can notice above that all the English and German texts form their sentences in fairly similar ways. If we look closely enough, in fact, we will also notice that Welsh, looked at syntactically, is not all that different from English and German (though it looked quite different when we only looked at words). Now Hungarian seems the sole "odd man out," clearly quite different from all the other languages in our example. Hungarian's use of the word 'in' as part of and after the noun 'heavens' and its use of 'the your name' are quite different structures from the other languages. And, indeed, Welsh is related to English and German, though more distantly than they are related to each other. Hungarian is not related to any of these languages.

Thus, we have argued that if two groups of people who speak the same language stop regularly communicating with one another, whether for social, political, or geographical reasons, the language they speak will change differently for each group. Two different dialects will appear, and eventually the change may lead to what will be considered two different languages. This happened to fifth-century Germanic, for instance, which eventually split into English and more modern varieties of German, as well as other languages. It happened to Latin as well. As the Roman Empire fell apart, the diverse and far-flung groups of people who spoke Latin began to diverge more and more from a common model. This eventually gave rise to the so-called Romance languages (Catalan, French, Italian, Portuguese, Provencal, Romanian, Spanish, and others).

Scholars can trace the changes that occurred in each case to turn Latin into each of these *daughter* languages. For example, for English 'dear', Italian, Spanish, and Protuguese all say *caro* [karo], while French says *cher* [ser]. The first three languages have retained the initial [k] from Latin (which said 'dear' as *carus* [karus]). French has undergone a change that changed initial [k] in a variety of words to [s].

Since oral language has been around much longer than written language, and since most of the earth's languages have not in the past, nor now, been written down, we have no direct evidence of the changes that created most languages. Thanks to the fact that we have written records of Latin, we can trace its evolution into the Romance languages. We can also do the same for the parent and daughter languages in other cases where written sources exist.

But this also gives us a way to make intelligent guesses about what happened in cases where no written records exist. Looking at cases like Latin, where written records do exist, we can get a good idea of what constitute typical, normal, or expected changes in language. We can then use this knowledge to "reconstruct" what may have happened in cases where no records exist to help us. For example, suppose we found a group of languages that had the following words for roughly the same or a similar concept (say 'honor'): language 1: *hono,* language 2: *hono,* language 3: *fono,* language 4: *vono;* and we found many other such correspondences in other words, that is, cases where languages 1 and 2 had [h], language 3 had [f], and language 4 had [v]. These similarities are unlikely to have happened by chance. In cases where we have direct evidence (based on written records or study of contemporary languages), a change of [f] or [v] to [h] is common, but a change of [h] turning into either [f] or [v] is not. Further, a change of [f] to [v] in front of vowels is very common. Thus, we could reconstruct a scenario in which some parent language, which has perhaps disappeared, has changed in languages 1 and 2 by having initial [f] go to [h] and in the case of language 3 by having initial [f] go to [v].

By such a method, used over many cases, we could even reconstruct a parent language we had no records of at all. In this case, if there was other supporting evidence, we would conclude that languages 1, 2, 3, and 4 were related as daughters to the parent language we had reconstructed via the changes we had hypothesized.

Such historical reconstruction has been very successful in linguistics. But there are pitfalls. There are cases where one language has borrowed so much from another one that it becomes nearly impossible to conclude that it was not originally related to the language it borrowed from, but rather to another language. Nonetheless, such methods have taught us that English, which together with German is the daughter of fifth-century Germanic, is related more distantly to such languages as Greek, Latin, and Russian, since all of these are "granddaughters" several times removed of a parent language we call *Indo-European,* a language that is long dead and for which there are no direct records. Indo-European was spoken about 6,000 years ago.

Indo-European gave rise to the Celtic languages (for example, Welsh, Scots Gaelic, Irish, and Breton), the Romance languages (Catalan, French, Italian, Portuguese, Provencal, Romanian, Spanish), the Germanic languages (Dutch, English, Flemish, Frisian, German, Yiddish), the Hellenic languages (of which Greek is the only remaining member), the Baltic languages (Latvian, Lithuanian), the Slavic languages (Bulgarian, Czech, Macedonian, Polish, Russian, Serbo-Croatian, Slovak, Slovenian, Ukrainian), and the Indo-Iranian languages (Bengali, Hindi, Punjabi, Urdu). Albanian and Armenian are also Indo-European languages. Thus, all these languages are related to each other as sisters or as cousins.

Of course, since people have moved all over the earth in rather chaotic ways, we cannot tell to what other languages a language is related by where it is spoken. Hungarian is spoken in Europe and is surrounded by Indo-European languages, but it is not an Indo-European language. Rather, it is in the Finno-Ugric family within the Uralic languages (together with Estonian, Finnish, and Lapp). Bengali, Hindi, and Marathi, spoken in India, are Indo-European. Kannada, Malayalam, Tamil, Telugu, also spoken in India, are not. Rather they are Dravidian languages, stemming ultimately from a different parent than the Indo-European languages. Of course, it may be that beyond languages like Indo-European, spoken 6,000 years ago, there was a parent language that gave rise to Indo-European and other ancient languages, which in turn gave rise to all the languages in the world today (save those that arose via creolization). However, we cannot prove this.

There are over 4,000 languages spoken today, and many have died (we can never know how many, since most died leaving no written record). Of course, there are many more non-Indo-European languages than Indo-European ones. The languages of the world fall into many families and larger groupings (like Indo-European), and we are by no means sure of the groupings in all cases. For example, there were hundreds of American Indian languages (many of which have died, thanks to the death of many American Indian groups), which fall into many families, and these families may or may not all have stemmed from the same parent language.

Finally, we should realize that what gets named as a single language is often a political matter. There are dialects of German and Dutch that are mutually intelligible (and, by the same token, dialects of German that are not). There is little linguistic reason to count Dutch and German as different languages rather than dialects of the same language. There is, however, a great deal of political reason for it, including a boundary between the two countries and the fact that Germany invaded Holland in the Second World War.

Figure 9-1 is a "family tree" diagram showing the relationship of some of the Indo-European languages to each other.

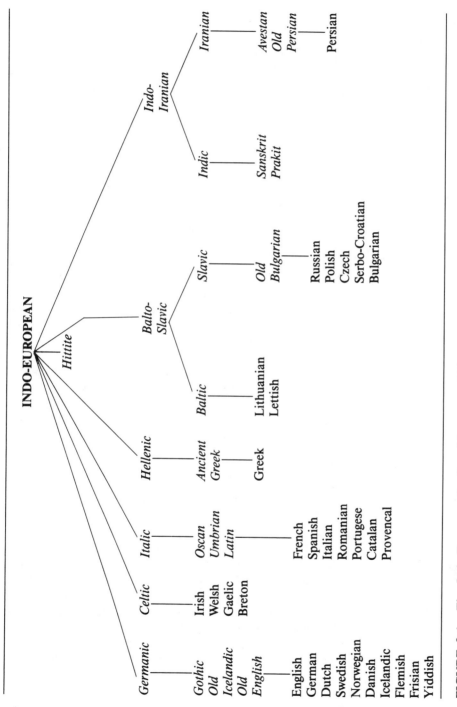

FIGURE 9-1. The Indo-European family of languges. Oldest attested languages are in italics; currently spoken languages are in roman type.

————————————— E X E R C I S E —————————————

Exercise J. English is a Germanic language and is more closely related to German than it is to Latin, since German and English have the same parent language (though Latin, German, and English are all Indo-European languages). In its history, however, English has borrowed quite extensively from both Latin and French (a daughter of Latin) thanks to the contacts it has had with Latin, the historic language of the Catholic church, and with French (the language of the Norman invaders; and in any case, France is close to England). Thus, many of its words are related to Latin or French words rather than to German ones. Using a German-English dictionary and a Latin-English dictionary, list twelve words in English that obviously are closely related to German words and twelve English words that are closely related to Latin words.

> EXAMPLE: Looking in my German-English dictionary, I see in the English section the word 'ride'. The German for 'ride' is listed as the verb *reiten* (for riding a horse) and *fahren* (for riding in a car). The first is obviously related to English 'ride', and the English and German words in all likelihood came from the same word in the past, becoming 'ride' in English and *reiten* in German. By the way, the 'en' on the end of the German verb is the marker of the infinitive (it functions like English 'to' in 'to ride'). Or, looking in the English section of my Latin-English dictionary, I see the English word 'offer'. The Latin for this word is listed as *offerre*. The two words are obviously closely related, and English 'offer' has in all likelihood come from borrowing the Latin word (and changing it a bit). The 're' form at the end of the Latin word is the marker of the infinitive form of the verb.

9.8. THE COMPLAINT TRADITION

It is not uncommon today to hear people complain that English is deteriorating and degenerating. They often blame this on the education system or (if willing to display their prejudices openly) on poor people and minority groups. However, people have been lodging this complaint for as long as we have written records in English. It is also a common complaint throughout history in the case of many other languages. It stems from the fact that all languages, whether we like it or not, change. They do not really change for the better or worse. At any one time they represent some balance—always good enough for communication—between the competing demands of quick and easy communication, on the one hand, and clarity and expressiveness, on the other. None of them are perfect, none are imperfect. They are all human languages; that is, they follow the dictates set by the human biological capacity for language, mixed inextricably with the nature of human culture, which everywhere makes intricate and complex demands for communication.

People will complain that one should not strand prepositions, but if asked they will readily acknowledge that 'Which schools did you give money to?' (with a stranded preposition) is correct and that 'To which schools did you give money?' is somewhat odd and sounds out of date. This change has virtually gone to completion, and the complainers are fighting a losing battle. Both forms communicate just as well.

In cases like 'good' for 'well' ('I did good on the test' instead of the traditionally correct 'I did well on the test'), or the less common, but still commonly heard, loss of 'ly' on adverbs ('They ran quick to the store' rather than the "correct" 'They ran quickly to the store'), the forms the complainers like as "correct" are often heard, and the change is less far along. One or both of these changes may not succeed, but then again they may.

But what if they did? If the 'ly' on adverbs was dropped from the language altogether, the position of the adverb would still signal its function, and meaning would in no way be impaired (adverbs modify verbs and adjectives, adjectives modify nouns; as long as one can tell verbs from nouns, then one can tell adverbs from adjectives—but in fact, since adjectives and adverbs are both modifiers, why shouldn't they have the same form?).

My point is not that 'quick' is better than 'quickly'. Rather, it is that which one is "correct" at any given time is simply a matter of social convention. Social conventions, whether in language or other aspects of society, must stay stable enough to allow for continuity and, at the same time, must allow for change to leave room for adaptation to new conditions. Language does this very well indeed. No one ever wakes up to hear their language so changed they can no longer understand it, and no living language ever failed to change enough to cope with whatever world it had to talk about. As the creoles show, humans do not need any particular education, or any advice from books or pedants, to create a perfectly good, indeed quite beautiful, language. In regard to language, we humans are equal, and we are masters.

RECOMMENDED FURTHER READING

BRICE HEATH, SHIRLEY (1983). *Ways with Words: Language, Life and Work in Communities and Classrooms.* Cambridge: Cambridge University Press. (A readable classic involving theory and practice that anyone interested in language, literacy, and education ought to read.)

CAZDEN, COURTNEY (1988). *Classroom Discourse: The Language of Teaching and Learning.* Portsmouth, N.H.: Heinemann. (Highly readable, and a good survey of the area.)

KOCHMAN, THOMAS (1981). *Black and White Styles in Conflict.* University of Chicago Press. (Very entertaining study of black/white differences in college classrooms.)

LABOV, WILLIAM (1972). *Language in the Inner City: Studies in the Black English Vernacular.* Philadelphia: University of Pennsylvania Press. (Contains, among much else, an excellent chapter on narrative.)

LABOV, WILLIAM (1972). *Sociolinguistic Patterns.* Philadelphia: University of Pennsylvania Press. (A classic by the founder of modern sociolinguistics.)

MILROY, JAMES & MILROY, LESLEY (1985). *Authority in Language: Investigating Language Prescription and Standardisation.* London & New York: Routledge & Kegan Paul. (An good, accessible, and entertaining introduction to sociolinguistics.)

MILROY, LESLEY (1987). *Language and Social Networks.* Oxford & New York: Blackwell. (The best current introduction to variation in language.)

MILROY, LESLEY (1987). *Observing and Analysing Natural Language.* Oxford & New York: Blackwell. (Readable guide to how sociolinguistic research is actually done in the field.)

PATTISON, ROBERT (1982). *On Literacy: The Politics of the Word from Homer to the Age of Rock.* Oxford: Oxford University Press. (Very entertaining and a good overview of politically and culturally situated approaches to literacy.)

ROMAINE, SUZANNE (1988). *Pidgin and Creole Languages.* London: Longman. (An accessible guide to work in the field; it cites a good deal of the relevant literature.)

SCOLLON, RONALD & SCOLLON, SUZANNE B. K. (1981). *Narrative, Literacy, and Face in Interethnic Communication.* Norwood, N.J.: Ablex. (Excellent and highly readable book.)

STEPHENS, JOHN & WATERHOUSE, RUTH (1990). *Literature, Language and Change: From Chaucer to the Present.* London: Routledge. (A highly readable introduction to changes in literary English.)

WOLFSON, NESSA (1989). *Perspective: Sociolinguistics and TESOL.* New York: Newbury House. (A good introduction to sociolinguistics in the context of work on teaching English to speakers of other languages.)

CHAPTER 10

Discourse

Language
in Context

10.1. THE NATURE OF DISCOURSE

Consider the meaning of a sentence like 1a below. The meaning of this sentence combines together several simple **propositions,** listed in 1b. A *proposition* is the simplest sentence-like unit of meaning. It combines a term for one simple action, process, or state of affairs (called a **predicate**) together with a term or terms for the participants in that action, process, or state of affairs. Since propositions are units of meaning, I will write them in small capital letters, to make it clear they are not English sentences. We can consider them 'simple sentences' made out of concepts or ideas in the *language of thought* (discussed in Chapter 1). In the propositions listed in 1b, 'x' is a variable for some unnamed individual object, a person in this case, and 'y' is a variable for another unnamed individual object, a physical entity in this case:

> *1a.* The tall man lit an awful cigar

> *1b.* x is KNOWN   (contribution from 'the')
>   x is TALL   (contribution from 'tall')
>   x is a MAN   (contribution from 'man')
>   x LIT y   (contribution from 'lit')
>   y is not KNOWN (contribution from 'an')
>   y is AWFUL   (contribution from 'awful')
>   y is a CIGAR   (contribution from 'cigar')

NOTE: KNOWN means that a thing referred to is assumed to be already known to the hearer based on the previous discourse, the context in which the communication occurs, or on the basis of mutual knowledge that the hearer shares with the speaker.

The simple propositions in 1b can, however, be packaged together in many different ways. For example, the sentences below also combine together the propositions in 1b:

2a. It was the tall man who lit an awful cigar

2b. It was an awful cigar that the tall man lit

2c. What the tall man lit was an awful cigar

2d. What the tall man did was light an awful cigar

2e. An awful cigar was lit by the tall man

2f. An awful cigar was what the tall man lit

2g. The man who was tall lit an awful cigar

2h. The tall man lit a cigar which was awful

2i. The tall man, he lit an awful cigar

Furthermore, the propositions in 1b could also be combined together using more than one sentence. For example, consider the ways of packaging the propositions in 1b given below (some of which also use the proposition 'x HAD y', which is implied by the sentence in 1a but not explicitly asserted):

3a. There was a tall man. He lit an awful cigar.

3b. The tall man lit something awful. It was a cigar.

3c. There was a tall man with an awful cigar. He lit it.

3d. There was an awful cigar which a tall man had. He lit it.

3e. There was a tall man. He had an awful cigar. He lit it.

3f. The tall man lit something. It was awful. It was a cigar.

3g. There was a tall man. He had something awful. It was a cigar. He lit it.

Notice here that when the propositions in 1b are combined together by using more than a single sentence, these sentences are connected by pronouns. For example, in 3a the pronoun 'he' in the second sentence ('He lit an awful cigar') refers back to 'a tall man' in the first sentence ('There was a tall man'). Thus, the pronoun connects the second sentence to the previous one. This is one of several ways English has of signaling that one sentence is talking about the same thing that a previous sentence was talking about. The pronoun here binds or links the two sentences together, and is said to be a **cohesive device** or a marker of **cohesion.**

Thus, we see that speakers or writers always have lots of choices about how they will combine the propositions they want to express. And all the sentences in 1a and 2a–i and the sets of sentences in 3a–g mean the same thing in the narrow sense of having the same truth value. That is, all of these sentences and sets of sentences are true or false under the same conditions. They all simply assert that all of the propositions in 1b are true. But then why does language allow all these options? Each of these options has a different *use* from the others; each is used in a different context. Each of these sentences or sets of sentences is a different sort of a *tool* used to communicate the propositions in 1b. And they differ from each other because the conditions of doing this job differs a bit depending on the context of communication (who you are communicating to, what they know, where you are communicating, and why).

We have brought up three topics here, topics with which this chapter will deal: (a) how propositions are packaged together in a single sentence or a set of them (*information packaging*); (b) how sentences are linked or connected (*cohesion*); and (c) how sentences are used, that is, how they are matched to different contexts or purposes of communicating (*contextualization*).

We will take up these topics as follows below: First, in Section 10.2 we will discuss how information is packaged inside sentences, an aspect of topic (a) above. In Section 10.3 we will discuss how sentences are fitted to their contexts of utterance, topic (c) above. In Section 10.4 we will take up the topic of cohesion directly, topic (b) above. However, a good deal of the discussion throughout this chapter will relate to how sentences are linked together in discourse. In Section 10.5 we return to packaging, topic (a), this time to discuss how information is packaged not just within sentences but across connected stretches of discourse such as stories.

Any discussion of how sentences are fitted to the contexts in which they are used, which is topic (c), brings up another major area of concern for the study of language in context. When we communicate, we are not just *talking* to people, we are also *acting on* and *with* them. Talk, in actual conversation, is *social action.* Thus, in this chapter we will also study the nature of conversation, social action, and speech acts. We will take up this topic at the end of the chapter, in Section 10.6.

─────────────── **E X E R C I S E** ───────────────

Exercise A. Following the model exemplified in 1a and 1b in Section 10.1, state what propositions are combined in the following English sentences:

1. Black cats like white cats.
2. Boys become men.
3. The pretty, black cat kissed the dog.

10.2. PACKAGING INFORMATION WITHIN SENTENCES

Left Dislocation: A Case Study

One of many ways English has of packaging information is called **left dislocation.** We will look briefly at how left dislocation functions in context. In this discussion I will call any single noun or any string of words functioning like a noun (by, for instance, serving as the subject of the sentence, or the object of the verb), a *noun phrase,* NP for short. Thus, in a sentence like 'The little cat likes John', I will call both 'the little cat' and 'John' noun phrases or NPs. Consider the sentences in 4a and 4b:

4a. I haven't seen my red sweater since I got it

4b. My red sweater, I haven't seen *it* since I got it

These are two alternative ways of packaging the same information. The sentence in 4a is a declarative sentence, the type of sentence that represents the usual pattern in English. 4b, on the other hand, is a special-purpose device, a special deviation from the normal pattern represented by 4a, used for more specialized tasks. Sentences like 4b are called left dislocations because they look as if the NP (in this case 'the red sweater') has been "dislocated" from its normal position (where the 'it' occurs) to the beginning of the sentence, leaving behind the pronoun to hold its old place.

The beginning of a sentence is a salient position, one where we can place information we want to draw special attention to. Linguists use the term **foregrounding** for devices that help bring special attention to information (like placing it at the front of the sentence, and other devices, such as adding special stress or emphasis to a word or phrase). In 4b, the phrase 'my red sweater' is foregrounded. Left dislocations may appear odd when written down, since they do not normally appear in expository writing. However, they are very common in speech (almost all speakers use them, even if they are consciously unaware of that fact).

Now, let's look at the actual discourse that 4b came out of.[1]

5. An' I got a red sweater, an' a white one, an' a blue one, an' a yellow one, an' a couple other sweaters, you know. And uh my sister loves borrowing my sweaters because they're pullovers, you know, an' she c'n wear a blouse under'em an' she thinks 'Well this is great'. (pause) *An' so my red sweater, I haven't seen it since I got it.*

[1] This example, and others used in this and the next section, are based on examples in "Foregrounding Referents: A Reconsideration of Left Dislocation," in Elinor Ochs and Bambi Schieffelin, eds., *Acquiring Conversational Competence* (London: Routledge & Kegan Paul, 1983), pp. 158–74.

The left dislocation here is used in a fairly typical way. Notice that the red sweater is introduced ('An' I got a red sweater . . .'), then dropped from the talk for some time as the girl talks about her other sweaters and her sister's love for borrowing them. At the end of the passage, the girl wants to again talk about the red sweater. The problem is that since it has not been mentioned for a while, it has dropped into the background of the listener's attention or consciousness (the listener is now focused on other things). Thus, the speaker uses left dislocation to place the phrase 'my red sweater' at the front of the sentence, and this foregrounds it. Left dislocation here has the function of bringing information back into the focus of consciousness or attention. This foregrounding ensures that the speaker and listener are mutually focused on the same information (her red sweater) when that information has not been recently mentioned and has dropped from avid attention.

Left dislocation has several other functions, but we will look at only one more. Imagine that a speaker wants to talk about a person named Pat McGee, that is, Pat McGee is going to be the speaker's topic of conversation. The speaker may be unsure what exactly the hearer already knows about this referent, Pat McGee. The speaker may, in fact, fear that the listener does not know enough about Pat McGee to be able to identify him well enough to understand what the speaker wants to say about him. In this case, the speaker can use left dislocation to focus the hearer's attention on Pat McGee and then say something about him that either checks on the listener's knowledge about Pat McGee or gives information that helps the hearer identify him sufficiently to understand what the speaker wishes to say about him. For example, consider the case below:

6. K: *Uh Pat McGee, I don't know if you know him, he, he lives in Palisades.*
   J: I know him real well as a matter of fact he's one of my best friends
   K: He used to go to the school I did, an' he
   J: No, no (hh)
   K: he was in the dorm with me, and I was over him, and he, he had a room. An' he
   J: No! (hh). Heh heh
   K: he despised me.

Here the speaker ("K") uses a left dislocation (*"Pat McGee,* I don't know if you know *him, he* lives in Palisades") to check on what the hearer ("J") does or does not know about the topic (Pat McGee). Everything between 'Pat McGee' and 'he despised me' (which is what the speaker wants to say about the topic) is "background information" used to get the hearer straight on who is being talked about or, better put, to assure that the speaker and hearer are focused on the same thing in the right way so that something new can be said about it. Here, then, left dislocation is used to introduce a new topic in such a way as to ensure that what the speaker intends to say about it will be properly understood.

Function Words and Content Words

Sentences *package information.* To understand how they do this, we need to draw a distinction between *content* words and *function* words. Content words (sometimes also called **lexical** words) belong to the major parts of speech: nouns, verbs, and adjectives. These categories are said to be **open categories** in the sense that they each have a large number of members, and languages readily add new members to these categories through borrowing from other languages or the invention of new words.

Function words (also sometimes called **grammatical** words) belong to smaller categories, categories that are said to be **closed categories** in the sense that each category has relatively few members and languages are resistant to borrowing or inventing anew such words (though they sometimes do). Such categories as determiners (for example, 'the', 'a/n', 'this/that', 'these/those'—these are also sometimes called articles), pronouns ('he/him', 'she/her', 'it', 'himself', 'herself'), prepositions ('in', 'on', 'to', 'of'), and quantifiers ('some', 'many', 'all', 'none') are function word categories.

Function words show how the content words in a sentence relate to each other, or how pieces of information within the sentence fit into the overall ongoing communication. For example, the definite determiner 'the' signals that the information following it is already 'known' to the speaker and hearer. Pronouns signal that their referents have been previously mentioned, or are readily identifiable in the context of communication or on the basis of the speaker and hearer's mutual knowledge. Prepositions link NPs to other words in the sentence (for example, in 'lots of luck', 'of' links 'luck' to 'lots'; in 'ideas in my mind', 'in' links 'my mind' to 'ideas'; and in 'look at the girl', 'at' links 'the girl' to the verb 'look'). I have not mentioned adverbs. Adverbs are messy and complicated. Often they function in a way that is mid-way between a function word and a content word. I will for the most part ignore them.

Since function words show how the content words in a sentence relate to each other, they can help us make guesses about what sorts of content words accompany them and what these words mean. To see this, consider the first stanza of Lewis Carroll's poem "Jabberwocky":

> <u>Twas</u> bryllyg, <u>and the</u> slythy tove<u>s</u>
> <u>Did</u> gyre <u>and</u> gymble <u>in the</u> wabe:
> <u>All</u> mimsy <u>were the</u> borogove<u>s</u>;
> <u>And the</u> mome rath<u>s</u> outgrabe.

I have underlined the function words. I have also underlined the plural affix ('es' and 's') since it functions just like a function word, though it is not a separate word. In this poem, Carroll uses real English function words, but nonsense content words (how do we know they are content words? By how they are placed in relation to the function words). Despite the fact that half the "words" in this text are nonsense, any speaker of English can use the function words to unravel the grammar of the sentences and to make good guesses about what content word categories (noun, verb, adjective) the nonsense content words belong to. The speaker of English can even make some good guesses about what the nonsense words might mean or what they might refer to. Thus, we readily interpret the stanza as a description of an outdoor scene with creatures of various sorts frolicking or moving about.

Function Words and Information

Since function words carry less of the real content of the communication (their job is to signal the grammar of the sentence), we can say that they tend to be *informationally less salient or significant* than content words. While they are certainly helpful, they are often dispensable, as anyone who has written a telegram knows.

Thus, let us make a distinction between two types of information in a sentence. Information that is relatively new and relatively unpredictable I will call **informationally salient.** The actual specific meaning of any content word in a sentence is unpredictable without knowing exactly what the content word means. In the Carroll poem, we vaguely know that 'toves' are probably active little animate creatures, but we have no idea what exactly they are. Thus, content words are usually informationally more salient than function words.

Information that is given, assumed already known, or predictable I will call **informationally less salient.** Often, even if you have not heard a function word, you can predict exactly where it should have been and what word exactly it would have been. For example, if you heard 'Boy has lots ideas', you could well predict that 'the' is missing in front of 'boy' and 'of' between 'lots' and 'ideas'. If, however, you heard 'The boy has lots of', you could not predict what content word should come after 'of' (though 'of' signals it will be an NP). Thus, function words are usually informationally less salient than content words.

In general, then, the distinction between content words and function words is between two types of information. However, beyond this gross dichotomy, the distinction between information that is more or less salient is one that can only be drawn in the actual context of communication.

Information and Stress

Consider the following dialogue:

7. A: I haven't read any good books lately.
   B: Well, I read an *interesting* book recently. (Goes on to describe the book)

The nature of the information in the response by "B" is partially set up by the remark made by "A," which here represents the context in which "B"'s response occurs. In this context, only the word 'interesting' is new information, is unpredictable, and is therefore informationally salient. The function words ('I' and 'a') are both totally predictable in this context. Considering the content words in the sentence, 'read' is predictable because it already occurred in "A" 's preceding remark. 'Book' also occurred in the preceding remark. 'Recently' was not directly mentioned in the preceding remark, but it is heavily implied by 'lately' in that remark.

Thus, in this response, the function words are least informationally salient, the content words 'read', 'book', and 'recently' are less salient than 'interesting', but more salient (as content words) than the function words. And 'interesting' is the informationally most salient word in the sentence.

English uses **stress** to mark degrees of informational saliency. Stress is a *psychological concept,* not a physical one. English speakers use and hear several different degrees of stress in a sentence, but this is not physically marked in any uniform and consistent way. Stress is physically marked by a combination of increased loudness, increased length, and by changing the pitch of one's voice (raising or lowering the pitch, or gliding up or down in pitch) on a word's primary (accented) syllable. Any one or two of these can be used to trade off for the others in a complicated way. In any case, English speakers unconsciously use and recognize stress, and it can be brought to conscious awareness with a little practice (some people are better than others at bringing stress differences to conscious awareness, though they can all unconsciously use and recognize it). A word with more stress than another word sounds more salient (it often sounds louder, though it may not really be louder, but just be longer or have a pitch change on it, both of which will make English speakers think it sounds louder).

Say the sentence in "B" 's response in 7 above (in a quick and normal way). In this context, 'interesting' has the most stress. The relatively unsalient content words 'read', 'book', and 'recently' have less stress than 'interesting', with 'recently' having a bit more than the others, being a bit less predictable. The function words have next to no stress, just enough to get them said at all. Thus, the stress reflects directly the informational saliency of the words in the sentence:

8. I	read	an	interesting	book	recently
|	|	|	|	|	|
least stress	third most stress	least stress	most stress	third most stress	second most stress

In English, often the word with the most stress in the sentence gets special treatment. The pitch change on this word (up or down) is the most dramatic, and this pitch change tends to be the center of the intonation contour of the sentence as a whole (if several words are equally salient and equally heavily stressed, the last one tends to constitute the intonational peak or center of the sentence).

The context in which an utterance is uttered, together with the assumptions that the speaker makes about the hearer's knowledge, determines the degrees of informational saliency for each word and phrase in a sentence. Thus, in a context in which little is assumed to be already given and known, like that in 9a below, several pieces of information may be quite salient:

9a. Guess what happened? A *friend* of mine *shot* her *husband.*

Here all three content words, 'friend', 'shot', and 'husband' are informationally salient and have a good degree of stress. If the context assumed more information as already given and thereby mutually known to speaker and hearer, some of these content words would have less informational saliency and therefore less stress. For example,

9b. A: What did your friend do?
    B: My friend *shot* her *husband.*
9c. A: Who did your friend shoot?
    B: My friend shot her *husband.*

In 9b, the context created by "A"'s question renders the friend known information and thus 'my friend' is now less informationally salient in the response. In the context created by "A"'s question in 9c, both the friend and the fact that a shooting took place are known, and therefore only 'husband' is informationally salient in the response.

Of course, in a given context, even a function word's information might become important, and then the function word would have a greater degree of stress. For example, consider the context below:

9d. A: Did Mary shoot her husband?
    B: No she shot YOUR husband!

In this context, the information carried by 'your' is unpredictable, new, and salient. Thus, it gets stressed (in fact, it gets extra stress because it is contrastive—*yours* not *hers*—and surprising).

E X E R C I S E

Exercise B. Tape record a conversation (for example, of people having dinner together). Transcribe several minutes of the conversation. Then underline the words that have the most stress (emphasis). Discuss why each word is salient or important in the context in which it occurs.

Information and the Mind (Consciousness)

We have seen that the more salient information is in a sentence, the more stress it receives. Now we want to relate our talk about information in sentences to a view of the mind as it plans how it will construct sentences in context. As a person is talking, he or she must consider how to package information into each sentence. Such considerations are, of course, largely unconscious. Decisions about packaging are based on the speaker's view of what is in the hearer's mind (what the speaker takes the hearer to know, believe, and currently to be paying attention to) and what effect (and affect) the speaker wants to have on the hearer.

If a piece of information has just been mentioned in the discourse, then the speaker can assume that such information is in the forefront of the hearer's attention or consciousness. Let's call such information *forefront* information. Such information is often placed in subject position and is often represented by a pronoun. This allows the speaker's sentence to tie directly to the preceding contribution and to the current focus of the hearer's attention. Thus, consider 10 below:

> *10.* My father's new gold watch got ripped off.
> Now *he*'s fit to be tied.

In 10 the pronoun 'he' names recent information, information that has just been mentioned (in the preceding sentence) and that is thus in the forefront of the hearer's consciousness. The pronoun form helps signal this fact and allows the hearer to easily attach the information in the sentence 'he's fit to be tied' to the preceding information that the hearer has already stored in his mind. Think of it this way: Hearing 'My father's new gold watch got ripped off', the hearer forms a 'hook' in his mind for the referents 'my father' and 'new gold watch', hooks on which he can then hang all subsequent information that will come up in the conversation about these referents. When he then hears 'he' starting the next sentence, this signals that the information to follow is to be placed on the 'my father' hook.

Notice that if a piece of information is in the forefront of the hearer's consciousness, is the focus of his or her awareness, then it certainly does not need to be foregrounded by the speaker. We saw above that left dislocation is a way to foreground information; that is, it is a device to bring certain information into the forefront of a hearer's consciousness when it is not already there. Thus, we would never use left dislocation for information that is already in the forefront of a hearer's consciousness, already the focus of their awareness. Thus, 'My father's gold watch got ripped off. My father, he's fit to be tied' is decidedly odd, since the left dislocation in the second sentence foregrounds 'my father', which thanks to the first sentence is already the focus of the hearer's consciousness.

If a piece of information has been mentioned in the preceding discourse, but is not recent (that is, it has been mentioned a ways back), then the speaker can assume that it is in the hearer's consciousness, but in the background of consciousness, not the forefront. It is not in the hearer's current active focus of attention. Thus, the speaker in this case needs to signal that the information is given, known, but not recent. The speaker needs to bring the information from the background of the hearer's consciousness to the forefront. The speaker needs to reactivate the information in the hearer's attention. In this case, the speaker uses a full definite NP (definiteness is marked by the determiner 'the', or a possessive pronoun, like 'my', or by use of a proper name like 'Mary'), rather than a pronoun. In some circumstances the speaker can use a left dislocation or a related form known as *topicalization* (like left dislocation, except the fronted noun phrase is not repeated as a pronoun later in the sentence, see 11c):

11a. A policeman gave me a ticket for speeding. My girlfriend was in the car and she ripped it up and threw it out the window. *The policeman* saw her and was fit to be tied.

11b. An' I got a red sweater, an' a white one, an' a blue one, an' a yellow one, an' a couple other sweaters, you know, and uh my sister loves borrowing my sweaters because they're pullovers, you know, an' she c'n wear a blouse under'em an' she thinks 'Well this is great' (pause). An' so *my red sweater,* I haven't seen *it* since I got it.

11c. I saw Mary the other day with her husband John. I can't really stand John. I certainly wouldn't want to spend any time with him. But *Mary, I really like.*

In all these cases the speaker uses something to signal that the referent has been mentioned but must be reactivated. In 11a the definite determiner 'the' and the full NP 'the policeman' (rather than the pronoun 'he') serves this function. In 11b the possessive pronoun 'my' definitizes the NP 'my red sweater'. This definitizing, together with the left dislocating of this NP and its being a full NP and not a pronoun, all signal the return of 'my red sweater' to the focus of attention. In 11c the use of a proper name ('Mary')—proper names are always definite—and the use of topicalization (putting 'Mary' in the front of the sentence) signals the job of reactivating information.

If information has not been mentioned in the discourse at all, but the speaker assumes that the hearer knows it anyway, then the speaker assumes the information is in the hearer's mind, but not in consciousness (forefront or background). The information is assumed simply to be in some long-term storage part of the mind. The speaker may assume the hearer knows the information because the speaker in fact knows the hearer does know it, or because the speaker assumes that anyone in the culture would, or because the speaker assumes that anyone in this conversation could have inferred such information from what has already been said. In this case, the speaker must signal that the information is known but must bring it from long-term storage into consciousness. Thus, consider

12. Hey, guess what? *The Russian guy who was on those Donahue Space Bridges* is speaking in *the Square* tonight.

Uttered in Boston or Cambridge, the speaker would assume that the hearer knows readily that 'the Square' is Harvard Square and that this is so obvious that no more need be said (despite the fact that there are many other squares in Boston and Cambridge). 'The' indicates that the information is given, assumed known. On the other hand, the long phrase 'the Russian guy who was on those Donahue Space Bridges' assumes that the hearer knows who Vladimir Posner is (though not necessarily by name), that in some way this man is in the hearer's mind. The speaker, assuming that the hearer has seen the Donahue Space Bridges on TV (simulcast conversations between Soviet and U.S. audiences moderated by Phil Donahue and Vladimir Posner), uses this information to help the hearer retrieve from long-term storage the person the speaker wants to speak about. The speaker gives enough information to bring this assumed known information out of the hearer's memory store and into consciousness. Once again, 'the' signals that the speaker takes the information to be known to the hearer, and in this case the length and complexity of the NP signals that the speaker assumes this information is not 'obvious' but must be actively searched for in the long-term memory store.

Finally, if information has not been mentioned in the previous discourse and is not assumed to be already known to the hearer in any fashion, the speaker assumes that the information is *new* information. The speaker must carefully mark new information because it is often the point of the communication, and, since it is new, it cannot be readily recovered or reconstructed if it is missed. New information is signaled by an indefinite determiner 'a/n' and/or by the presence of a fair degree of stress signaling that such information is informationally salient. It often is placed at or near the end of the sentence, where it will be hard to miss and easier for the hearer to remember and retain. Thus, consider

13a. Who did Mary shoot? She shot her *husband.*

13b. Who did Mary shoot? She shot a *man* she had been *seeing* for the *last year* or so.

13c. What does Mary do for a living? She *sells running shoes.*

In 13a the stress on 'husband' signals that this is new information. Since the connection of a husband to Mary is clear to anyone and Mary is known information, no more than 'husband' need be said. In 13b the indefinite determiner 'a' in the NP 'a man she had been seeing for the last year or so' signals that the referent is new information. The NP is much longer because the speaker needs to set up this referent in the hearer's mind and there is no clear and obvious connection like 'husband'. Various words in this NP are marked as new and salient information by the presence of stress.

In 13c the stress on the verb 'sells' and on the components of the NP

TABLE 10-1.   Types of Information and Their Relation to Previous Discourse and to the Hearer's State of Mind

DISCOURSE	THE MIND	STATUS OF INFORMATION	FORMS
Recently mentioned	Forefront of consciousness	Given/Old	Pronoun
Mentioned, but not recently	Background of consciousness	Given/Old	Definite determiner with noun
Not mentioned, but known	In mind, but not in consciousness	Given/Old	Definite determiner with noun and often modifiers
Not mentioned, or known	Not in mind	New	No definite determiner, stressed

'running shoes' mark these as new pieces of information. English has no indefinite determiner (like 'a/n') for plural NPs; the absence of any determiner is taken to signal that the NP is indefinite (not already known, though in some cases 'some' can be used as the plural indefinite determiner).

Table 10-1 sums up our discussion in this section.

─────────────────── E X E R C I S E ───────────────────

Exercise C.   Below is a passage from Walker Percy's essay "Notes for a Novel about the End of the World."[2] I have organized the first paragraph of the essay diagrammatically. Each sentence is numbered, and its subject is separated from the rest of the sentence. If material precedes the subject of the sentence, this is listed. Say why each subject has the form it does in terms of the information it conveys, where it occurs in the text, and the assumptions the author may be making about what is and what is not in the hearer's mind (and where in his or her mind it is—long-term storage, foreground of consciousness, background of consciousness). The phrase 'the wounded man' is somewhat odd—why doesn't the author use 'a wounded man'? Why does he use 'the wounded man' instead? What does the way in which the author apportions information to "first

─────────────────────────────

[2]From his book *The Message in the Bottle: How Queer Man Is, How Queer Language Is, and What One Has to Do With the Other* (New York: Farrar, Straus and Giroux, 1978), pp. 101–18.

position," or subject position, and the position following the subject contribute to the effectiveness and artistry of the passage?

	First Position	Subject	Rest
1.		A serious novel about the destruction of the U.S. and the end of the world	should perform the function of prophecy in reverse
2.		The novelist	writes about the coming end in order to *warn* about present ills and so avert the end
3.	Not being called by God to be a prophet	he	nevertheless pretends to a certain prescience
4.	If he did not think he saw something other people didn't see or at least didn't pay much attention to	he	would be wasting his time writing and they reading
5.		This	does not mean that he is wiser than they
6.	Rather might	it	testify to a species of affliction which sets him apart and gives him an odd point of view
7.		The wounded man	has a better view of the battle than those still shooting

	First Position	**Subject**	**Rest**
8.		The novelist	is less like a prophet than he is like the canary that coal miners used to take down into the shaft to test the air
9.	When the canary gets unhappy, utters plaintive cries, and collapses	it	may be time for the miners to surface and think things over

10.3. WHAT SENTENCES ARE ABOUT

We have now discussed at some length the issue of how information is packaged to communicate. Now we turn more directly to the issue of how information is crafted to fit the contexts in which we communicate. We all use language differently in different contexts, and members of different sociocultural groups use language somewhat differently in what appear to be similar contexts. We will first take up the issue of how we signal what we are talking about (and we will see that there are several different senses to the phrase 'what we are talking about'). Then we will turn to different styles of language, styles found in different contexts of use and among different social groups.

We have progressed far enough now to take up an interestingly complex question: What role does the subject of a sentence play in discourse? We saw in Chapter 2 that subjects are often ACTORS, but that they are not always ACTORS. For example, In 'Mary hit John', 'Mary' is both the subject of the sentence and an ACTOR, but in 'John was hit by Mary' or in 'John received a blow to the head', while 'John' is the subject, it names not the ACTOR, but rather the PATIENT (the participant who is affected or "done to"). In fact, subjects have no one consistent meaning in terms like ACTOR or PATIENT (semantic roles).

Many linguists have claimed that the subject of a sentence names the TOPIC of the utterance the sentence is used to make, that is, it names what the utterance is about. And there is no doubt that this is true in many languages. It is not clearly true of English, however, where the matter is far from simple.

Consider the following context. A person "A" knows both "B" and "B"'s sister Mary. A knows that Mary has been applying to colleges, though let us assume that "A" doesn't know exactly which ones. In the course of the conversation, Mary's name comes up, and "A" says to "B": "How'd Mary do on her college applications?" This sort of context invites a response in which Mary is the topic. She is mentioned in the preceding remark ("How'd *Mary* do on her college applications?"), and since this question essentially asks about her, is asking for information about her; it clearly invites the respondent to talk about Mary. Now both the responses below are possible and appropriate in this context (the word that has the main stress in the sentence is underlined):

14a. She got into <u>Stanford</u>

14b. <u>Stanford</u> admitted her

In 14a the pronoun 'she' signals that Mary is given information (information, in fact, that has been recently mentioned—namely, in the question 'How'd Mary do on her college applications?'—and that is therefore assumed to be in the forefront of the hearer's consciousness). 'Got into' is known information, being part of "A" and "B"'s mutual knowledge about Mary (that she has been applying to colleges and that they are discussing whether she got into any and which they were). It thus gets less stress than 'Stanford' (though a bit more than the function word 'she'). 'Stanford' receives main stress as the new information in the sentence. 14a is clearly about Mary, and 'she', the pronoun for Mary, is the topic of the sentence as well as the subject.

14b is equally about Mary in the sense that it appropriately answers the question 'What happened to Mary?' In 14b, however, the pronoun for Mary ('her') is not in subject position (but object position). 'Stanford', which is new information and stressed, is in subject position. Thus, in this sentence, 'her' is the topic of the sentence (the question asked about Mary, and 'her' stands for Mary), but 'Stanford' is its subject.

English does, however, supply a way to have your cake and eat it too. If speakers want the topic in subject position and the new information at the end of the sentence—which is the norm across languages—they can use 14a (using 'got into' instead of 'admit'). Even if the speaker wants to use 'admit', the speaker can passivize the sentence and say

14c. She was admitted by *Stanford*

Note that the passive allows the topic (Mary's pronoun) to get into subject position and the new information to move to the back of the sentence. This is one of the discourse functions of the passive. Its other function is to suppress mention of the subject of the active sentence (often the ACTOR), as when we say something like 'He was killed in Viet Nam' where we do not have to mention who or what killed him (because we don't know or don't want to say).

Topicality

Let's reconsider 14b, reprinted below:

14b. (What happened to Mary?) *Stanford* admitted her

We said in the last section that in this sentence the topic is 'her' (the response must be construed to be about Mary, if it is to be an appropriate response to the question, which is about Mary). The new information is 'Stanford'.

While it is clear that given the question 'How'd Mary do on her college applications?' 14b can be construed to be about Mary, English speakers also feel there is a sense too in which it is about its subject 'Stanford'. In 14b 'Stanford' is highlighted, it is the *psychological center of attention* in a way in which it is not in 14a, where it is not in subject position:

14a. (What happened to Mary?) She got into *Stanford*

It is difficult to say exactly what 'psychological center of attention' means, and the concept clearly needs more research. But we can say that subjects, if they have any uniform function, are the psychological "launching off" points of sentences, the dock from which the "boat" (information in the sentence) departs. They represent the perspective from which the speaker has chosen to view the event or state described by the sentence. Somehow, 14a sees Mary getting into Stanford from her perspective, while 14b sees the same event from Stanford's perspective. Note in this respect the contrasts below using symmetrical verbs that allow either participant as subject:

15a. John left his wife (Sue)
John married Sue
John met Sue for lunch
John bought a bike from Sue
John gave Sue a book

15b. Sue left her husband (John)
Sue married John
Sue met John for lunch
Sue sold a bike to John
Sue got a book from John

All the sentences in 15a seem to empathize with John, and all those in 15b to emphasize with Sue. Yet each pair in 15a and 15b "mean" the same thing, describe the same event. The event is simply viewed from different angles, and the subject determines the angle.

Unfortunately, the term 'topic' and associated terms have been used in many different, and sometimes inconsistent, ways in linguistics. So I will clearly explicate the terminology I will use here. I will call information that is new (and thus receives the highest degree of stress in a sentence) **highlighted** information.

Placing stress on such information is an invitation for the hearer to focus on this information, to place it in the forefront of his or her consciousness. Thus, such information can thereafter be mentioned by using a low degree of stress or a pronoun, signaling that it is now in the focus of the hearer's attention.

Words that represent given information (in the sense that they have been mentioned in the preceding discourse) or are known information (in that they are part of the hearer's knowledge or can be readily inferred from the context or general knowledge) I will call **topically relevant** information. Thus, in 16 below, the underlined words are highlighted, and the other words are *topically relevant* (that is, relevant to what is being talked about in the dialogue between speaker and hearer).

16. Well, I read an <u>interesting detective</u> novel recently

The topically relevant material ties back to the preceding context (though as we have seen we can distinguish between pieces of this information that are more or less informationally salient).

The subject of a sentence I will call the **psychological (or perspectival) topic,** the **P-topic** for short. Sometimes the P-topic is given or known information (as in 14a above), and thus topically relevant. Sometimes it is new and focused information (as in 14b above), and thus not topically relevant (that is, it doesn't serve to tie back to the preceding discourse, but moves the discourse ahead by introducing new information). Saying it is the psychological or perspectival topic, but not topically relevant, means that it represents the perspective one is taking on the information in the sentence, but that it is not topically related to what has gone before. Of course, something else in the sentence then must be topically relevant (unless this is the first sentence in a discourse) or the sentence would not fit with its context, would seem irrelevant to it.

Finally, let me repeat a constraint on conversation already mentioned above: One must speak *topically.* That is, in any context, one does not have to use a P-topic (subject) that directly ties to the context, but the sentence must have topical material that does tie to the context. Thus, 14a is topical because its P-topic is old information in the context; but 14b is also topical even though its P-topic is new and does not therefore tie directly to the context. However, 14b does have given information in it that ties to the context, that is, it contains information that is topically relevant in the context (namely, 'her').

In fact, speaking topically without having a P-topic that is topically relevant, as in 14b above, is one way in which to have your cake and eat it too in conversation. The context really requires that I talk about Mary ('How'd Mary do on her college applications?'), but I want to talk about Stanford. So I say 14b. I have honored your topic (Mary) by speaking topically (including given information about Mary, namely 'her'), but have in fact not used 'Mary' as my P-topic as you might have wished (wanting to talk about Mary) but rather introduced my own P-topic, 'Stanford'. Now I can, if I wish, go on to talk about Stanford, and you cannot accuse me of having not honored your "bid" to talk about Mary, despite the fact that you may find yourself talking about Stanford—what I want to talk about, but not necessarily what you wanted to talk about.

First Position in the Sentence

The first and last positions in a sentence are psychologically salient positions. Humans tend to notice and pay attention to the beginnings and ends of things. English allows certain material that normally comes later in a sentence to be "preposed" (placed) in front of the subject, thereby co-opting the subject's normal salient position in the front of the sentence. Thus, consider the following examples. In 18a–g below, material occurs at the front of the sentence that otherwise normally occurs later in the sentence (see 17a–g).

17a. Mr. Jones was delightful yesterday

17b. Mr. Jones was delightful on the film set

17c. I don't like Mr. Jones unfortunately

17d. I don't like Mr. Jones

17e. I think Jones will win, even though I don't claim to be an expert

17f. Jones scored a goal while I wasn't looking

17g. He stood up when I came in

18a. Yesterday, Mr. Jones was delightful

18b. On the film set, Mr. Jones was delightful

18c. Unfortunately, I don't like Mr. Jones

18d. Mr. Jones, I don't like him (left dislocation)

18e. Even though I don't claim to be an expert, I think Jones will win

18f. While I wasn't looking, Jones scored a goal

18g. When I came in, he stood up

Such material that is placed in front of the sentence constitutes a **frame** for the sentences that follow. The sentence material that follows is interpreted "in light of," in the framework of, in the context of (however you want to put it) the material that is placed in front of the sentence. 17a says that Jones was delightful yesterday and does not seem to imply any more than this. 18a, on the other hand, seems to imply that there was something special about yesterday that helps us to interpret or evaluate the claim that Jones was delightful then. Perhaps he is not so delightful on other days, or perhaps recently he's been a bore, but yesterday was an exception. Thus, 18a means something like 'in the context or framework of *yesterday* being significant in regard to the claim I am about to make, about Mr. Jones (my psychological topic), he was delightful.' Of course, the hearer must infer what exactly it is about yesterday that helps interpret the claim that Jones was delightful. And the hearer will do this based on his or her knowledge of the context, of Jones, and of the speaker.

On the other hand, 17a means 'About Mr. Jones (my psychological topic), he was delightful yesterday'. That is, all 17a says is that it happens that Jones's delightfulness occurred yesterday. Normally, in a sentence like 17a, 'delightful' will receive the most stress (be most highlighted), since temporal and spatial phrases at the end of a sentence are usually downplayed (it is their neutral position in English). That is, we normally say: 'Jones was DELIGHTFUL yesterday', with 'delightful' most highlighted. If, however, we place extra stress on 'yesterday' and say 'Jones was delightful YESTERDAY', then, we produce a sentence that is, in fact, very similar to 21a where 'yesterday' is preposed to the front of the sentence. Stress and positioning often "trade off" in English.

E X E R C I S E S

Exercise D. Consider the following two interchanges, where I have underlined the words in "B"'s response that get the most stress and are, thus, most highlighted. In saying these sentences to yourself, be sure you say them in a quick and normal way, stressing the words I have underlined and downplaying the others:

1. A: How'd Mary do on her college applications?
   B: Well, she got into <u>Stanford</u> yesterday.

2. A: How'd Mary do on her college applications?
   B: Well, <u>yesterday</u> she got into <u>Stanford</u>.

3. A: How'd Mary do on her college applications?
   B: Well, <u>Stanford</u> admitted her yesterday.

4. A: How'd Mary do on her college applications?
   B: Well, <u>yesterday Stanford</u> admitted her.

For each response to A above, give (a) the psychological topic of the sentence, (b) topically relevant information, and (c) the frame of the sentence, if any. Then discuss the possible differences in meaning of each response.

Exercise E. Package the following simple sentences in at least three relatively "loose" ways and three tighter ways. (HINT: 'My old radio broke' tightly packages the two simple sentences 'My radio is old', and 'My radio broke'; 'My radio, which is old, broke' is a somewhat looser packaging of these two sentences, and 'My radio is old and it broke' is a very loose packaging.) You can add little words to help combine the sentences (for example, in the phrase 'from drinking milk', the little word 'from' lets one get 'drinking' into another sentence).

1. My cat is small.
2. My cat is black.
3. My cat drank milk.
4. The milk was bad.
5. My cat got sick.

10.4. HOW GRAMMAR HELPS US TO FIT SENTENCES TO THEIR CONTEXTS

In this section we are going to study how certain grammatical devices allow utterances to fit their contexts and to connect together with preceding and following utterances. Every main verb (that is, not helping verbs) defines the nucleus or center of a **clause**. A clause is a main verb and its associated arguments (the NPs and PPs that go with it) and other modifiers. Thus, the sentence below is made up of three clauses, each of which is numbered and enclosed in brackets:

19. While ₁[John was eating his dinner], ₂[Mary said that₃[she liked cats]]

Clauses

1. John was eating his dinner
2. Mary said that she liked cats
3. She liked cats

The verb 'eat' defines the first clause, with its subject 'John' and its object 'his dinner'. The verb 'say' defines the second clause, with its subject 'Mary' and its object 'that she liked cats'. The object of 'say' is itself a clause. The verb 'like', with its subject 'she' and its object 'cats', constitutes this clause. The little grammatical words 'while' and 'that' help signal how the clauses fit together both structurally and semantically.

The syntactic devices of a language allow clauses to be more or less tightly *integrated* with each other. The clauses in a sentence can be loosely put together, or tightly bound to each other. Consider, for instance, the three simple sentences below (composed of only one clause each):

20a. The king died
20b. The queen got sick
20c. The queen died

The loosest association of these three sentences would be not to integrate them at all, but to just string them together in a discourse. Next, we could integrate them ever so slightly, by placing 'and' and 'and then' in front of the second and the third. They would still be simple sentences, not part of a single sentence, but at least the 'and' and 'and then' would connect them and to a small extent signal how they relate to each other:

21a. The king died.   The queen got sick.   The queen died.
21b. The king died.   And the queen got sick.   And then the queen died.

In 21a, the hearer must infer what exactly is the connection between the three sentences. The most likely inference a hearer would draw would be that the queen got sick and died *after* and *because* the king died. However, this is not explicitly said, and there are other possibilities; for example, the three events could have happened more or less simultaneously. Even in 21b, where the 'and then' explicitly signals that the queen's death took place some time after her illness, her illness could have occurred either at the same time or after the king's death, and her illness and death could have had no causal relation to the king's death, though without further information we readily try to infer such a relation.

Next, we can choose to integrate our three sentences a bit more tightly by placing two of them into one sentence:

22a. After the king died, the queen got sick.   And then she died.
22b. The queen got sick after the king had died.   And then she died.

Here the word 'after' explicitly signals that the event of the king dying preceded the queen's illness. Since 'after' has the function of explicitly telling us how one event is temporally ordered with another, the order of the events need no longer be said in the same order they occurred in the real world; that is, 22b can talk about the queen's illness before the king's death, even though the events happened in the real world in the opposite order.

The two clauses connected by 'after' ('the queen got sick', 'the king died') are part of one sentence now, but they are still not all that tightly integrated, not as tightly as English will allow. Such subordinate clauses as 'after the king died' are called *adverbial subordinate clauses,* and they are relatively loose ways to combine one clause with another while also signaling how the clauses fit together semantically.

Let's look at yet tighter ways to integrate clauses. Consider the following cases:

23a. After the king died, the queen got sick and—died.
23b. The king's dying caused the queen to get sick and—die.
23c. I know that the queen got sick and—died because the king died.

Here we see several different devices for tightly bonding clauses to each other. In 23a, the subject of 'the queen died' is elided (left out) because it is identical to the subject of 'the queen got sick'. This allows us to integrate the two clauses tightly. In 23b we have used a participle to make the clause 'the king died' into the subject of the verb 'cause'. This tightly integrates 'the king died' into the overall sentence, and together with the ellipsis of 'the queen' in 'the queen died' integrates all three clauses into one sentence in a very tight way. Finally, 23c introduces the verb 'know', which allows the two integrated clauses 'the queen got sick and died' to be embedded as its object. In 23c the clause 'the king died' is once again fairly loosely integrated to the whole sentence through an adverbial subordinate clause, this time with 'because', which overtly signals the causal relation that was only inferred in 22a and b.

As we use tighter and more integrative devices, our clauses look almost to disappear into the whole sentence. However, we can go one step further. By turning the verbs of these clauses into nouns (something English often allows), we can really make them disappear and get our most integrated example:

24. The king's death caused the sickness and death of the queen.

Here we have changed the verb 'die' into the noun 'death' and the verb + adjective 'got sick' into the noun 'sickness'. Our clauses are completely gone now. We once again have a simple sentence, a sentence composed of only one clause, defined by the only verb in the sentence ('caused'). However, the sentence still communicates the same information as the three clauses we started with (it communicates the same propositions that they did). Our three clauses have structurally fallen into the "Black Hole" of syntax, though they have left their information behind (something that Black Holes in physics don't allow!).

We have moved along a continuum of integration, where at each step the syntactic devices of the language allow more and more tight integration of information. In general, there is an important trade-off between the amount of integration a speaker uses and the amount of inferencing the hearer must engage in to understand the semantic connection between the clauses. They are inversely related: The more integration, the less inferencing; the less integration, the more inferencing that is required.

Pragmatic Mode Versus Syntactic Mode

We can use the concept of integration (how tightly packaged material is in a sentence) to make an important distinction about different ways of using language. This distinction turns out to play an important role in dealing with various issues, including characterizing the relation between writing and speech, and studying language acquisition, language change, and social interaction in language as well as the relationship between language use and success in school.

Let's set up a continuum of different ways of using language (whether in speech or writing). At one end of the continuum the language used is highly integrated. That is, the speaker uses a good number and variety of integrative devices to package information tightly into sentences. At the other end of the continuum is language that is much less integrated.

Below I represent this continuum and give a name to each pole. I call language toward the highly integrated end of the continuum **syntactic mode language.** I call language toward the less integrated pole **pragmatic mode language.** Syntactic mode language uses overt signals that guide the hearer or reader in interpreting the sentences of the discourse. It thus leaves less work for the hearer or reader to do in drawing inferences (making educated guesses) about what the speaker or writer meant. Pragmatic mode language uses less of these overt syntactic signals and thus demands that the hearer or reader draw more inferences about what is meant and about how various pieces of information hook up to each other.

Since these inferences are based on the hearer or reader's knowledge of the speaker's beliefs and values, as well as knowledge about context and content that the hearer or reader shares with the speaker or writer, pragmatic mode language tends to be used among people who know each other fairly well (have a good deal of mutual knowledge and experience). Syntactic mode language, which trades less on inferences about what is meant and how information is connected, can more readily be used between strangers, people who share less common knowledge and common experience (and who thus may be less good at drawing the appropriate inferences about what the speaker or writer actually means, about how the speaker or writer's information is connected).

SYNTACTIC MODE	PRAGMATIC MODE
High integration	Low integration
Explicitly signals meaning, leaving less to inferences made by hearer/reader	Leaves more to inferences made by hearer/writer based on shared knowledge
Public language language between strangers	More private language language between peers or intimates
More formal	Less formal

The distinction between pragmatic mode and syntactic mode can be readily related to a more general distinction concerned with the degree to which speakers or writers rely on *context* to make their meaning clear. Syntactic mode language, with its overt signals of how information is to be combined, is used when speakers or writers want to rely as little as possible on the context to carry their meaning. That is, they want to rely as little as possible on inferences drawn by the hearer or reader based on the previous discourse, mutual knowledge shared with the speaker or writer, or overall knowledge of the content being spoken or written about. Pragmatic mode language, on the other hand, is used when speakers and writers want to rely heavily on the hearer or reader to draw such inferences.

We can say, then, that the syntactic mode is used in what we can call *low context* settings or situations; the pragmatic mode is used in *high context* situations. Note that this distinction is *not* one between speech and writing. Lectures are speech, but low context and personal letters are writing, but high context. However, most uses of writing in school and public settings is indeed low context.

We can see then that the distinction between syntactic mode and pragmatic mode is about how tightly or loosely information is packaged in sentences. The distinction between low context and high context is about how little or how much the speaker or writer relies on context to carry his or her meaning. But the two are related in that syntactic mode language is associated with low context language and the pragmatic mode with high context language.

To see the contrast between low and high context uses of language, let's first look at two instances of rather high context language.[3]

25. A: Y'have any cla— y'have a class with Billy this term?
    B: Yeah he's in my Abnormal class.
    A: Oh yeah, how.
    B: Abnormal Psych.
    A: Still not married?
    B: Oh no definitely not, no.

26. A: Ohh I g'ta tell ya one course
    B: Incred—
    A: The mo— the modern art the 20th Century Art, there's about eight books.

In 25 speaker "B" first says 'Abnormal', assuming the hearer can infer that it refers to her Abnormal Psychology class. Later, not sure the hearer can actually draw this inference, she explicitly says 'Abnormal Psych.'. When speaker "A" says 'still not married', she is assuming that "B" can retrieve from the discourse the fact that it is 'Billy' she is talking about. In 26 the relationship between the '20th Century Art' course and the number of books is not stated overtly (that is, it is not explicitly said that the eight books are required for the course). Rather, the context of the discourse and the hearer's knowledge of how courses work is used to make the relationship clear.

The example in 26 could be rephrased in a low context way by building in explicitly the inferences that the hearer is invited to make in the original version.

---

[3]Examples taken from Elinor Ochs, "Planned and Unplanned Discourse," which appears in Elinor Ochs and Bambi Schieffelin's book *Acquiring Conversational Competence*, pp. 129–57, cited in footnote 1.

Thus, 27 below relies much less on context and inferences drawn on the basis of context:

27. There's about eight books required for the 20th Century Art course I'm taking.

What we assume about what the hearer or reader knows or doesn't—how much knowledge the hearer or reader shares with us—normally determines whether we will use low or high context language. It is important to realize, however, that certain circumstances may require one type of language or another, even if either would in reality be equally effective. That is, speakers and writers can use low or high context language to signal their attitude toward the hearer or reader and the context, even if the other type of language would in reality have communicated equally well.

Consider the following case (which we first looked at in Chapter 1): A young college woman was reporting an experiment she had been in to her boyfriend and later to her parents at dinner. The experiment had asked her to rank the moral offensiveness of several characters in a story. In the story a woman named Abigail has an amorous episode with a riverboat captain named Sinbad, which he has required of her to take her to her lover Gregory, whom she could not reach otherwise. When she reaches Gregory, he disowns Abigail because of what she has done. The college woman said the following about Gregory to her boyfriend:

> What an ass that guy was, you know, her boyfriend
> I should hope if I ever did that to see you, you would shoot the guy
> He uses her and he says he loves her
> Sinbad never lies, you know what I mean?

On the other hand, to her parents she says about Gregory

> Well, when I thought about it, I don't know, it seemed to me that Gregory should be the most offensive. He showed no understanding for Abigail when she told what she was forced to do. He was so callous. He was hypocritical, in the sense that he professed to love her then acted like that.

Since both these excerpts are speech to intimates, they both rely to a fairly good extent on the hearer's being able to draw inferences based on context and mutual knowledge. However, clearly the example to the parent's does so less that the example to the boyfriend. In the latter, the speaker explicitly spells out that Gregory (whom she overtly names) is the most offensive (something inferred in the previous example from 'What an ass that guy was'). Further, the latter excerpt clearly says that what she has against Gregory is that he is a hypocrite who claims to love Abigail but mistreats her. In the example to the boyfriend, the whole line of argument is left for the hearer to infer from 'he (= Gregory) says he loves her' and 'Sinbad never lies, you know what I mean?'.

Obviously, both the boyfriend and the parents could have understood either excerpt. So what determines which one gets which sort of language? The woman is signaling *solidarity* with her boyfriend by high context language and *deference* and *respect* to her parents by low context language. This example also shows how such uses of language can vary with various social groups. In the social group this woman comes from (Anglo, upper middle class), it is not uncommon to use a fairly low context and syntactic mode language with parents in certain contexts. In many other groups, such language would not be used to parents. In these groups parents are equally respected, but such respect can not in general override the need to signal solidarity to the parents as members of one's family.

There are, of course, many ways of using language that lie between these two extremes. And, in fact, all of us are good at modulating our use of language between the two extremes so that our language will appropriately fit the context we are in and purposes we have. But we can characterize different uses of language by how close or how far away they are from each pole (syntactic mode/low context versus pragmatic mode/high context). For instance, a college essay on the history of physics is likely to be close to the syntactic mode/low context end of the continuum. An intimate conversation or a personal letter would lie further away from this pole, much closer to the pragmatic mode/high context pole. It is also the case that people with a good deal of practice and success in interacting with public institutions (schools, government agencies, businesses) will develop greater skills in using syntactic mode/low context language of more extreme sorts.

Neither pole is "better" than the other; each is appropriately used in different settings. All language has some syntactic signals in it, and all language relies to some extent on context (even written essays, where the reader must still know something about the subject matter or the essay would be inexplicable). The crucial issue is how much syntax one will choose to use and how much one will choose to rely on context. And this, as we have seen, is both a matter of realistically assessing what the hearer or reader does or does not know and of choosing the degree to which one wants to signal solidarity or deference or some combination of the two.

An Example of Syntactic Mode and Pragmatic Language

We will now look at two children doing the same task. For this task, one child uses language more toward the syntactic mode end of the continuum; the other child uses language more toward the pragmatic mode end.

These two examples come from a study in which children were asked to view a short film and then report to someone who had not seen the film what they had seen. The linguistic problem we will focus on is this: At the beginning of the film, a man is seen picking pears in a tree. As the film goes on, the pear picker is no longer seen, and various things follow—a man goes by with a goat, a boy steals a basket of pears and goes off on his bike, sees a girl ride by on another bike, hits a rock, spills the pears, and is helped by three other boys. The boy with the bike gives his helpers some of his pears, and then the three boys walk by the pear picker eating the stolen pears. The child reporting on the film must first identify the pear picker and then at the end *reidentify* him in such a way that the pear picker is distinguished from all the other characters that have been in the film since he was first seen at the opening of the film.

The first child, a ten-year-old girl, starts her report as follows:

28a. . . . there was a man that was picking some pears

Here the child uses the form 'there is a . . .' to introduce the man and to signal that he is a new character that the hearer does not know about. This is precisely one of the signaling functions of the syntactic form 'there is a . . .'. She then appends a relative clause to the NP 'a man', namely, 'that was picking some pears'. This clause gives information in terms of which the hearer can mentally identify and later reidentify (as we will see) the character. This is a prime function of this syntactic form (relative clause). Thus, the child has used certain syntactic signals to alert the hearer to her meaning and has packaged all her information into one sentence.

This child, after she has reported the rest of the film, concludes with

28b. . . . then they [the boys] walked by the man who was picking the pears

Here she once again uses a relative clause ('who was picking pears'). The relative clause, because it is identical to the one through which she originally identified the pear picker, works to clearly reidentify him, distinguishing him from all other male characters that have been in the film since he last appeared. Once again, she packages several propositions into one sentence ('they walked by the man/the man was picking pears' = 'they walked by the man who was picking pears').

The second child we will look at is a ten-year-old male. This child starts as follows:

29a. It was about this man.
He takes some pea:rs off the tree.

This child does not use the 'there was a . . .' form. He does, however, use a different syntactic form that equally signals new information/new topic. He uses the form 'it was about . . .' and furthermore uses the demonstrative 'this', which in this vernacular (and relatively new, but rapidly, spreading) use signals "new referent." Beyond this, however, he simply juxtaposes two simple sentences, each of which encapsulates a single proposition, next to each other. He does not package them together (by a relative clause, for instance). He does not signal how the information in these two sentences is connected, relying instead on the hearer to connect them together.

Note also that this child shows in other ways that he is relying on the hearer to draw inferences based on knowledge he or she shares with the speaker. He says 'it was about . . .', relying on the hearer to know that he is describing a film (which the hearer does know), and he uses 'the tree' (rather than 'a tree'), signaling that he takes the hearer to know about the tree (either on the basis of knowing that the film has a tree in it or on the basis of the obvious inference that if someone is picking pears, then there must be a tree from which they are being picked). It is possible that the child's 'it' and 'the' are "egocentric" references to his own mental picture of the film rather than to the hearer's assumed knowledge and inferencing abilities. But the point remains: The child can only successfully use this sort of language if he assumes—however unconsciously—that the hearer can make the correct inferences, and indeed the hearer can.

After describing the rest of the film, the child concludes

29b. . . . and when when he pa:ssed by that m͡a:n

the m͡a:n came out of the tree

Here the child uses 'when' to explicitly signal how the clause 'when he passed by the man' is connected to the clause 'the man came out of the tree'. However, he seems to have failed to have reidentified the pear picker. He uses the phrase 'the man'. 'The' signals that the man is known but does not distinguish him from other men that have been in the film since the pear picker was last seen (for example, the man with the goat). There is, however, no real chance of misunderstanding here. The child is relying on the hearer to draw the obvious inference that if a man is coming out of a tree and the man is old/known information (as 'the' indicates), then it must be the pear picker, since he was in a tree.

We can deepen our understanding of the contrast between syntactic mode and pragmatic mode by considering the fact that the first child is a white middle-class girl, the second a black working-class boy. In his reidentification of the pear picker (29b above), the second child uses a *prosodic device* that is typical of black English, though not mainstream dialects (standard English). Prosody has to do with the pitch, rhythm, and duration of the words in a sentence. The second child elongates the vowel on 'man' (/ma:n/) and places a rising and then falling intonation (pitch movement) on the word. This signals something like 'the referent of this phrase is old information, though not recently mentioned'. This helps the hearer identify the referent since the hearer is signaled to search past the most recent referents, though it does not explicitly identify the referent the way a relative clause would have. Note, then, that the child *does* consider the hearer's task, but at the same time he leaves the hearer some work to do on his or her own.

Further, he trades on a prosodic device where the first child used a syntactic device. One reason some black children have a somewhat harder time adapting to writing in the early grades is that such prosodic devices do not readily translate into written language. They must learn to substitute for them other devices (like relative clauses) that can do much the same work.

There are a number of things we can learn from these two children. The first child is more toward the syntactic mode end of the continuum, and the second child is more toward the pragmatic mode end. However, the second child does use some syntactic devices to package information. Few uses of language are "pure pragmatic mode"; almost all uses of language make some use of syntactic devices. The issue is not whether (usually) but how much.

These two uses of language make rather different interpretational demands on the hearer. They make different assumptions about the hearer. They also signal what sort of context the child takes himself or herself to be in. The first child treats the hearer as more distant, as if the hearer shares little knowledge with her, and explicitly does much of the interpretive work for the hearer through her overt and explicit packaging devices. The second child leaves more for the hearer to do and treats the hearer as less distant and as sharing knowledge with him. Note that the issue is *not* which assumption is correct—both assumptions are correct. In cases like these, the speaker creates the context and in a sense creates the hearer as well.

The second child's assumptions work perfectly well—any hearer can draw the inferences that he demands and do so relatively effortlessly. We can ask why the first child signals to the hearer what the hearer surely knows or can rather easily get for him or herself just as easily as we could have asked why the second child fails to explicitly signal what the first child did. As the sociolinguist William Labov has pointed out, "explicitness" is not an unmitigated good—it can also be condescending and pedantic. In the case above, neither child is right or wrong. They simply make different assumptions, create different hearers, and construct different contexts.

However, it is important to note that the style adopted by the first child is rewarded more by schools than the style adopted by the second child. This is perhaps because it "translates" more easily into writing, or the sorts of writing that schools value and reward (see Chapter 9).

_____ **E X E R C I S E** _____

Exercise F. The following oral text occurred as part of a friendly conversation among a group of friends and relatives. The speaker is making an argument as to why she believes in "fate."[4]

---

[4]This text is taken from Deborah Schiffrin's book *Discourse Markers* (New York: Cambridge University Press, 1987), pp. 49–50. It is good example of normal everyday speech.

I believe in that. Whatever's gonna happen is gonna happen. I believe that y'know it's fate. It really is. Because my husband has a brother, that was killed in an automobile accident, and at the same time there was another fellow, in there, that walked away with not even a scratch on him. And I really feel—I don't feel y'can push fate, and I think a lot of people do. But I feel that you were put here for so many years or whatever the case is, and that's how it is meant to be. Because like when we got married, we were supposed t'get married like about five months later. My husband got a notice t'go into the service and we moved it up. And my father died the week after we got married. While we were on our honeymoon. And I just felt that move was meant to be, because if not, he wouldn't have been there. So y'know it just seems that that's how things work out[5]

Read the oral text above several times. Then write a version of the argument in your best "school-based" writing (that is, in low context, syntactic mode language). After you have done so, compare the two texts (the oral one and your written version) in terms of a variety of features that distinguish them. In particular (though you can discuss other sorts of features as well), contrast several low context, syntactic mode features of the written text with several high context, pragmatic mode features in the oral text. Explicate the same contrast for the oral text above and the written text by Walker Percy in Exercise C above. How does Percy's text compare to your written version of the oral argument?

10.5.   COHESION

Integration involves using syntactic devices to package material within a *single* sentence. It naturally goes with **cohesion. Cohesive devices** link *separate* sentences in a discourse together. They signal to the hearer the connections between the sentences that make up a discourse. Cohesive devices have in common with integration this function of explicitly signaling to the hearer how the linguistic material is to be understood. Both integrative devices and cohesive devices cause the hearer to make less inferences based on context and knowledge shared with the speaker (though some inferencing is always necessary; no piece of language is totally explicit).

There are six major types of cohesive devices. Examples of each of them (numbered in reference to the following discussion) are seen in the discourse below:

---

[5]A period = falling intonation followed by noticeable pause; a comma = continuing intonation: may be slight fall or rise in contour; may be followed by a short pause.

30. The Federal Government expected Indian Nations to sign treaties.

However, though	=	6
most of	=	2
them	=	1
had *in fact*	=	6
done so,	=	3
the	=	2
Seminoles	=	5
would not __.	=	4

Each of the numbered words or phrases is a cohesive device that signals to the hearer how the second sentence is linked (or how it coheres) with the preceding sentence. Below I list the six major classes of cohesive devices and show how the member of that class represented in our example above functions. The numbers below correspond to those used in the example.

COHESIVE DEVICES

1. *Pronouns.* In the example, the pronoun 'them' links back to the preceding sentence by picking up its reference from a phrase in that sentence ('Indian Nations').

2. *Determiners and quantifiers.* The quantifier 'most' links to the preceding sentence by indicating that we are now talking about a part ('most') of a whole that was talked about in the preceding sentence ('Indian Nations'). The determiner 'the' in front of 'Seminoles' links to the preceding sentence by indicating that the information it is attached to ('Seminoles') is assumed to be predictable or known on the basis of the preceding sentence. In this case, it is predictable because the preceding sentence mentioned Indian Nations, and Seminoles are an Indian Nation.

3. *Substitution.* The words 'done so' are a dummy phrase that substitutes for (stands in for) 'signed treaties' in the previous sentence. This allows us both not to repeat this information and to signal that the second sentence is linked to the preceding one.

4. *Ellipsis.* The blank after 'would not' indicates a place where information has been left out (elided) because it is totally predictable based on the preceding sentence (the information is 'sign a treaty'). Since we reconstruct the left-out information by considering the preceding sentence, this ellipsis is a linking device.

5. *Lexical cohesion.* The word 'Seminoles' is lexically related to 'Indian' since Seminoles are Indians. This links the two sentences together through the fact that they contain words that are semantically related.

6. *Conjunctions and other conjunction-like links.* The word 'however' signals how the hearer is to relate the second sentence to the first. It signals that

there is an adversative relation between the two sentences. 'In fact' also links the second sentence to the first, though in a way that is subtle enough and hard enough to describe that it is possible that only native speakers would get its placement just right in a variety of cases. Related to this category are "discourse particles," words like 'so' and 'well' that also help tie sentences together into meaningfully related chains of sentences that "sound" like they go together.

There is an interesting trade-off between integration and cohesion. If one packages information that could have been in several sentences tightly into one, then one doesn't need cohesive devices to link these separate sentences together. However, all discourse is made up of separate sentences, however tightly packaged each of them is, and must have some cohesive devices to link them together.

There have been a large number of studies of the use of cohesive devices in writing. It is important to note that good writers don't necessarily use a lot of cohesive devices. It isn't a case of "the more the better." Good writers use a variety of such devices and choose them carefully to signal exactly the meaning they intend.

_____ E X E R C I S E S _____

Exercise G.   Identify a variety of cohesive devices (several of each type, if they exist in the text) in the oral text in Exercise F above and in the written text in Exercise C above. Compare the way in which cohesion is used in these two texts.

Exercise H.   Consider several (two or three) paragraphs from any short story or novel by Henry James and several paragraphs from any short story or novel by Ernest Hemingway. Compare and contrast James and Hemingway in how they use syntactic devices for integration and in how they use cohesive devices. How would you compare them in terms of the syntactic mode/pragmatic mode continuum?

10.6.   PACKAGING BEYOND THE SENTENCE:
THE ORGANIZATION OF CONNECTED DISCOURSES

When people speak, speech comes out of their mouths in little spurts. Unless we pay close attention, we don't usually hear these little spurts, because the ear puts them together and gives us the illusion of speech being an unbroken and continuous stream. Each little spurt out of which speech is composed has one salient piece of new information in it. This information carries the most stress in the spurt and is also marked by a salient movement in the pitch of the voice (either rising, falling, rising-then-falling, or falling-then-rising). There is often a pause or slight break in tempo after the little spurt.

Focuses of Consciousness

Speaking metaphorically, we can think of the mind as functioning like the eye. For example, consider a large piece of information that I want to communiate to you, such as what happened on my summer vacation. This information is stored in my head (in my long-term memory). When I want to speak about my summer vacation, my "mind's eye" (the active attention of my consciousness) can only focus on one small piece of the overall information about my summer vacation at a time. Analogously, when my eye looks at a large scene, a landscape or a painting for example, it can only focus or fixate on one fairly small piece of visual information at a time. The eye rapidly moves over the whole scene, stopping and starting here and there, one small focus or fixation at a time (watch someone's eye as they look over a picture, a page of print, or at a scene in the world). The "mind's eye" also focuses on one fairly small piece of information at a time, encodes it into language, and puts it out of the mouth as speech. Each small chunk in speech represents one such focus of the mind's eye and usually contains only one piece of new information. I will call each such chunk a **focus of consciousness.**

To see these focuses of consciousness operating, consider the following example, taken from the opening of a story told by a seven-year-old black girl. Each focus of consciousness is numbered separately. Within each one, the word or phrase with the most stress and carrying the major pitch movement, and which thus carries the new and most salient information, is underlined:

1. last yesterday
2. when my father
3. in the morning
4. an' he . . .
5. there was a hook
6. on the top of the stairway
7. an' my father was pickin me up
8. an' I got stuck on the hook
9. up there
10. an' I hadn't had breakfast
11. he wouldn't take me down
12. until I finished all my breakfast
13. cause I didn't like oatmeal either

Each underlined word or phrase is said with a major pitch movement (rising, falling, rising-falling, or falling-rising—in all the above cases, except the chunk in 13, the pitch movement is rising or falling-rising; 13 is said with a fall in pitch). When a whole phrase, rather than a single word, is underlined, this pitch marking works as follows: Each content word in the phrase has a fair degree of stress, and the last one in the phrase gets the most stress and is where the salient pitch movement occurs. So in 'the top of the stairway', the content words 'top' and 'stairway' are stressed, and the function words are not. The last content word, 'stairway', has a salient pitch movement on it (in this case the child's voice falls on 'stair' and then rises on 'way'). In 'he wouldn't take me down', the major pitch movement is distributed over 'take' (which starts it) and 'down' (which ends it), which is common with English verb + particle combinations.

Notice that each underlined word or phrase (minus its function words, which are necessary glue to hold the phrase together) contains new information. The first chunk (1 above) tells us when the events of the story happened (in this child's language 'last yesterday' means *in the recent past*). The second one introduces the father, a major character in the story to follow. The third tells us when the first event of the story (getting stuck on a hook) took place. The fourth is a speech disfluency showing us the child planning what to say (all speech has such disfluencies). The fifth introduces the hook; the sixth tells us where the hook is. The seventh introduces the action that leads to getting stuck. Thanks to having been mentioned previously in 2, the father is now old information and thus 'my father' in 7 has little stress. Therefore, 'my father', now being old information, can be part of the overall focus 'my father was pickin' me up', which contains only one piece of new information (the action of picking up). The eighth focus of consciousness gives the result of the previous one, that is, the result that the narrator gets stuck. The rest of the focuses of consciousness work in the same way, that is, one new piece of information at a time. Adults, of course, can have somewhat longer focuses of consciousness (thanks to their increased ability to encode the focuses into language), but not all that much longer.

Notice too that once the child gets going and enough information has been built up (and thus, some of it has become old information), then each focus of consciousness tends to be one clause long. After focus 6 all the focuses of consciousness are a single clause, except for 9. And as the child continues beyond the point I have cited, more and more of her focuses are a single clause. Most focuses of consciousness in all speech (regardless of age or dialect) are one clause long. In fact, there is evidence in the psychology of language that speech is planned and output one clause at a time.

Stanzas and Higher-Order Organization

The information embraced within a single focus of consciousness is, of course, often too small to handle all that the speaker wants to say. It is necessary usually to let several focuses of consciousness scan a body of information larger than a single focus. This is to say that the speaker has larger chunks than single focuses of consciousness in mind, and that several such focuses may constitute a single unitary larger block of information.

Consider again the beginning of the young girl's story in the last section. These focuses of consciousness (1 through 13) constituted the opening or setting of her story, the background material one needed to know to situate and contextualize the main action of the story that then followed. That is, these focuses constituted a unitary block of information within the story as a whole.

If we reprint these focuses of consciousness in a slightly different form, a pattern emerges that shows ways in which this information is organized beyond the small focuses of consciousness. Below I place each clause on a separate line (except for the adverb that states the time of the story as a whole) and remove the normal disfluencies that indicate planning but that may obscure from our analytic view underlying patterns in the information.

SETTING OF STORY

Stanza 1

1. Last yesterday in the morning
2. There was a hook on the top of the stairway
3. An' my father was pickin' me up
4. An' I got stuck on the hook up there

Stanza 2

5. An' I hadn't had breakfast
6. He wouldn't take me down
7. Until I finished all my breakfast
8. Cause I didn't like oatmeal either

We see here that the child has built her story setting or opening out of eight clauses (really seven clauses and the opening adverbial phrase). These eight clauses fall into two groups, four clauses about getting stuck and four about having to finish breakfast. This is typical also of speech. These two groups of clauses are each about one important event (getting stuck and having to finish breakfast, respectively). Such groupings of clauses I will call **stanzas.** Each stanza is about one important event, happening, state of affairs, or character, at one time and place. When time, place, character, or event changes, we get a new stanza. I use this term (stanza) because these chunks are somewhat like stanzas in poetry.

Connected speech is like a set of boxes within boxes. The focuses of consciousness, most of which are a single clause, are grouped together as one larger, unitary body of information, like the setting for a story. This larger body of information is composed of stanzas, each one of which takes a single perspective on an event, state of affairs, or character. Presumably, this distribution of information has something to do with how the information is stored in the speaker's head, though speakers can actively make decisions about how to group or regroup information as they plan their speech.

EXERCISE

Exercise I. Organize the oral text in Exercise F above into stanzas (groups of clauses or sentences that go together by being about a single character, event, or state of affairs, or, in the case of this text, that go together as a single "move" in the argument). Do the same for the written text in Exercise C. Discuss the reasons for your analysis in both cases (what led you to make the choices you did?).

Macrostructure

Larger pieces of information, like a story about my summer vacation, an argument for higher taxes, or a description of a plan for redistributing wealth, have their own characteristic, higher-level organizations. That is, such large bodies of information have characteristic parts much like the body has parts (the face, trunk, hands, legs, etc.). These parts are the largest parts out of which the body or the information is composed. They each have their own smaller parts (ultimately, body parts are composed of skin, bones, and muscles, and the parts out of which a body of information is composed are ultimately composed themselves of stanzas and focuses of consciousness). The setting of the child's story we have been discussing is a piece of the larger organization of her story. It is a "body part" of her story.

Below, I reprint this child's story as whole. The story is printed with each clause on a separate line. The clauses are organized into stanzas. Each larger "body part" of the story is numbered with a Roman numeral and labeled in bold capitals. These larger "body parts" of the story as a whole can be called its **macrostructure,** as opposed to its lines and stanzas, which constitute its **microstructure.**

A SEVEN-YEAR-OLD CHILD'S STORY

I. SETTING

Stanza 1

1. Last yesterday in the morning
2. there was a hook on the top of the stairway

3. an' my father was pickin' me up
4. an I got stuck on the hook up there

Stanza 2

5. an' I hadn't had breakfast
6. he wouldn't take me down
7. until I finished all my breakfast
8. cause I didn't like oatmeal either

II. CATALYST

Stanza 3

9. an' then my puppy came
10. he was asleep
11. he tried to get up
12. an' he ripped my pants
13. an' he dropped the oatmeal all over him

Stanza 4

14. an' my father came
15. an he said "did you eat all the oatmeal?"
16. he said "where's the bowl?"
17. I said "I think the dog took it"
18. "Well I think I'll have t'make another bowl"

III. CRISIS

Stanza 5

19. an' so I didn't leave till seven
20. an' I took the bus
21. an' my puppy he always be following me
22. my father said "he—you can't go"

Stanza 6

23. an' he followed me all the way to the bus stop
24. an' I hadda go all the way back
25. by that time it was seven thirty

26. an' then he kept followin' me back and forth

27. an' I hadda keep comin' back

IV. EVALUATION

Stanza 7

28. an' he always be followin' me

29. when I go anywhere

30. he wants to go to the store

31. an' only he could not go to places where we could go

32. like to the stores he could go

33. but he have to be chained up

V. RESOLUTION

Stanza 8

34. an' we took him to he emergency

35. an' see what was wrong with him

36. an' he got a shot

37. an' then he was crying

Stanza 9

38. an' last yesterday, an' now they put him asleep

39. an' he's still in the hospital

40. an' the doctor said he got a shot because

41. he was nervous about my home that I had

VI. CODA

Stanza 10

42. an' he could still stay but

43. he thought he wasn't gonna be able to let him go

This girl's story has a higher-order structure made up of a **setting,** which sets the scene in terms of time, space, and characters; a **catalyst,** which sets a problem; a **crisis,** which builds the problem to the point of requiring a resolution; an **evaluation,** which is material that makes clear why the story is interesting and tellable; a **resolution,** which solves the problem set by the story; and a **coda,** which closes the story. Each part of the story (except the evaluation and coda) is composed of two stanzas.

This is the structure of all stories regardless of what culture or age group is telling them. However, there are also aspects of story structure that are specific to one cultural group and not another. For example, devoting a block of information to an evaluation prior to a story's resolution is more common in black culture than in some other cultures in the U.S. Many other social groups tend to spread such evaluation material throughout the story or to place it at the beginning.

Another aspect of this story that is more specific to black culture is the large amount of parallelism found in the way language is patterned within the stanzas. Note, for example, how Stanza 3 says 'an' then my puppy came' and gives four things about the puppy, and then Stanza 4 says 'an then my father came' and says four things (all of them speech) about the humans involved. This parallel treatment of the father and the puppy forces the hearer to see the story as in part about the conflict between the puppy as a young and exuberant creature and the adult world (home and father) as a place of order and discipline. As a seven-year-old child, the teller of the story is herself caught in the conflict between her own urges to go free and her duty to go to school and ultimately enter the adult world.

Notice that the part of the story labeled "evaluation" makes clear that the essential problem with the puppy is that he wants to freely *go* places where he cannot go, just as, we may assume, a child often wants to go where she is not allowed to go and must go where she doesn't want to go. In line 21, the child says 'My puppy he always be following me', and repeats this in the evaluation. This bare 'be' form in black English means that an action is habitual (regularly happens). Here it indicates that the puppy's urge to follow and go with the girl is not just a once or sometime thing, but a regular and recurrent event that follows from the nature of the puppy. It is a problem that must be resolved. The resolution of the conflict between the puppy and the adult world takes place at a hospital where a doctor (an adult) gives the puppy a shot and puts him to "sleep." Thus, the adult world dictates that in the conflict between home and puppy, the adult norms must win. The child is working through her own very real conflicts as to why she can't have her puppy and, at a deeper level, why she must be socialized into the adult world of order, duty, and discipline. This, in fact, is the basic function of narrative: Narrative is the way we make deep sense of problems that bother us, the way we make sense of the world of our social experience.

Linguists and psychologists have proposed many other approaches to the higher-order structure of stories and other connected sorts of language (exposition, argument, description). But they all agree that such connected blocks of information are stored in the mind in terms of various "body parts" and that in telling or writing such information we often organize the information in terms of these parts, though of course we can actively rearrange the information as we produce it and can often actively discover structure in information as we produce it.

E X E R C I S E

Exercise J.   Organize the story below (told by a twelve-year-old white middle-class girl to a woman in her thirties) into clauses and stanzas, as I did for the story about the puppy above (I have rather randomly put in commas and periods; you can ignore these if you like). Analyze the *macrostructure* of the story, that is, organize the story into its larger "body parts," using any labels you want for these parts. You do not need to follow the analysis of the puppy story. After you give an analysis of the story's macrostructure, give an analysis of what you take to be the story's meaning(s) (the way you would a piece of literature). What title would you give to this story, and why?

STORY

Well see, we have this park near our house. And it really stinks, but me and my friend Sarah were over there, and we were playin on the swings. And this other kid was over there. We call him "tin head cans," or whatever, because he goes around through garbage and stuff and picks up cans and brings em to the store to get the money. And so we're playin, and he starts callin us names, and so we call him names back, and then he starts talkin about our mothers. So I take a rock and I threw it at him. It missed him. I made sure it missed him. It just banged on the slide. And then he started throwing rocks at us, and now he was throwin rocks, and he was spittin and everything else. He wouldn't dare have hit us with it though. And my mother was going down the street, okay? And she saw him spittin at us, so my mother was trying to go over to his house, but she couldn't find 'im. And instead she went to Jeremy and Erica's house, they're brats, they do everything he does, except they get buckets and they dump 'em on people, and stuff like that. And so then him and my mother went over there, and she went up to where he was sittin, and I was telling my mother that he was up to the tree, and I told him that my mother was coming. And my mother came up, and she goes: "What's your name?". And he goes: "I'm not gonna tell you, you're not my mother." And my mother started calling him names and stuff like that, and then it turns out that he has this problem, like cause he's got some disease or somethin, and he doesn't quite know how to make friends, or anything like that. And one day we went over there, another day, he starts swingin chains around, okay? And he whips Sarah with a chain, and whipped me with a padlock that was on the chain. And I didn't do anything, but I grabbed him, okay? And I go: "You hit me again and you're gonna be in so much trouble you're not gonna believe it." So instead he starts swinging a swing. He wasn't on it, he just started swinging it. He swung it into me. I go up to him and I kicked him so hard he was like ahhhhh. And he fell after I kicked him. I kicked him in both of his shins so it really hurt, and he'd get big bruises on his shins. And the mark I had from the padlock was about a lump, it was about like that, and the mark went—oohhhh, and it was all black and blue, and you could see the shape of the padlock. And then, let's see, Sarah's mother starts talkin to his mother, and the mother said: "I'll be glad to pay any hospital bills and anything like that." And Sarah goes: "All I want him to do is apologize." And he goes, like this: "I *did* apologize." And Sarah, yeah, like, "Oh you wanna be my friend, after you whipped me with a chain?". He whipped her in the neck, he whipped once in her leg, and once in her arm, and once on her stomach. And then I go like this, after he yells at her like: "I'm sorry, I'm sorry," and I go like this: "Oh yeah that's a great way to make friends, whip people with chains and say 'hi I wanna be your friend', that's dumb." And so then the next day we went over there, he was up in the tree, and he has a bunch of rocks and a bucket of sand up there, kay? And he started throwin sand at us. And Debbie got sand thrown at her. She goes up to the tree, she took the bucket of sand, and dumped it over his head. And he went home screamin and cryin. He's thirteen, and he went home screamin and cryin, and told his mother. And everybody ran, cause they didn't want to get in trouble. And then he doesn't cause any trouble anymore, cept when people start with him.

10.7. SPEECH AND CONVERSATION AS SOCIAL ACTION

Having dealt with how information is packaged within and across sentences, as well as with how speakers communicate in ways that are appropriate to social contexts, we now reach our final topic. We take up the ways in which language is a form of *social action* in terms of which we act on and with other people.

The Cooperative Principle in Conversation

One of the chief functions for which we use language and engage in conversation is to convey information. Conveying information is not the only reason we talk; often we talk just to keep the social bond between ourself and our hearer or hearers alive and well. But it is often an important part of why we talk to others. The philosopher H. P. Grice has pointed to four simple rules that govern "rational" exchanges of information. Grice proposed his rules as "universal," true of all cultures; but notions like "relevance," "true," and "clear," which appear in the rules, are so culture bound that I will restrict my discussion to mainstream Western culture. Grice's four rules are as follows:

1. Say as much as necessary and no more.
2. Tell the truth.
3. Be relevant.
4. Be clear.

At the very least, you must pretend that you are obeying these rules if you are to be accepted as a cooperative conversational partner. Consider Rules 2, 3, and 4: If I cannot assume that the majority of messages I will receive in conversation are true, relevant, and clear enough to be understood, then I would cease to engage in conversation. And, as far as the first rule goes, if people consistently said less than was necessary, then conversations would be unclear (and violate the fourth rule), and if they consistently said more than was necessary, then this material would be irrelevant (and the conversation would violate the third rule). These four principles together are often referred to as the **cooperative principle.**

The rules of the cooperative principle allow us in everyday communication to convey information that we have not explicitly said. Since, in a conversation, we all mutually assume that everyone is adhering to these rules, a speaker can communicate more than what he or she has explicitly said or even strictly implied or entailed. This "more" is called **implicature.** For example, if you ask me "Did you see Peter and Joan yesterday?" and I answer "I saw Peter," you can conclude that I did not see Joan, even though I have not explicitly said so. The rules require me to give just the right amount of information in answer to your question. Since I did not say 'Yes' or something like 'Yes, I saw both Peter and Joan yesterday', but singled out my seeing Peter, you can infer that I cannot sincerely assert that I saw Joan as well (otherwise the rules would require that I say so). You can conclude that I did not see Joan. Thus, the rules of the cooperative principle allow us to communicate successfully without explicitly having to say everything we intend.

One can also flout (break) these rules of the cooperative principle, while still intending to be cooperative, and thereby *exploit* the rules to produce a particular communicative effect, often *irony.* If Professor Jones writes the following job recommendation for one of his philosophy graduate students, Bill Smith, "Mr. Smith writes quite well, and attended all his classes regularly," he has said true and relevant things. But he has violated Rule 1 in that clearly he has said too little. There is obviously more that should be said about a viable candidate for a job in philosophy, and Professor Jones knows it. In this case, the recipient asks why Professor Jones did not obey the rule he broke (Rule 1). The only reason that Jones has not obeyed Rule 1 and said more must be that Jones has nothing positive to say on the matter of Smith as a philosopher. Rather than come out and say "Smith is no good at philosophy," he has left it to be inferred from his violation of Rule 1. Thus, Jones has communicated that Smith is no good at philosophy *indirectly,* without having to actually say this, and has also achieved a certain degree of irony.

We manage to communicate more than we have said explicitly so regularly that we don't really notice the matter. Consider another example: We are roommates, and you, a strong and able-bodied person, are on your way out for the evening. I say to you, "Can you take out the garbage on your way out?" What I have said literally means *Do you have the ability, are you able, to take out the garbage?*. But since you are clearly able bodied, I know that you have this ability. So I have broken Rule 3 ("be relevant"), asking something that I obviously already know the answer to. Since you know I am not stupid, and that I know you are able bodied and capable of carrying out the garbage, you will know that I have purposely broken Rule 3 and that I know you will realize this. You will conclude that I must not want to know whether you are capable of taking out the garbage, but rather I must want the garbage taken out and want to know if you will take it out—otherwise why am I interested in garbage at all here and why am I asking you questions to which I obviously know the answer? So I have really asked you to take out the garbage, but without having said so directly.

Why would I do this—engage in this indirect strategy? In the example where I answered "I saw Peter" to your question about whether I had seen Peter and Joan, I simply did not want to have to say explicitly all that could have been said. It was easier just to say "I saw Peter." But ease of communication is not the only reason we are often less explicit than we otherwise could be. Even when we convey information to each other in conversation, we still have to remember that conversation involves a *social relationship* between two or more people. In addition to conveying information, we have to monitor this social relationship. And this social relationship often requires us to be indirect, rather than explicit, for reasons of politeness, the maintenance of solidarity with others, and the need to respect others' rights. To see this more clearly, we need to discuss the fact that talking to people is not just talk, but also a form of *social action* we perform on them or with them.

EXERCISE

Exercise K. In each of the cases below, state what the second speaker wants to communicate beyond what is explicitly said (that is, what conversational implicatures are involved in the second speaker's response). In each case, give a reason why the second speaker may have formulated his or her response as he or she did. Further, in the second case, do you think that the second speaker lied?

1. (Husband and wife at home)

   Husband: I feel even sicker today.
   Wife: You have a doctor.

2. (Joe saw Betty, his former girlfriend, two weeks ago and Peter yesterday. He is now talking to his new girlfriend Ann, who knows both Peter and Betty):

   Ann: Have you seen Peter or Betty recently?
   Joe: In fact, I saw Peter just yesterday.

3. (Overweight husband and his not overweight wife)

Husband: Let's go out for some ice cream?
Wife: There's some great fruit salad in the box.

Speech Acts

When I utter words in a conversation, I do more than *talk,* I also *act.* By uttering words, I can accomplish various actions such as asserting, promising, apologizing, inviting, forgiving, offering, agreeing, rejecting, or denying, and many others. All of these, and many more, are called **speech acts,** actions performed by uttering words.

Some of the speech acts I can perform by uttering words are "official" actions, backed up by various social institutions. Thus, if I utter the words "I baptize you in the name of . . ." or "I pronounce you man and wife" or "I christen this boat the *Mary Jane,"* I have performed the action of baptizing, marrying, or christening only if the church, the state, or the government (some official body) has given me the right to perform these actions by uttering these words. In addition, in some cases, I have to do other things beyond uttering words to bring off the action. For example, in baptizing, I have to pour water on you and make the sign of the cross (in some religions).

Other speech acts performed by uttering words do not require any official organization to back them up. The action is performed simply by uttering the words. Thus, if I say, "I promise you to do X" or "I offer to do Y," or "I forgive you for Z" or "I invite you to do W," I have engaged in the action of promising, offering, forgiving, or inviting. Anyone can do these actions and needs no official sanction (though I can't promise you, offer you, forgive you, or invite you for anyone other than myself, unless they have empowered me to do so).

Sentences that involve verbs that name actions (like 'I *claim* . . .', 'I *promise* . . .', 'I *forgive* . . .', 'I *swear* . . .', 'I *baptize* . . .', 'I *pronounce* you man and wife') are called **performative sentences.** They both name an action (claiming, promising, forgiving, swearing, baptizing, and pronouncing) and actually perform that action at the same time, so long as the performative verb (the verb naming the action, like 'claim', 'promise', 'forgive', 'swear', 'baptize', 'pronounce') is in the present tense and has a first-person subject ('I' or 'we'). If I use such a performative verb in the past tense (for example, 'Yesterday, I promised John to help him'), I am reporting an action I performed in the past, not doing one in the present. If I use a subject other than the first person (for example, 'John promised Mary he would help her'), I am reporting an action that someone else took, not doing one myself. Of course, reporting is itself an action, and so I am engaging in the action of reporting, though I am not naming it (by using the verb 'I report . . .') and I am not engaging in the action of promising.

Now, to perform any action named by a performative verb, I do not actually have to use that performative verb. Thus, I can promise to help you by saying (31a) below, using a performative verb ('promise'), or I can just say (31b), which does not actually contain the word 'promise':

31a. I promise to help you

31b. I will help you

31b can be used to make a promise, though it does not use the word 'promise'. Whereas the action performed in 31a is made explicit by the use of the word 'promise', that action is not named in 31b but left to be inferred by the hearer. Such speech acts as 31b are called **indirect speech acts** because they do not explicitly and overtly name the action they are performing as performative sentences do. Nevertheless, 31a and 31b perform the same action (promising).

For any speech act, there is always more than one way to perform it; often there are several ways. For example, I want to request you to take out the garbage. I can perform this with a performative (as in 32a below), or through several different indirect speech acts, as in 32b–i:

32a. I request you to take out the garbage.

32b. Will you take out the garbage?

32c. Could you take out the garbage?

32d. Would you take out the garbage?

32e. Please take out the garbage.

32f. The garbage needs to go out.

32g. Are you able to take out the garbage?

32h. Do you want to take out the garbage?

32i. Could I ask you to take out the garbage?

In the right circumstances, all of the above could be interpreted as requests to take out the garbage. All of them are slightly different from a direct order ('Take the garbage!'), which is a speech act that requires that some social institution or organization has given one the power to give orders (like being parent or being in the army). At the same time, on other occasions, in other contexts, the sentences 32b–32i (the indirect requests) could be used to perform speech acts other than requesting. For example, in another circumstance, 32f might be not a request to have the garbage taken out but a simple statement or claim, and 32g might be not a request but a real question about your desires (though, given that these sentences are about something as trivial as taking out the garbage, it is hard to imagine contexts where they are not requests to have the garbage taken out).

It is important to see this last point: A given sentence can often be interpreted as performing different speech acts, depending on the context in which it is uttered and what we assume about the intentions of the speaker. Thus, if a police officer who has picked up a suspected drunk driver asks him "Can you stand on one leg?", the officer is not asking whether he is merely capable of doing this act; he is asking him to try and do it. He is not requesting information, he is requesting action. On the other hand, if a doctor is asking an elderly man over the phone which skills he is losing and which he has retained, and the doctor says "Can you stand on one leg?", he is making a request for information, not a request for action. The elderly man can say yes to the doctor; the suspected drunk driver cannot just say yes to the police officer.

Or consider that "Do you want to take out the garbage?" is probably a request for you to take out the garbage; "Do you want to go to the movies?" is probably either a request for you to go to the movies with me or an invitation; "Do you want to get your face slapped?" is a threat (not an invitation or a request); and "Do you want to have a massage?" is an offer to give you something, not a request for you to do something. So the 'Do you want . . .' form can perform (indirectly) many different speech acts, depending on the context and what exactly is mentioned in the sentence.

Face and Politeness

There are many ways to perform any speech act, either using a direct (performative) form or one or more indirect forms. Any indirect form can be used to perform different speech acts, depending on the context of utterance and the content mentioned. Why does all this variety exist, and what determines which form we actually use? The answer lies in the fact that all forms of communication, including giving and getting information, are *social activities*. When humans engage in social activity with others, they bring with them two paramount needs. Unfortunately, these needs often conflict with each other.

First, we all need to get close to each other, to have a sense of community, to feel we're not alone in the world; we need to feel accepted and involved, to achieve rapport with others. But second, we also need to keep our distance from each other, to preserve our independence and protect our privacy so others don't impose on us or engulf us. This duality reflects the human condition: We humans are both social creatures and individualists at one and the same time.

Sociologists often discuss these two needs in terms of the technical concept of **face**. They say that each person has a **positive face** that they face toward others and that represents their need for involvement with others. At the same time, each person has a **negative face** that they face away from others and that represents their need for independence and privacy. We can "violate" peoples' positive face by failing to involve them; we can "violate" their negative face by over-involving them and imposing on them. In the social activity of conversation, speakers do not want to "lose face" by having either their positive or negative face hurt, and speakers must also take care not to hurt the positive or negative face of their hearer or hearers. Thus, sociologists say that conversation, and social interaction generally, involves a lot of "face work" (work to save our own face and not offend other people's face).

We all keep balancing the needs for involvement and independence, but individuals as well as cultures place different relative values on these needs and have different ways of expressing them. Some people in a given culture and some cultures as a whole care more about positive face (involvement) or negative face (independence) in given types of social interaction. For example, for many Americans, if two strangers are waiting a long time at a bus stop, they must exchange some form of small talk. The needs of positive face (involvement) take precedence. In many other cultures, however, such small talk to strangers would impose oneself on them inappropriately and would violate the strangers' negative face. Therefore, in these cultures, negative face takes precedence in this circumstance.

Our needs for involvement and independence are not sequential but simultaneous. We must serve both needs at once in all we say. And this often creates a certain tension. Anything we say to show we're involved with others is in itself a threat to our (and their) privacy and individuality. And anything we say to show we're respecting other people's privacy, keeping our distance from them, is in itself a threat to our (and their) need for involvement. Whatever we do to serve one need necessarily causes a certain tension and risks violating the other. But we can't step out of the process altogether. If we try to withdraw by not communicating at all, we violate our need, and the need of others, for involvement.

Because of this tension, communication will never be perfect. We have no choice but to keep trying to balance independence and involvement. And we use the great variety of different ways in which the language allows us to form speech acts to achieve this balance. The care and work it takes to achieve this balance constitutes **conversational politeness.** The different forms available for speech acts are then resources for politeness in conversation.

When you have to choose a particular form of a speech act—for example, you want to ask for change for a dollar—what sorts of factors go into this decision? The decision involves a rather complex computation, though one we usually all pull off quickly and unconsciously in real speech (but in certain circumstances we become aware of the complexity and have to give the matter some conscious effort and worry). To make a decision about the form in which I will enact a speech act, I have to ask myself the following questions:

1a. How socially close or distant am I and the hearer (for example, are we close friends, is the hearer older than me, are we social equals, and so forth)?

1b. How much or little power does the hearer have over me (for example, am I talking to my boss or my employee, to a policeman who has pulled me over for a ticket, to a service employee, to a judge)?

1c. How significant (to me; to the hearer) is the act I want to engage in (for example, am asking for change for a dollar, for a large loan, to borrow a car)?

1d. How much emphasis do you and I (and our culture or cultures) place on positive face needs as against negative face needs in circumstances like this one?

1e. How does the actual context I am in affect the answers to the above questions (for example, asking for money on the street when I am dressed in a suit is different from when I am obviously down and out, and asking for money in an emergency is different than in more normal circumstances)?

1f. Would the hearer compute the answers to the above questions the same as me in a circumstance like the one we are in?

Based on the answers to these questions, I may say any of the following to ask you for change for a dollar: 'Give me change for a dollar', 'Got any change?', 'Hey Harry, have you got any change?', 'Would you happen to have change for a dollar?', 'I'm sorry to trouble you, but do you have change for a dollar?', 'Do you know where I can get change for a dollar?', 'It's so embarrassing, but I don't have enough change, may I ask you for change for a dollar?', and so on through many more variations.

No matter what we say in conversation, it is always both words and a social act subject to conventions of politeness. Thus, any speech act must be formed to honor the face demands of both the speaker and the hearer. It is a subtle process, fraught with possibilities for insulting or hurting others if we even inadvertently violate their face needs. The problems and dangers obviously get worse in the case of people communicating across different cultures and different social groups in our own culture.

--------------------- E X E R C I S E ---------------------

Exercise L. Formulate at least two versions of an appropriate speech act for each situation below. Discuss the factors that are involved in each case to utter an appropriate speech act, and compare the two or more versions you have made up. SUGGESTED FURTHER PROJECT: Tape record several non-native, second-language speakers of English role playing the situations below (get only one response for each case). Also tape record several native speakers of English. Compare the speakers within and between groups, as well as to the answers you gave (paying attention to whether they sound too polite or not polite enough in each case, as well as to other factors that you find of interest).

1. You and a close friend are in a car together. Your friend is driving, and you want him or her to put the window up because it is too cold for you.

2. You and your boss (the boss is not a close friend and is older than you) are in a car. The boss is driving, and you want him or her to put the window up because it is too cold for you.

3. Your teacher gives you a lower grade on a paper than you think you deserve. You go to the teacher's office and try to get the teacher to reconsider the grade.

4. You are in a restaurant. The soup is cold (it is supposed to be hot) and you want the waiter or waitress to bring you another bowl.

RECOMMENDED FURTHER READING

BOLINGER, DWIGHT L. (1986). *Intonation and Its Parts: Melody in Spoken English.* Stanford: Stanford University Press. (Everything you ever wanted to know about intonation by the master of intonation.)

BROWN, GILLIAN & YULE, GEORGE (1983). *Discourse Analysis.* New York: Cambridge University Press. (Good, substantive, but dry overview of the field.)

COULTHARD, MAX (1977). *An Introduction to Discourse Analysis.* London: Longman. (Very readable. Deals with conversational analysis and speech acts.)

EDELSKY, CAROLE (1991). *With Literacy and Justice for All: Rethinking the Social in Language and Education.* London: Falmer. (A well argued book with special relevance for those interested in English as a Second Language teaching and learning.)

GEE, JAMES PAUL (1990). *Social Linguistics and Literacies: Ideology in Discourses.* London: Falmer. (Discusses the role of discourse analysis in dealing with social, cultural, educational, and political issues germane to language and society.)

GIVON, TALMY (1979). *On Understanding Grammar.* New York: Academic Press. (Deals well with the interaction of syntax and discourse.)

GUMPERZ, JOHN J. (1982). *Discourse Strategies.* New York: Cambridge University Press. (Readable discussion of cross-cultural communication, contextualization cues, and conversational analysis.)

HALLIDAY, M. A. K. & HASAN, RUQAIYA (1976). *Cohesion in English.* London: Longman. (Useful as a reference work.)

LEVINSON, STEPHEN C. (1983). *Pragmatics.* New York: Cambridge University Press. (Excellent but rigorous review of conversational implicature, speech acts, and conversational structure.)

SCOLLON, RONALD & SCOLLON, SUZANNE B. K. (1981). *Narrative, Literacy, and Face in Interethnic Communication.* Norwood, N.J.: Ablex. (Excellent and highly readable book. Deals with cross-cultural communication, lines and stanzas, narrative, and development of literacy.)

Index

A

Accents, 333
Action, 56, 218 (*See also* Actor)
  goal of, 51
  goal structures of, 284
  recipient of, 51
  source of, 51
  theme of, 51
Actor, 51, 56, 218
Affix, 162, 167, 174, 175, 219
  inflectional, 175
Affricates, 121, 122
Allophones, 94, 96, 97, 127
Alveolar stops, 115
Ambiguity, 190, 192, 268
American Sign Language (ASL), 6–7, 65, 73
Analogical thinking, 289
Animal communication. *See* Communication
    systems
Argument, 40
  deductive, 32
  inductive, 34
  obligatory, 229
  optional, 229, 230
  premises in, 32
  structure, 228, 233, 236, 265
  valid, 32, 34
Arguments of the predicate, 40–41, 228
Aristotle, 33
Article, 187

Articulation:
  manner of, 119, 122
  place of, 119, 122, 123
Artificial intelligence, 253
Aspects of language. *See* Language, aspects of
Aspiration, 95, 126
Athabaskan Indians, 352–54

B

Basic forms, 82, 85 (*See also* Lexical forms)
Basic systematic sounds, 86
Belief worlds, 39 (*See also* Possible worlds)
Bilabial sounds, 95, 115
Bilabial stops. *See* Stops
Binary notation, 247
Black vernacular English (BVE), 336–37,
    339–40, 341, 355–59
Blocking, 174
Brown, Roger, 319
Budwig, N., 310

C

Canonical forms. *See* Lexical forms
Canonical patterns, 198, 209, 214

Case, 224, 227, 369
  system of Latin, 224–25
Case assignment rule, 227
Catalan, 15
Categorical oppositions, 306
Causatives:
  analytic, 61, 62, 299, 300, 303–4
  lexical, 61, 62, 299, 300, 301, 302, 303–4
Chomsky, Noam, 294
Clause, 399, 401
  adverbial subordinate, 400
Closed categories, 384
Cognition, 305, 309
  nonlinguistic, 308
Cognitive processes, 248
Cognitive science, 246
Cohen, Steven, 249–50
Cohesion, 381, 409
  marker of, 380
Cohesive device, 380, 409
  classes of, 410–11
Communication, as social activity, 425
Communication systems, 65–68, 69, 70, 76, 77
  animal, 2–4
  bounded discrete, 4–5
  differences between human and animal, 5–7
  point-by-point (unbounded analog), 2–4
  properties of, 67–69
Communicative competence, 349
Complementary distribution, 87
Complementizer, 216
Compound nouns. *See* Words, compound
Connotation, 38
Consciousness, 388, 389, 390
  focus of, 412, 414
Consonants, 115–16, 118
  deletion rule, 78–80, 85
  fricative, 124
  nasalized, 84, 85, 87, 182–83
  stop, 95, 124
  voiced vs. voiceless, 88–89, 183
Content questions (wh-questions), 210–11, 212, 214, 215 (*See also* Wh-question generalization)
  relative clauses in, 214
Contextualization, 381
  cues, 351
Continuants, 119–20
Conversation, 420–21
  cooperative principles of, 421
  politeness in, 426
  as social relationship, 422
Creole languages, 163, 359, 363–64
Cross-modal naming, 256
Culture, influences on syntax, 11–13

D

Dative generalization, 236
Decreolization, 366
Deduction. *See* Argument, deductive
Denotation, 32, 35, 45
Derived sounds, 86
Derived structure. *See* Structures
Determiner, 187
  definite or indefinite, 188
Deutsch, W., 310
Dialect, 128, 129, 163, 182, 333, 341
  nonstandard, 81–82
Diphthong, 116, 130, 133
Direct causation, 274
Discourse patterns, 352–53, 400, 411
Diversity. *See* Language, difference
Do rule, 206
Dutch, 307

E

Encapsulation, 258
English:
  distinctive features of, 126
  nondistinctive features of, 127
Ergative languages, 220
Events, 52
  causatives, 58–59
  directed actions, 57
  go type, 56
  simple actions, 56
Experiencers, 55, 62

F

Face, 425–26
"Family resemblance" terms, 275
Forefront information, 388, 389
Foregrounding, 382
French, 15, 17, 130, 309
Fricative, 92, 95, 120, 121, 122

Fricative *(cont.)*
 types of, 121
Functors, 23

G

Garden-path sentences, 261–62, 265
German, 15, 17, 308–9
Glides, 116, 117, 118, 120
Goal, 62
Grammar:
 generative, 200
 morphological component of, 165, 172
 overgeneralization in, 297–98, 299, 300
 phonological component, 178
 syntactic component, 172
 universal, 294, 295
Grammatical devices, 399
Grammatical relations, 157–58, 218, 221,
  224, 226, 227
Greek, 17, 18
Greenlandic Eskimo, 16, 17

H

Hawaiian, 360, 361
Hesitaters, 159
Highlighted information, 395
Holophrases, 314, 316–17
Hungarian, 149

I

Idioms, 160
Implicature, 421
India, 1
Indonesian, 181, 182
Infinitives, 216
Inflection rule, 205
Information packaging, 381, 382, 384
Innate knowledge, 293, 294
Instrument, 63
International Phonetic Alphabet, 74
International Phonetic Association (IPA), 110
Intonation:
 focus, 104, 105, 106, 107, 108, 128
 pattern or contour, 105–6
Italian, 15, 130

J

Japanese, 360, 361
Jargon, 359, 360 (*See also* Trade jargons)

K

Kaluli, 311, 329
Korean language, 1–2, 10–11
 kkita, 1, 10

L

Language (*See also* Speech)
 agglutinative, 147
 analytic, 18
 aspects of, 143, 144, 340
  imperfective, 340
  perfective, 340
 changes in, 18, 367, 372
 competence, 26
 cultural distinctions, 7–10
 definiteness of, 143, 144
 difference, 8, 344
 fusional (inflectional), 17, 147
 isolating (analytic), 17
 lexifier, 361
 overgeneralization, 297–98, 299, 300
 performance, 26
 polysynthetic, 17, 18
 production, 277, 278
 prototype, 8
 reconstruction, 370, 372–74
 social uses of, 342
  deference, 405
  formal vs. informal, 342
  solidarity, 405
  status, 342
 social variables of, 355
 substrate, 361
 superstrate, 361, 366
 terms, 153–54
  focus, 8–9
  prototype, 8–9
 of thought, 37, 47, 49, 52, 274, 379
  events in, 52, 137
  objects in, 137, 138, 139
  states in, 52, 138, 139
 universals, 8

Language *(cont.)*
  vs. metalanguage, 36–37
Language acquisition:
  device (LAD), 294
  generalization in, 290
  stages of, 312–13
Latin, 15, 17, 18, 161, 219, 220
Left dislocation, 382, 383, 389
Lexical causatives, 298
Lexical entries, 234, 265, 271
Lexical forms, 80
Lexicon. *See* Mental lexicon
Linguistic communication system, 313
Linguistic knowledge, 77
Linguistic theory, 13
Linguistic typology, 15
Liquids, 116, 117, 118, 120
Location, 62
Logical properties, 49–50

M

Manipulative action scene, 311–12
Meaning, 35, 273 *(See also* Denotation)
  characteristic features, 274
  defining features, 274
  as perspective, 63, 64
Mental language. *See* Language, of thought
Mental lexicon, 80, 172, 195, 229, 231–32,
    252, 253, 255, 260, 271
Mental locations. *See* Experiencer
Mental model, 272–73, 275
Mental processes, 246 *(See also* Cognitive
    processes)
Mental states. *See* State
Minimal attachment, 264
Morphemes, 15–17, 18, 100, 140, 141,
    145–49, 160–64, 177–81 *(See also*
    Affix; Prefix; Suffix)
  bound, 161
  definition of, 160
  derivational, 152–53, 161, 166, 172
  Eskimo, 15, 17
  free, 161
  Greenlandic Eskimo, 16, 17
  inflectional, 153, 161, 166, 172
  morphological cases, 140
  possessive, 179
  Russian, 17
  Vietnamese, 16–17
Morphological case. *See* Case

Morphology, 13
Morphophonemic alternation, 278
Morphophonemic rules, 279, 280
Morpho-phonological rule, 180, 181
Morse code, 247

N

Nasal sounds, 75, 83
Nasals, 83, 117, 118
Navajo, 11–13
Negative sentence rule, 208–9
Neuroscience, 253
Nominals, 41, 321
  critical attributes account, 321
  prototypes account, 321, 322
Noun phrase (NP), 168, 187, 188
  NP movement, 241

O

Object. *See* Parts of speech
Object language, 37
Obstruents, 121
Oral sounds, 75, 83
Overextension, 321–22

P

Packaging information. *See* Information
    packaging
Papua New Guinea, 163 *(See also*
    Kaluli)
Parsing, 260, 263–64, 265
Parts of speech, 156
  object, 157, 187, 196, 215, 220, 221, 222,
    226, 229
  subject, 157, 187, 196, 220, 221, 222, 226,
    229
Passives, 242, 324–25
Paths, 62
Patient, 62
Philippines, 181
Phonemes, 92, 94, 96, 97, 127
  detection device, 251–52, 253, 255, 256,
    257
  recognition device, 251

Phonetics:
   defined, 111
   features of English, 134–35
Phonological component (module), 86,
      178
Phonology, 13
   rules, 77–81 (*See also* Consonants, deletion
      rule)
   optional vs. obligatory, 82–83
Phrase structure diagram. *See* Phrase
      structure tree
Phrase structure rules, 25, 194–97, 199, 200,
      209
Phrase structure tree, 193
Phrases, 145, 159, 187–88
Physical location. *See* State
Pidgin languages, 163, 361–62, 363, 364
   expanded, 362
Pitch, 99, 105, 106, 107, 108, 412–13
Plot motifs, 283
   types of, 283–84
Portuguese, 15, 293, 361, 366
Possession. *See* State
Possessor, 54, 62
Possible worlds, 38, 39, 40, 45, 48
Pragmatic mode, 401–2, 405, 407–8
   language, 402
Predicate-argument structure, 44
Predicates, 41, 52, 59–60
Prefix, 162, 173
Prepositional phrase, 187, 195, 198,
      260
   fronting rule, 198–99
Productivity, 174–76
Pronunciations:
   prestigious, 356, 367
   stigmatized, 357
Properties. *See* State
Proposition, 44, 379
Prosodic device, 407, 408
Provençal, 15
Psycholinguistics, 245
Psychological center of attention, 395
Psychological topic (P-topic), 396

Q

Quantifiers, 48
Questions:
   embedded (indirect), 217
   formation of, 206–7

R

Recipient, 62
Relative clause construction, 265, 292
   reduced, 266
Representation, 246
   phonetic (surface), 90, 91
   underlying, 90, 91
Rhythm of sentences, 103
Romance languages, 15
Romanian, 15
Roots, 161
Russian, 17, 18, 311

S

Sanskrit, 1, 17
Schwa, 102, 130, 131, 369
Scollon, Ronald and Suzanne, 352–53
Segments:
   basic, 86–87, 90 (*See also* Representation,
      underlying)
   complementary distribution of, 87
   derived, 86–87
   voiced vs. voiceless, 88–89
Semantic expansions, 327–28, 329
Semantic fields or networks, 274
Semantic representation, 42, 235–36
Semantic roles, 51, 52, 61–62, 227, 235, 240,
      241
   assignment of, 233, 234, 238
Semantics, 13
   concepts, 222
   of predicates, 52
Semantics/discourse processor, 267, 268, 269,
      270–71, 272–73
Sense, 36, 38, 45 (*See also* Meaning)
Sentences, 185–86, 393
   embedded, 215–16, 217, 238, 239
   parts of:
      names, 21–22
      predicates, 21–22
   performative, 423
   reflexive, 222
      reversible vs. irreversible, 324–25
Shires, Linda, 249–50
Sibilants, 177
Simplified Predicate Language (SPL), 21
   lexicon of, 22–23
   recursive rules of, 26
   semantics of, 27–30

Simplified Predicate Language *(cont.)*
  problems with, 31
  syntax of, 23–25
  translation from English to, 46, 49, 50
Singapore, 338
Slobin, Dan, 367–68
Sonorants, 120
Sound symbols, 73–76
Sounds:
  alveo-palatal, 122
  classification of, 124–26
  features of, 112, 115
  nasal and oral, 114–15, 181
  stop, 180
  voiced and voiceless, 92, 112–14, 177–78, 183
Source, 62
Spanish, 15, 102, 121, 130
Speech *(See also* Language)
  child-directed, 326
  errors, 277–79
  organs of, 75
  planning process, 278, 279–80
  as social action, 420, 422
  variability patterns in, 343
Speech acts, 423
  indirect, 424
Standard English, 334–35, 337
Stanzas, 414
State, 52, 150–51
  mental, 54–55
  physical location, 53
  possession, 54
  properties, 53–54
Stop aspiration rule, 96
Stops, 92, 95–96, 118–19, 121, 122
  alveolar, 119
  aspirated, 95, 96
  bilabial, 119, 180
  nonaspirated, 95, 96
  velar, 115, 119, 180, 181
Story structure, 417–18
Stress, 104, 128, 386
  as psychological property, 99
Structural knowledge, 72
Structures:
  derived, 199
  surface, 199, 213, 233
  underlying, 199, 213, 233
Subject. *See* Parts of speech
Suffix, 162, 173
Surface structure. *See* Structures
Syllables, 98–101, 116, 117

  open vs. closed, 101
  stress on, 99–100, 102, 103–4, 128
Syllogism, 33
Symbols, 65, 66–69, 71, 246, 247, 249–50
  systems of, 247, 250
Syntactic frame, 279
Syntactic mode, 401–2, 405, 407–8
  language, 402
Syntactic processor, 254–57, 259, 261, 263–64, 265, 269, 270, 271, 273
Syntax, 5–6, 13, 148
  influence of culture on, 11
  Navajo, 11–13

T

Tagalog, 181, 182
Tense, 142, 144, 226
Terms. *See* Language
Theme, 51, 53–55
Theory of grammar, 172
Tok Pisin, 163, 362, 363, 364, 368
Tone group, 105, 106, 108
Topicalization, 389, 395–96
Trade jargons, 359
Transformation (transformational rule), 199, 200, 205–6, 209, 214, 239, 241
Translation, problems in, 46
Turkish, 17, 18

U

Underlying structure. *See* Structures
Uniformity. *See* Language, universals
Universe of discourse, 27, 28, 48–49
U-shaped development, 296

V

Validity, 32 *(See also* Argument)
Velum, 95, 114, 115
Verb phrases, 168, 189–90
Verbs:
  dative, 236
  denominal, 323
  helping, 201, 204, 211
    modals, 201, 202, 204

Verbs *(cont.)*
   main, 201, 202
   regular or irregular, 202
Vietnamese, 16–17
Vocal chords, 75, 78, 112
Vowels, 115–16, 118, 129–30
   nasal form, 83, 85, 87, 127
   oral form, 85, 87
   reduction, 102
   regular (lax), 130, 131
   tense, 130, 132
   vowel-lengthening rule, 89–90
   vowel-nasalization rule, 85

W

Wh-movement, 214–15
Wh-question generalization, 291
Wittgenstein, Ludwig, 275
Word formation rules, 164, 165, 174, 176

Word order 218, 219
   free vs. fixed, 294–95
Word recognition, 251–53
Word recognition device, 253, 254, 255, 256,
   257–59, 260, 264, 265, 266, 267, 268,
   269
Word structures, 168
Words:
   compound, 159, 160, 166–67, 171
     rules, 167, 172, 173
   definition of, 158
   grammatical (function), 103, 140, 151, 384,
     385
   lexical (content), 103, 141, 151, 384, 385
     as theoretical entities, 186

Y

Yes/no questions, 206–7, 209, 211, 212,
   214